139

Anaesthesiologie und Intensivmedizin
Anaesthesiology
and Intensive Care Medicine

Herausgeber:
H. Bergmann · Linz (Schriftleiter)
J.B. Brückner · Berlin   R. Frey · Mainz
M. Gemperle · Genève   W.F. Henschel · Bremen
O. Mayrhofer · Wien   K. Peter · München

Band 1
ZAK 1979 Innsbruck
Begrüßungsansprachen, Festvortrag
Panel III: Präoperative Anaesthesieambulanz
Freie Themen: Allgemeinanaesthesie,
Postoperative Nachsorge
Panel V: Anaesthesieletalität

Zentraleuropäischer Anaesthesiekongreß

Prae- und postoperativer Verlauf
Allgemeinanaesthesie

Herausgegeben von
B. Haid und G. Mitterschiffthaler

Mit 106 Abbildungen und 86 Tabellen

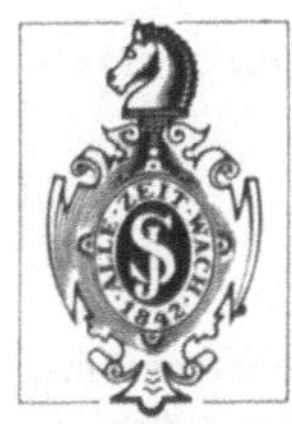

Springer-Verlag
Berlin Heidelberg New York 1981

Univ.-Prof. Dr. med. Bruno C. Haid und
OA Dr. med. Gottfried Mitterschiffthaler
Klinik für Anaesthesiologie der
Universität Innsbruck
Anichstraße 35, A-6020 Innsbruck

CIP-Kurztitelaufnahme der Deutschen Bibliothek
ZAK <1979, Innsbruck>:
Zentraleuropäischer Anaesthesiekongreß/hrsg. von B. Haid u. G. Mitterschiff-
thaler. – Berlin; Heidelberg; New York: Springer
(Anaesthesiologie und Intensivmedizin; . . .)
NE: Haid, Bruno [Hrsg.]; HST
Bd. 1. Prae- und postoperativer Verlauf. Allgemeinanaesthesie. – 1981
(Anaesthesiologie und Intensivmedizin; 139)

ISBN-13: 978-3-540-10942-6   e-ISBN-13: 978-3-642-68188-2
DOI: 10.1007/978-3-642-68188-2

NE: Beigef. Werk; GT

Inhaltsverzeichnis

Panel V
Anaesthesieletalität
(Vorsitz: E. Rügheimer)

Verzeichnis der Referenten und Vorsitzenden

Balogh D., Dr. med., Klinik für Anaesthesiologie der Universität Innsbruck, A-6020 Innsbruck

Benke A., Prof. Dr. med., Institut für Anaesthesiologie der Krankenanstalten Rudolfstiftung, A-1030 Wien

Bergmann H., Prof. Dr. med., Institut für Anaesthesiologie (Blutzentrale) des Allgemeinen Krankenhauses, A-4020 Linz

Belopavlovic M., Dr. med., Instituut voor Anaesthesiologie, Rijksuniversiteit, Groningen, Niederlande

Bläss J., Dr. med., Institut für Anaesthesiologie der Universität Basel, CH-4004 Basel

Brenken U., Dr. med., Instituut voor Anaesthesiologie, Rijksuniversiteit, Groningen, Niederlande

Brosch F.R., M.D., Department of Anesthesiology, Medical Center University of Alabama, Birmingham, Alabama, USA

Daub D., Dr., Abteilung für Anaesthesiologie der Technischen Universität Aachen, D-5100 Aachen

Dick W., Prof. Dr. med., Department für Anaesthesiologie des Zentrums für Interdisziplinäre Medizinische Einheiten der Universität Ulm, D-7900 Ulm

Enzenbach R., Prof. Dr. med., Institut für Anaesthesiologie der Universität München, D-8000 München

Feurstein H.V., Prof. Dr. med., Institut für Anaesthesiologie der Landeskrankenanstalten Salzburg, A-5020 Salzburg

Günter P., Dr. med., Abteilung für Anaesthesie, Stadtspital CH-2300 Interlaken

Hack G., Priv. Doz. Dr. med., Institut für Anaesthesiologie der Universität Bonn, D-5300 Bonn

Harnoncourt K., Doz. Dr. med., II. Medizinische Universitätsklinik Graz, A-8036 Graz

Hartung H.-J., Dr. med., Abteilung klinische Medizin Mannheim der Universität Heidelberg, Theodor-Kutzer-Ufer, D-6800 Mannheim

Henriksen H., Ass. Prof. M.D., Department of Anesthesiology, University of California, Los Angeles, USA

Hudabiunigg K., Dr. med., Institut für Anaesthesiologie der Universität Graz, A-8036 Graz

Ishii S., Dr. med., Department of Anesthesiology, National Hospital, Kyoto, Japan

Jeretin St., Prof. Dr. med., Institut für Anaesthesiologie der Universitätskliniken Ljubljana, Ljubljana, Jugoslawien

Kapferer J.M., Dr. med., Anaesthesieabteilung, Sanatorium der Barmherzigen Schwestern, A-6020 Innsbruck

Kessler G., Dr. med., Abteilung für Anaesthesiologie des Universitätskrankenhauses Eppendorf, D-2000 Hamburg

Kurka P., Dr. med., Institut für Anaesthesiologie, Wilhelminenspital, A-1050 Wien

Langrehr D., Prof. Dr. med., Instituut voor Anaesthesiologie, Rijksuniversiteit, Groningen, Niederlande

Lenz G., Dr. med., Zentralinstitut für Anaesthesiologie der Universität Tübingen, D-7400 Tübingen

List W.F., Prof. Dr. med., Institut für Anaesthesiologie der Universität Graz, A-8036 Graz

Lutz H., Prof. Dr. med., Institut für Anaesthesiologie und Reanimation der Städtischen Krankenanstalten, D-6800 Mannheim

Momose T., Dr. med., Department of Anesthesiology, National Hospital, Nagoya, Japan

Necek St., Dr. med., Institut für Anaesthesiologie (Blutzentrale) am Allgemeinen Krankenhaus, A-4020 Linz

Opderbecke H.W., Priv. Doz. Dr. med., Anaesthesieabteilung des Städtischen Klinikums, D-8500 Nürnberg

Paravicini D., Dr., Klinik für Anaesthesiologie und Operative Intensivmedizin der Universität Münster, D-4400 Münster

Purschke R., Prof. Dr. med., Anaesthesieabteilung St. Johannes Hospital, D-4330 Dortmund

Rothe K.F., Dr. med., Zentralinstitut für Anaesthesiologie der Universität Tübingen, D-7400 Tübingen

Rügheimer E., Prof. Dr. med., Institut für Anaesthesiologie der Universität Erlangen, D-8250 Erlangen

Salehi E., Dr. med., Abteilung für Anaesthesiologie der Technischen Universität Aachen, D-5100 Aachen

Silvay G., Prof. M.D., Department of Anesthesiology, Mount Sinai Hospital, New York, USA

Spiess CH. K., Dr. med., Klinik für Anaesthesie und Allgemeine Intensivmedizin, A-1090 Wien

Scheible G., Dr. med., Department für Anaesthesiologie des Zentrums für Interdisziplinäre Medizinische Einheiten der Universität Ulm, D-7900 Ulm

Schüttler J., Dr. med., Institut für Anaesthesiologie der Universität Bonn, D-5300 Bonn

Schwerd W., Prof. Dr. med., Institut für Rechtsmedizin der Universität Würzburg, D-8700 Würzburg

Stoeckel H., Prof. Dr. med., Institut für Anaesthesiologie der Universität Bonn, D-5300 Bonn

Striebel J., Priv. Doz. Dr. med., Facharzt für Anaesthesie, Rudolstadter Weg 6, D-6800 Mannheim 31

Tolksdorf W., Dr. med., Institut für Anaesthesiologie und Reanimation der Städtischen Krankenanstalten, D-6800 Mannheim

Vadon P., Dr. med., Institut für Anaesthesiologie der Universität Graz, A-8036 Graz

Weis K.H., Prof. Dr. med., Institut für Anaesthesiologie der Universität Würzburg, D-8700 Würzburg

Weissauer W., Ministerialdirigent, Dr. jur., D-8000 München

Begrüßungsansprachen

Offizielle Begrüßungsrede des Kongreßpräsidenten, Herrn Univ. Prof. Dr. med. Haid
Begrüßungsrede des Präsidenten der Europäischen Sektion des Weltbundes der Anaesthesie-
gesellschaften, Herrn Prof. Lassner
Begrüßungsrede des Rektors der Universität Innsbruck, Herrn Prof. Dr. Fliri
Begrüßungsrede des Bürgermeisters der Stadt Innsbruck, Herrn DDr. Lugger
Begrüßungsrede des Landeshauptmanns, Herrn Dr. Salcher

Offizielle Begrüßungsrede des Kongreßpräsidenten, Univ. Prof. Dr. med. Haid
Sehr geehrter Herr Landeshauptmannstellvertreter Dr. *Salcher*!
Sehr geehrter Herr Bürgermeister und Präsident des Tiroler Landtags DDr. *Lugger*!
Sehr geehrter Herr Rektor der Universität Innsbruck, Magnifizienz Prof. Dr. *Fliri*!
Sehr geehrter Präsident, Prof. Dr. *Lassner*!
Hochverehrter Prof. Dr. *Bonica*!
Sehr geehrte Kolleginnen und Kollegen!
Liebe Freunde aus Fern und Nah!

Als Leiter der 16. gemeinsamen Tagung der Deutschen, Schweizerischen und Österreichischen Gesellschaft für Anaesthesiologie, Reanimation und Intensivtherapie ward mir die
ebenso ehrenvolle wie angenehme Aufgabe zuteil, Sie alle, die Sie in so großer Zahl aus 21
Ländern und 3 Kontinenten zu diesem Kongreß nach Innsbruck gekommen sind, begrüßen
zu dürfen. Ich tue dies mit größter Freude und aufrichtigem Herzen!

Gleichzeitig möchte ich allen amtlichen Stellen sowie Mitarbeitern und Helfern, die zum
Gelingen unseres Kongresses beigetragen haben und noch beitragen, vor allem dem Organi-
sationskomitee sowie den 203 Referenten herzlich danken, daß sie zum Teil den weiten Weg
hierher nicht gescheut haben.

Rückblickend hätte Innsbruck eigentlich schon viel früher der Bestimmungsort dieses
gemeinsamen Treffens sein sollen, aber leider stand uns ein entsprechendes Kongreßhaus
nicht zur Verfügung. War es doch die Medizinische Fakultät der Universität Innsbruck, welche 1959 als erste die Schaffung eines selbständigen Institutes mit Lehrkanzel für Anaesthesiologie und vom Bundesministerium für Unterricht die Genehmigung ihres Ansuchens erhalten hatte.

Über die Errichtung dieses ersten unabhängigen Univ. Institutes durften wir uns doppelt
freuen, nicht allein, weil wir es in Innsbruck „endlich geschafft" hatten, sondern weil damit
der Anstoß gegeben war für die Nachfolge weiterer Universitätsinstitute in Österreich und im
ganzen Deutschen Sprachraum bzw. am Europäischen Kontinent.

Mit dem Inkrafttreten des Universitätsorganisationsgesetzes im Jahre 1975 wurde zu guter letzt das Institut ex lege auf Grund unserer mit dem gemeinsamen Neubau errichteten

und praktisch 1969 betriebenen Bettenstation in „Klinik für Anaesthesiologie" umbenannt.

In dieser feierlichen Stunde ist es mir ein echtes, innerstes Bedürfnis, meine sehr verehrten Damen und Herren, jene Institutionen und Persönlichkeiten kurz zu erwähnen und zu bedanken, die an der Entwicklung der Klinik entscheidend mitgewirkt haben:

Als ersten meinen verehrten Lehrer in Anaesthesiologie, Prof. Dr. Stuart C. *Cullen*, der mit in seiner damaligen Universitätsstadt Iowa City jenes erste Rotary-Stipendium vermittelt hatte, das die Erlangung einer kompletten, amerikanischen Anaesthesieausbildung mit allen erreichbaren Degrees ermöglichte. Zu seinem größten Bedauern fühlte sich Dr. *Cullen* schon im heurigen Frühjahr nicht in der Lage, zu uns zu kommen, weil sein Gesundheitszustand längere Reisen nicht mehr zuließe. Er sandte uns die besten Grüße und wünschte dem Kongreß einen erfolgreichen Verlauf. Vor 3 Wochen ereilte mich die Trauernachricht, daß er am 11. August plötzlich verstorben ist. Alle, die ihn kannten, werden Dr. *Cullen*, der auch Ehrenmitglied unserer Gesellschaft war, ein stets ehrendes Gedenken bewahren.

Der 81jährige Sir Robert *Macintosh* aus Oxford, Inhaber des ersten Lehrstuhls für Anaesthesiologie in Europa, bedauerte insistierend, wegen seiner Schwerhörigkeit nicht zu uns kommen zu können; umsomehr aber wünschte auch er unserem Kongreß einen glänzenden Verlauf. Sir Robert hatte im Jahre 1958 anläßlich einer Sitzung der Österreichischen Gesellschaft für Anaesthesiologie in Innsbruck Mitglieder der Medizinischen Fakultät unter Dekan Prof. *Heinz* empfohlen, doch auch an den Innsbrucker Kliniken eine selbständige Institution ähnlich dem Nuffield Department of Anaesthetics in Oxford zu installieren; vermochte doch nur diese die an allen operativen Abteilungen erforderlichen Anaesthesien in derselben unabhängigen Weise auszuführen, eine Forderung, welche die Professoren *Tapfer* und *Hörbst* mit Zustimmung Prof. *Hubers* vehement erhoben hatten.

Indessen hatte Prof. *Breitner*, mein unvergeßlicher Lehrer in Chirurgie, gemeinsam mit Assistenten diese Notwendigkeit schon 1947 anläßlich einer Goodwilltour mit praktischen Demonstrationen durch amerikanische Ärzte, unter ihnen auch Dr. *Cullen*, erkannt und zunächst die Einführung der modernen Anaesthesiologie als eine unabdingbare Voraussetzung unterstützt, um mit ihr ehestens die Errungenschaften vor allem der operativen Medizin auch an unseren Kliniken nützen und verwirklichen zu können. Durch Intervention bei Unterrichtsminister Dr. *Kolb*, hatte er 1951/52 den ersten Lehrauftrag für Anaesthesiologie in Innsbruck erwirkt und darüberhinaus wertvolle Vorarbeit für die Errichtung des selbständigen Universitätsinstitutes geleistet.

Dem Institut für Anaesthesiologie wurden dann allerdings bei der Errichtung im Jahre 1959 vom Bundesministerium für Unterricht nur eine Assistenten- und eine Sekretärinnenstelle zugebilligt. Erst als das Amt der Tiroler Landesregierung unter Landeshauptmann *Wallnöfer* und zuletzt auch mit Hilfe von Landeshauptmannstellvertreter Dr. H. *Salcher* schrittweise 20 Ausbildungsstellen zur Verfügung stellte, gewährte der an sich dafür zuständige Bund bislang insgesamt 14 Assistentenstellen. Wegen der ständig zunehmenden Anaesthesieanforderungen und der zusätzlichen, reanimatorischen und intensivmedizinischen Aufgaben leidet unsere Klinik noch immer an einer oft unerträglichen Unterdotierung, die nicht nur große organisatorische Schwierigkeiten und immer wieder Beschwerden von Seiten der überforderten Mitarbeiter verursacht, sondern mitunter auch nicht länger überhörbare Nachteile und erhöhte Risiken für die Patienten mit sich bringt. Ohne die Festesstimmung zu trüben, dürfen wir hier ganz im Geiste Prof. Breitners die Bitte um Hilfe, bzw. Abhilfe dieser Notsituation aussprechen.

Mit diesem Wunsche im Herzen sei es mir anschließend, meine sehr verehrten Damen und Herren gestattet, zum Andenken Prof. *Breitners* eine Büste zu enthüllen, die im Jahre

1950 von *Gustinus Ambrosi* modelliert worden war, wegen stets steigender Kostensumme jedoch nie zur Ausführung gelangte. Es war wohl ein glücklicher Zufall, als diese im Ausgeding befindliche Gipsbüste vor einem Jahr vom Sockel stürzte und zerbrach, aus den Bruchstücken jedoch, dank der sofortigen Hilfsbereitschaft und durch die hervorragende künstlerische Arbeit von Frau Prof. Ilse *Glaninger-Balzar* unter Weglassung der thorakalen Basis wieder zusammengesetzt und ergänzt, die nunmehrige Bronzebüste entstehen konnte.

Mit der späten Gestaltung dieses Kunstwerkes und seiner Enthüllung zum heutigen, festlichen Anlaß soll Prof. *Breitner*, dem frühen Wegbereiter der Anaesthesiologie nochmals gedankt und sein Bemühen gewürdigt werden. Gleichzeitig aber mag damit auch die von ihm stets ausgestrahlte, echt fröhliche und verbindliche Atmosphäre ohne Nostalgie wachgerufen werden und dieselbe Stimmung Säle und Hallen des Kongreßhauses während unserer Tagung belebend durchfluten. Ich danke schön.

Als nächster wird Herr Prof. *Lassner* aus Paris, der Präsident der Europäischen Sektion des Weltbundes der Anaesthesiegesellschaften einige Worte an uns richten!

Begrüßungsrede des Präsidenten der Europäischen Sektion des Weltbundes der Anaesthesiegesellschaften, Herrn Prof. Lassner
Herr Landeshauptmann, Herr Bürgermeister, meine Herrn Präsidenten.
Meine lieben Kollegen, Damen und Herren!

Ich freue mich sehr, Ihnen 3 Grüße überbringen zu können. Zunächst den der französischen Anaesthesiegesellschaft, dann den der Europasektion des Weltbundes der Anaesthesiegesellschaften und 3. den der Europäischen Akademie für Anaesthesiologie. Es ist mir besonders lieb, meinen alten Freund Bruno *Haid* zu dem guten Gelingen, das ja schon als sicher angesehen werden kann, gleich zu gratulieren und allen seinen Mitarbeitern für die viele Mühe, die so ein Kongreß macht. Ich möchte nur ganz kurz zwei Worte noch über den Titel Ihres Kongresses sagen, der seit vielen Jahren ja immer wieder stattfindet und in seiner Art ein Muster darstellt. Er heißt nämlich „Zentraleuropäischer Kongreß", das kommt gelegentlich so in den Hintergrund; denn das Wort „zentral" steht davor. Ich meine aber der Akzent soll auf „europäisch" gelegt werden und Europa geht vom Atlantik bis zum Ural. Nun, daß der Anspruch auf Ausdehnung Europas den Organisatoren und insbesondere den Tiroler Organisatoren bewußt ist, das habe ich mit Vergnügen festgestellt und zwar dadurch, daß ich erfahren habe, daß der Festvortrag von einem Europäer gehalten wird, meinem alten Freund John *Bonica*. Gleichzeitig habe ich auch bemerkt, daß der Anspruch Tirols auf seine Ausdehnung nach dem Süden jetzt noch größer geworden ist, denn es schließt auch Sizilien ein, wo Herr *Bonica* herkommt. Das alles ist schön, denn das ist europäisch gesehen und daher die vielen Gründe, Ihnen alles Gute zum Kongreß zu wünschen.

Ich darf nun den Rektor der Universität Innsbruck, Herrn Prof. Dr. *Fliri* um seine Begrüßungsworte bitten!

Begrüßungsrede des Rektors der Universität Innsbruck, Herrn Prof. Dr. Fliri
Herr Landeshauptmann, Herr Bürgermeister und Präsident des Tiroler Landtages, hohes Tagungspräsidium, sehr geehrte Damen und Herren!

Dem Rektor der Leopold-Franzens-Universität zu Innsbruck, die den Eintritt in ihr 4. Lebensjahrhundert vor wenigen Jahren gut hinter sich gebracht hat, wird die Ehre zuteil, dem „Zentraleuropäischen Kongreß für Anaesthesie" den gesammelten Gruß aller Mitarbeiter und Angehörigen zu übermitteln.

In wenigen Jahrzehnten ist unsere Alma Mater Oenipontana personell fast auf das zehnfache angewachsen und stellt mit mehr als 14 000 Studenten, 200 Professoren, 600 Assistenten und zahlreichem, zusätzlichen Personal schon quantitativ eine wichtige Größe in dieser Stadt und im Zentrum der Alpen dar. Andererseits ist der räumliche Wirkungsbereich, abgesehen von der ökonomischen Dimension unserer biologischen Fakultät, eher kleiner geworden. Zumal, die Studenten wechseln den Studienplatz im Gegensatz zu früher nur selten und an der Medizinischen Fakultät, der in jeder Hinsicht größten von unseren 7 Fakultäten, besteht für alle außer Österreicher, Südtiroler (nicht bis Sizilien), Liechtensteiner und Luxemburger eine strenge Aufnahmesperre. Umso wichtiger sind unsere internationalen, wissenschaftlichen Beziehungen, ohne die eine Universität verdorrt.

Umso mehr Dank verdient daher jeder, der sie pflegt. Ich danke daher den Organisatoren dieses Kongresses, daß sie gerade unsere Universitätsstadt gewählt haben und ich bin überzeugt, daß nicht nur die Teilnehmer, sondern auch unsere hohe Schule großen Gewinn haben werden. Gleich, ob sie nun die grundlegend ethischen, die biologisch physiologischen, die praktisch technisch ärztlichen oder wohl auch die organisatorisch wirtschaftlichen Fragen aus der Sicht der Anaesthesie in ihrem weitesten Sinne behandeln werden. Wir von der Universität sind Ihnen für die Arbeit dieser Tage sehr verbunden. Ich wünsche daher dem Kongreß im Namen der Alma Mater Oenipontana in jeder Hinsicht einen erfreulichen Verlauf.

Begrüßungsrede des Bürgermeisters der Stadt Innsbruck, Herrn DDr. Lugger
Herr Präsident! Magnifizenz! Herr Landeshauptmann! Festlich versammelte Kongreßteilnehmer!

Ich hatte zwar schon gestern die Ehre, kurz „Grüß Gott" sagen zu dürfen. Heute darf ich das noch einmal offiziell machen und Sie alle herzlich begrüßen in der Universitätsstadt Innsbruck! Wir haben ja einige schmückende Beiwörter für unsere Stadt: Wir sind Olympiastadt, wir sind Europastadt, aber wir sind insbesondere eine Stadt der Begegnung, denn der Name Innsbruck kommt von Innbrücke und das Wappen von Innsbruck zeigt eine alte Brücke von oben gesehen. Die jüngste Stadt sind wir auch nicht mehr. Das kommende Jahr werden wir nämlich „800 Jahre Innsbruck" feiern. Durch die Kongreßsituation und dieses Haus, das vor fünf Jahren fertiggestellt werden konnte, haben wir jetzt immer mehr die Auszeichnung, aus aller Welt hervorragende Persönlichkeiten aus Wissenschaft, Wirtschaft, Kunst und Politik bei uns zu haben und in gemeinsamer Arbeit Zielsetzungen zu erreichen, die sich der jeweilige Kongreß vorgenommen hat. Und gerade durch die Ausführung Ihres Präsidenten, Ihres internationalen Präsidenten, der doch im Namen Europas im Rahmen Ihrer Organisation gesprochen hat, hat man das Über-Grenzen-Greifen ja gespürt und dahinter die Absicht von heute, über staatspolitische, gesellschaftspolitische Grenzen hinweg immer mehr den Menschen zu sehen. Und den Menschen auch als Persönlichkeit zu achten und die Toleranz als etwas Selbstverständliches hinzustellen, daß jemand also andere Gedanken hat, als man sie selbst kennt, auch in seiner gesellschaftlichen Auffassung. Und so begrüßen wir die Persönlichkeiten, die zu Kongressen kommen und über alle Länder und Grenzen hinweg sich bei uns frei fühlen im Sinne der Tradition, die wir haben, im Sinne auch der Berge, die uns der Herrgott geschenkt hat. Wenn wir nämlich auf unseren hohen Bergen stehen, führt unser Blick ungehindert in alle Gebiete unserer schönen, europäischen Heimat!

Daß wir stolz sind auf die Universität, habe ich gestern gesagt. Daß wir glücklich sind, einen Bruno *Haid* mit den Mitarbeitern zu haben, habe ich auch schon betont. Was wir noch besonders sagen möchten, ist, daß Ihre Disziplin immer den ganzen Menschen, den Patienten als eine einheitliche Persönlichkeit sieht. Daß man also wiederum von der reinen Spezifizierung im Rahmen der Medizin, wie wir Laien sagen, auf die Allgemeinmedizin übergeht, d.h. mit dem Patienten die Ganzheit zu sehen trachtet. Daß dies wiederum ein moderner Weg ist, das zeigt auch gerade die Entwicklung Ihrer Wissenschaft, Ihres Könnens und Ihres Strebens. Und so darf ich Sie im Namen der Stadt noch einmal herzlich begrüßen. Ich würde mich glücklich preisen, wenn Sie bald einmal wiederkommen würden; sonst bitte ich jedenfalls um eine gute Nachrede für Innsbruck.

Nun darf ich Herrn Landeshauptmann Dr. *Salcher* bitten, zu uns zu sprechen und abschließend den Kongreß zu eröffnen.

Begrüßungsrede des Landeshauptmanns, Herrn Dr. Salcher
Meine sehr geehrten Damen und Herren!

Aus eigener Kongreßerfahrung weiß ich, daß man die vielen Begrüßungsreden aus purer Höflichkeit über sich ergehen läßt. Deshalb möchte ich eine gute Nachrede, um die auch der Herr Bürgermeister gebeten hat, durch eine sehr kurze Begrüßungsrede provozieren.

Aber erlauben Sie doch bitte, daß ich Sie recht herzlich begrüße namens des Landes Tirol und dies aus mehreren Gründen: Einmal weil Tirol Gäste gern hat. Tirol ist ein Land, das die Gastfreundschaft seit vielen Jahrzehnten auch wirtschaftlich ausnützt, denn ohne die Gäste könnten wir nicht leben. Eine Zahl nur: Auf jeden Tiroler entfallen 60 Übernachtungen von Gästen. Umgerechnet auf die Bevölkerungszahl der Bundesrepublik Deutschland würde das bedeuten 3,6 Milliarden jährlich; als ich vor 2 Jahren in der Volksrepublik China war, habe ich das verdeutlicht damit, wenn Ihr uns da einholen wollt, müßts 60 Milliarden Übernachtungen zustande bringen.

Meine sehr geehrten Damen und Herren, warum ich das sage, weil Tirol aus dieser Situation eine Reihe von Problemen zu bewältigen hat, nicht zuletzt auch in der Krankenanstaltenplanung, wo wir in der Auslegung unserer Krankenhäuser ungefähr 35% Betten zulegen müssen, um diesen Berichten die erforderliche medizinische Behandlung zu geben. Also herzlicher Gruß in einem Land, das Gäste gern hat und hoffentlich auch gut betreut. Es gibt aber auch einen zweiten Grund, warum ich mich freue, daß Sie hier sind: Das ist die wissenschaftliche Bedeutung dieses Kongresses. Anaesthesiologie, Reanimation und Intensivtherapie, das sind jene Bereiche ihres Fachgebietes, die in den letzten 20 Jahren eine gewaltige wissenschaftliche und praktische Entwicklung durchgemacht haben. Wir haben im Tiroler Krankenanstaltengesetz vor wenigen Jahren sichergestellt, verpflichtend sichergestellt, daß auch das kleinste Krankenhaus in Tirol einen Anaesthesisten als Primararzt haben müßte. Wir haben in der Klinik *Haid* ein Forschungszentrum, das sicherlich internationalen Ruf hat, sonst wären Sie ja nicht hierhergekommen und wir haben in der Medizinischen Fakultät eine Einrichtung geschaffen, die gerade in den letzten Jahren sehr stark ausgebaut wurde. Und jetzt bitte ich um etwas Bedauern, die politische Verantwortung für die Summe der Universitätskliniken habe ich und wenn dieser Kongreß jene Aufmerksamkeit in der Öffentlichkeit erlangt, die ich ihm wünsche, dann wird Herr Prof. *Haid* bei den nächsten Dienstpostenplanverhandlungen auf Grund Ihrer Unterstützung sicher leichteres Werk haben, als in der Vergangenheit. Und etwas 3. noch was ich erwähnen möchte: In der Politik ist es sehr häufig der Fall und auch unter medizinischen Kollegen, das weiß ich. Man nimmt Leistungen für selbstverständlich hin, man kritisiert, wenn irgend etwas schief geht, aber man vergißt sehr häufig zu danken und dieser Unterlassung möchte ich mich nicht schuldig machen und hier vor diesem Kongreß Ihnen, lieber Professor *Haid*, für all das zu danken, was Sie uns in Ihrem Fachgebiet hier in Innsbruck geleistet haben! Herzlichen Dank! Dabei erlaube ich mir noch eine Fußnote anzubringen: Herr Prof. *Haid* stammt aus dem Ötztal. Das ist ein wunderschönes Tal in Tirol und die Leute, die da herstammen, zeichnen sich aus durch Hartnäckigkeit, durch Klugheit, durch Einsatzbereitschaft und ich möchte Ihnen noch als Fußnote sagen: Ganz leicht haben wir Politiker es mit ihm nicht. Aber er ist so überzeugend in seiner Art, daß er für sein Fach sicher noch im Land sehr viel leisten wird. Das wollte ich zur Begrüßung sagen.

Möge dieser Kongreß wissenschaftliche Auswirkungen für Ihr Fach haben, um es in der Zukunft noch weiter auszubauen; um auch die praktische-ärztliche klinische Tätigkeit die notwendigen Auswirkungen zu bringen. Denn sehr häufig — und das möchte ich als Kritik anbringen — sind solche Kongresse allzu einseitig wissenschaftlich orientiert und für die Praxis bleibt zu wenig. Ihr Programm beweist das Gegenteil. Möge dieser Kongreß einen guten Erfolg haben, mögen Sie hier im Land Tirol einen guten Aufenthalt haben, damit Sie wiederkommen! Der Kongreß ist hiermit eröffnet!

Festvortrag

J.J. Bonica

Development and Current Status of Anesthesiology

Dear Rector of the University, Prof. Fliri, Bürgermeister Lugger, Prof. Lassner, Landeshauptmann Salcher, Prof. Haid, Prof. Rügheimer, Dr. Guenter, Prof. Benke, Prof. Mayrhofer, Prof. Killian,
colleagues, ladies and gentlemen!

Introduction

At the outset I wish to apologize to you for speaking in English and not in German. I will attempt to speak slowly with the confidence that most of you, if not all of you, will understand.

I'm very pleased to return to Innsbruck for the fifth time in the past quarter century because it has given me an opportunity to see long time friends and meet so many new ones, including many bright young people who show the great potential of anesthesiology in this part of the world.

I'm also pleased to attend, for the first time, the Central European Congress of Anesthesiology sponsored by the three German speaking anesthesiology societies which represent among the most important segments of world anesthesia. I'm especially pleased that the Congress is being held here in Innsbruck for very personal reasons that have been mentioned by others.

As Secretary General of the World Federation of Societies of Anesthesiologists. I'm pleased and privileged to bring the warm congratulations and best wishes of President Quintin Gomez and other officers, of Dr. Douglas Howat, Chairman of the Executive Committee, and the nearly 50,000 members of W.F.S.A. As Past President of the American Society of Anesthesiologists, I take the liberty of conveying the best wishes of President Jess Weiss and the other 16,000 members of the A.S.A.

I wish to warmly congratulate the organizers of the Congress and the officers of the three societies for developing outstanding scientific and social programs, for attracting this impressively large audience and for holding the Congress in these excellent facilities.

The title of my talk is: "Development and current status of anesthesiology". I plan to give an overview of the subject worldwide. I will begin by reviewing the history of anesthesia, because I believe that one has to review the past in order to appreciate the present. I am confident that all of the anesthesiologists in the audience know this history, but I will repeat some of the highlights because they deserve repetition, and also because there are so many spouses in the audience who may not know this — one of the most exciting segments of the history of medicine.

Development of Anesthesiology[1]

Ever since the beginning of humankind, prevention and treatment of pain has been one of
the foremost reasons for the practitioner of the healing arts. An important aspect of this
task was the prevention of pain in one of the potentially effective therapeutic modalities —
surgical operations. The history of surgical anesthesia can be divided arbitrarily into 7
periods: 1) Pre-Anesthesia; 2) The First Great Discovery; 3) The Dark Ages of Anesthesia;
4) The Second Great Discovery; 5) The Renaissance of Anesthesia; 6) The Period of Growth
and Maturity.

Pre-Anaesthesia

In prehistoric and ancient times, attempts to prevent the pain of surgical operations included pressure on major nerves to produce regional analgesia, pressure on the carotid vessels
(strangulation), or blow on the head (concussion), to produce temporary unconsciousness;
the use of electricity (the electric fish applied to the part to be operated on); psychologic
analgesia (in the form of suggestion, incantation, rutuals, etc.); and the use of chemicals
such as opium, imbiding of alcohol to the point of unconsciousness, or the inhalation of
fumes of the "soporific sponge". These were very crude methods, were often ineffective or
caused a profound drugged sleep which all too infrequently resulted in death.

When emergency surgery was done without anesthesia, the pain inherent in the operation always caused great suffering which required restraint of the patient by four to six
people and heart rending screams which were usually drowned by the ringing of church bells.
Moreover, the pain often caused shock, which not infrequently progressed to death. In the
late 1850s, Sir James Simpson, the great Scottish obstetrician, who first used anesthesia for
childbirth and who introduced chloroform into clinical practice, carried out a study of
the records of London and Paris hospitals for the decade before and the decade after discovery of anesthesia, and concluded that 30% of deaths during or after surgery were caused
by the shock of the surgical pain. Consequently, although many operations had been conceived decades and even centuries earlier, only a few urgend procedures were carried out before
the advent of ether anesthesia.

The First Great Discovery

The successful demonstration of the anesthetic properties of ether by William T.G. Morton
on October 16, 1846 in Boston, Massachusetts, U.S.A., is considered one of the greatest
milestones in the history of medicine and the first and most important factor in the early
development of surgery. This event, which Sir William Osler, the famous physician, later
described as "medicine's greatest single gift to suffering humanity", culminated man's long
search for the prevention of pain during surgery. As with most discoveries, the stage for the
event was prepared by many studies during the preceding half century, including those of
Priestley, Davy, Hickman and others, who in the course of experimental studies noted the

---

1 References to the extensive bibliography are omitted, but can be found in the books by T.E. Keys,
   History of Surgical Anesthesia (N.Y. Shuman 19450, by Bonica, *Management of Pain* (Philadelphia,
   Lea & Febiger, 1953), *Faulconer and Keys Foundations of Anesthesiology* (Springfield, C. Thomas,
   1965), and in *Synopsis of Anaesthesia* (by Atkinson), Rushman and Lee (Bristol I. Wright, 1977).

anesthetic effects of nitrous oxide and ether. Moreover, in 1842 Crawford Long used ether successfully for removal of a tumor and W.E. Clarke used it for dental extraction, and two years later Horace Wells began to use nitrous oxide for dental procedures. Since none of these events provoked widespread interest, the credit for the "discovery" of anesthesia rightly belongs to Morton, because it was his illustration that convinced the world of the value of general anesthesia for surgical operations, and was followed by the immediate, widespread use of the procedure. Thus, it is noted that three days after a verbal report of Morton's successful use of ether by William Fraser reached England on 16 December 1846, which was given by Fraser and William Scott and two days later was given by William Squire for an operation done by the famous English surgeon, Robert Lister. Within a few weeks the news reached the continent, and ether anesthesia became used for the first time in France by Malgaigne and 12 January 1847 and subsequently by Heyfelder of Erlangen, Germany.

The new discovery interested not only surgeons but other physicians, some of whom began serious scientific study of ether, and later chloroform. Foremost of these was Dr. John Snow of London, the first full-time anesthesiologist, and Sir James Simpson, the obstetrician, who carried out brillant investigations that defined the therapeutic efficacy, but also the side effects of ether and subsequently, chloroform. Snow duly emphasized the hazards from improper use of these potent agents. Snow's precocious scientific studies of the pharmacology of ether and subsequently, chloroform together with his extensive clinical experience, prompted him to admonish the medical profession to restrict the administration of these potent agents to individuals with proper scientific knowledge and preceptorship training. Soon after Snow's premature death in 1858, Joseph T. Clover assumed Snow's mantle and carried out the work so ably begun. Others, including the famous physiologist Claude Bernard, carried out scientific studies of the pharmacology of these agents.

The Dark Ages of Anesthesia

Despite the obvious importance of anesthesia and its very promising beginning affected by Snow, Simpson, Clover and others, for the ensuing six decades, anesthesia went through its own "Dark Ages". In America and most other European countries, the administration of anesthesia was considered beneath the dignity of trained physicians and surgeons, and the task was relegated to totally untrained personnel — orderlies, nurses or medical students. Pleas by some American surgeons that only trained physicians should administer anesthetics fell on deaf ears. Even in Britain, Snow's admonitions and teachings were not fully effective, for although only physicians were permitted to administer anesthesia, many did so without the acquisition of the available knowledge and the necessary preceptorship training. Consequently, during this period anesthesia was one of the most important causes of death or complications among surgical and obstetric patients. Indeed, in some countries, particularly Britain and France, the problem developed into such magnitude as to become a major national issue. Review of these deaths often revealed that they were due to incorrect administration of the anesthetic.

This serious problem of anesthesia — related deaths during the latter half of the 19th Century, prompted several major developments. One was the frenetic search for safer anesthetic agents and techniques, which led tp the clinical use of ethyl chloride by Johann Heyfelder of Erlangen in 1849; the improvement of anesthetic apparatus by Clover and others in Britain and the combined use of oxygen with nitrous oxide by Andrews of Chicago. In addition, several important contributions were made by German surgeons and physicians. In 1869, Trendelenburg introduced a cuffed tracheostomy tube, and two years later administered anesthetics via such tubes. Soon thereafter, Heidenhain described the antisalivary effects of atrophine. In 1882 Freund, another synthesized cyclopropane, and two years later Carl Koller demonstrated the anesthetic properties of propane, which will be detailed in the next section.

Another development that occured about the same time was the decision by some surgeons, including the Mayo brothers, Crile, and several surgeons in America the continent, to train nurses in the administration of anesthesia because of their convictions that a trained nurse could administer these potent agents more safely than untrained physicians or other personnel.

The Second Great Discovery

Carl Koller's discovery of the local anesthetic properties of cocaine in 1884 can be considered the second great milestone in the history of anesthesia because in initiated a modern era of local and regional anesthesia. Like the discovery of general anesthesia, this event was not the result of serendipity, accident or an isolated discovery, but the combination of several technical advances and the acquisition of scientific konwledge during the preceding four decades. The first critical development was the invention of the needle and syringe, first in 1845 by Rynd of Dublin, who used it to inject analgesic substances near major nerves to treat neuralgia — a technique very popular during the 19th Century. Seven years later, Charles Pravaz of France devised a similar instrument to inject the sac of aneurysm to induce clotting as a therapeutic modality. Subsequently, in 1855 Wood of Edinburgh, apparently not congnizant of Rynd's or Pravaz's work, reported the invention of a similar instrument, which he also used to inject drugs near affected nerves to relieve neuralgia. This report prompted many others in Britain to use the technique, but especially the famous surgeon, Charles Hunter, whose strong support of Wood's work prompted the foremost men of Europe to adopt this method of pain therapy and caused Wood to be given the credit for the invention of the needle and syringe.

Another group of events which set the stage for Koller's epochal discovery were the extensive chemical and pharmacologic studies of the alkaloid of coca leaves, which was first isolated by the German Gaedicke in 1855, who gave in the name of erythroxylon. Five years later, another German Niemann, effected the process of isolating the pure alkaloid, which he renamed cocaine, and for the first time reported its tongue-numbing effects. It is of interest to note that in 1862, Moreno y Maiz published a monograph containing all of the knowledge on the chemistry, physiology, pharmacology, and toxicology of cocaine. Moreover, all of the investigators beginning with Niemann and including Demarle and Schroff, Percy, Bennett and Von Anrept, who, in the 1870s noted and reported the anesthetic effects of cocaine and suggested its use as a surgical anesthetic. Unfortunately, all of the aforementioned suggestions for its use for anesthesia were ignored until Koller's report, which was made at the Heidelberg Ophthalmologic Congress on September 15, 1884.

A little known fact is that Carl Koller, who had been born in Schuettenhofen, Bohemia in 1858 and graduated from the University of Vienna in 1882, made his discovery while serving as an intern and resident in ophthalmology at the Allgemeinen Krankenhaus in Vienna. Realizing the serious disadvantage of general anesthesia as then administered, he had searched for an agent with specific local anesthetic action, and like many others before him had tried all of the central acting narcotics, such as morphine injected near major nerves, only to fail.

Several months after Koller abandoned the search, Sigmund Freud, later to become the world famous psychoanalyst, asked Koller to do some physiologic studies on cocaine, which Freud had used as a nerve tonic and in the treatment of morphine addiction. Koller, on tasting the drug and feeling its numbing effect on the tongue, at once realized its possibilities and began extensive studies in Stricker's laboratory, first by instilling the drug on the eye of animals and subsequently on his own eyes and those of his colleagues, and later on patients for eye surgery. Because he could not afford the expenses of going to Heidelberg, he had Dr. Brettauer of Triest then Austria read the report.

Koller's report was received with incredible enthusiasm, and prompted the extensive use of cocaine, because this procedure held promise of producing anesthesia locally without the deleterious effect on vital organs inherent in general anesthesia as administered at the time. The report prompted further laboratory studies and extensive clinical use of cocaine as a topical anesthesia for surgeries of the eye and later the nose, throat, larynx and bladder, and soon thereafter was injected subcutaneously and intracutaneously to produce local analgesia. To give an example of how rapidly the procedure was applied clinically, I cite the fact that Dr. C.S. Bull, a well-known New York ophthalmologist, used cocaine for eye surgery on October 8, 1884, a little over three weeks after Koller's report was carried to New York by Dr. H.T. Noyes, who had attended the Congress in Heidelberg. Equally important is the fact that within a week of the arrival of the news of Koller's report, William Halstead, who later became the famous American surgeon, and his colleague Hall, began experimenting and developing techniques for blocking major nerves and nerve trunks.

The Renaissance of Anesthesia

Near the turn of the century, relatively small groups of physicians recognized the great legacy of Snow, Simpson, Koller and others and accepted the challenge provoked by the medical revolution, which took place at the time and decided to initiate the specialty of anesthesiology. These, together with the discovery of local anesthesia and other events, ushered in the Renaissance of Anesthesia, which was characterized by major development of the specialty. Interestingly, direction of the development of anesthesiology in continental Europe differed from the direction taken in Britain and the United States. On the continent, the great developments which contributed to the growth of the specialty involved primarily regional anesthesia. For fourteen years after Koller's demonstration, the use of cocaine was limited to infiltration and subcutaneous infiltration and topical application. However, during this period the stage was being set for the marked development in regional anesthesia which took place during the first three decades of the present century. In addition to the intensive studies of the pharmacology of cocaine and the development of regional techniques by Halstead and Hall, Corning in 1885 was the first to produce both subarachnoid and extradural block with cocaine, thus antidating Bier by fifteen years and Pages and Dogliotti by forty and fifty years, respectively. Next was the work of Quincke of Germany, who, in 1891 began to establish lumbar puncture as a safe procedure in routine neurologic examination. Seven years later August Bier, the German surgeon, gave the deliberate spinal anaesthetic.

Bier's demonstration of the efficacy of spinal anesthesia for surgery, initiated what I like to call the *Golden Age of Regional Anesthesia* because during the first three decades of the present century most of the local and regional anesthetic techniques we know today were conceived and developed, and a significant number of new and safer local anesthetics were synthesized and introduced into clinical practice. These developments were prompted by the conviction that properly applied regional analgesia — anesthesia afforded significant advantages over general anesthesia as then administered. This conviction was further enhanced by the lack of trained anesthesiologists on the continent. Moreover, many of the regional techniques were first used as research tools to study pain and subsequently as aids in diagnosis and therapy of nonsurgical pain and other medical disorders. Since most of these scientific activities took place in the German-speaking countries, they deserve special emphasis here.

Soon after its introduction, the systemic toxicity of cocaine became appreciated and prompted a frenetic search for a less toxic local anesthetic. Of the many synthesized, only tropocaine, halocaine and stovaine became used in many medical centers. Moreover, the German Heinrich Braun, who is often called the father of local and regional anesthesia, in 1901 introduced the addition of epinephrine to local anesthetic solution to produce local vasoconstriction, and thus prolong anesthesia and decrease toxicity. Another German, Alfred Einhorn, in 1899 synthesized and began to study procaine (Novacaine) proved to be clinically much safer than other local anesthetics, and replaced them for all techniques except topical anesthesia. During the ensuing fifty years, procaine was the most widely used local anesthetic, and became the standard of reference, but its short action prompted the search for longer acting agents. Of the many synthesized and given clinical trial, only two survive — tetracaine (Pontocaine) and dibucaien (Nupercaine), both developed in the late 1920s in Germany, where they were used extensively for every regional anesthetic techniques with excellent results.

The introduction of spinal anesthesia by Bier in 1898 and its subsequent widespread use by Tuffier of France, Matas and Tait and Cagliari in the United States, Barker in England and many other clinicians throughout the world were followed be the development and subsequent refinement of other regional techniques. Although Halstead, Matas and other Americans had devised and used clinically block of the branches of the trigeminal nerve and peripheral nerves to the extremities, most of the regional techniques were developed on the European Continent. In 1901 Cathelin and Sicard of Paris independently developed and used caudal epidural block by injecting the local anesthetics into the sacral canal. Several years later, it was widely employed by Stoeckel and Läwen, of Germany, who applied it to obstetrics and surgery respectively. In 1905 Sellheim of Germany introduced the technique of paravertebral somatic nerve block for surgery, and this was subsequently refined by other Germans Läwen, Kappis and Von Gaza and the Austrians Finsterer and Brunn and Mandl. In 1908 Mueller of Germany first described pudendal nerve block, which was subsequently widely used in obstetrics by Illman and Sellheim, Ilmer and other Germans, and later by obstetricians in other countries. In 1909 transsacral block, a form of paravertebral block in the sacral region, was introduced by Läwen and Von Gaza, and two years later, brachial plexus block by the supraclavicular and axillary percutaneous technique was described by the Germans Kulenkampff and Hirschel. After the original studies by the Americans Halstead and Matas during 1885–1898, the techniques of blocking the gasserian ganglion and the major branches of the trigeminal nerves were developed and refined by the Germans Härtel, Offerhaus, Schlosser and the French Pitres and Verger and Levy and Boudouin. Other techniques were developed and refined by German surgeons included the posterior approach to the celiac plexus by Kappis, Läwen and others during the period 1915–1925 and paracervical block for relief of labor pain by the German Gellert in 1926. Lumbar epidural (peridural) anesthesia for surgery was first described by Pages, a Spanish military surgeon in 1921, who called it metameric anesthesia, but the technique did not gain widespread use until after the publication in 1931–33 by the Italian surgeon Dogliotti.

Although most of these techniques were developed to produce surgical anesthesia, many of them were also applied for the management of nonsurgical pain. The use of diagnostic and therapeutic nerve blocks were first suggested by Corning, but it was not until 1900 when Schlosser began to experiment with the injection of alcohol into or around of the trigeminal nerve or the Gasserian; ganglion for the treatment of neuralgia, particularly tic doloureux, that this method became used widely by others mentioned above. The excellent results of pain relief in this condition led others to employ alcohol nerve blocks to other pain problems. In 1911 Lewy injected the superior laryngeal nerve with alcohol and a year later Luekens performed alcohol block of the internal laryngeal nerve to provide relief to patients with intractable pain due to advanced tuberculosis and cancer. Subsequently paravertebral alcohol block was used to relieve severe visceral and somatic pain.

One of the most brilliant chapters in the history of regional anesthesia was the use of paravertebral somatic nerve block and paravertebral sympathetic nerve block by Austrian and German physicians as a research tool for the study of pain pathways of various viscera, including the stomach, intestines, kidney, liver, spleen and other abdominal viscera. This procedure was used to confirm the findings from animal experiments carried out during the latter part of the 19th Century by Langley, Sherrington, Herz and others and by the human studies carried out by Henry Head. During the third decade of this century Läwen, Kappis, Von Gaza and Brunn and Mandl among others carried out extensive experimental and clinical research on the visceral pain pathways in humans. Subsequently this procedure was used as a diagnostic tool in visceral pain disease and to help differentiate, for example, epigastric pain due to cholecystitis or a gastric lesion from that caused by a disease of the thoracic viscera. Later, these and other German and Austrian physicians employed paravertebral sympathetic block as a therapeutic measure in certain visceral disease associated with severe pain. In 1925 Mandl gave an account of the application of this technic, especially in the treatment of angina pectoris – a procedure which subsequently became widely used in Europe and in America. This chapter of diagnostic and therapeutic block can be considered one of the most important contributions that German-speaking physicians and surgeons made to science and medical practice.

Very important contributions to the Golden Age of regional anesthesia were the comprehensive textbooks by a number of continental European authors. The first of these was by Braun published in 1905 and subsequently translated into English. In 1915, Pauchet and other French authors published beautifully illustrated and very instructive monographs depicting the various techniques of regional anesthesia. An extremely important source of information was the monograph published by Mandl in 1925 on the technique and clinical use of Paravertebral Sympathetic Block for the diagnosis, prognosis and therapy of various painful and nonpainful diseases. This was revised and published in English two decades later.

It is important to note that during this period, and indeed until after World War II, surgeons on the continent of Europe continued to administer their own regional anesthesia. This was due to the fact that with few exceptions, surgeons wished to dominate every aspect of surgery, including anesthesia. Consequently, the development of European anesthesiology was delayed until after World War II. One of the few surgeons who was an exception was Prof. Hans Killian, who is in the audience today. In 1928 Professor Killian traveled to the United States, and among other things, attended one of the meetings of the American Society of Anesthetists. This visit reaffirmed his conviction that a specialty of anesthesiology was needed, but unfortunately, upon his return to Germany he was not successful to help develop the specialty for some time. Nevertheless, we are still grateful to you, Prof. Killian, for your precocious foresight and for the help you have given the specialty in recent years.

Renaissance of Anaesthesia in Britain and the United States

In contrast to what occurred on the European continent and probably most other parts of the world, in Britain and the United States the development of anesthesia took a totally different direction. Emphasis was placed on the training of physicians as specialists in anesthesia and in the development of new techniques and refinement of older methods of general anesthesia.

In 1893 the "Society of Anaesthetists" was founded by J.F. Silk of Kings College Hospital, London and 40 other anaesthetists. As far as can be determined, this was the first society of anaesthetists in the world, which had as its objective the advancement of the science and art of anesthesia. In the same year, Hewitt published his textbooks, *Anaesthetics and Their Administration,* which dealt primarily with general anesthesia. Five years later the Society published the first volume of transaction, and in 1908 it was incorporated into the Anaesthetic Section of the new Royal Society of Medicine. A year earlier, H. Boyle had published the first edition of *Practical Anaesthetics.*

Across the Atlantic, nine American physicians met on October 6, 1905 to form the Long Island Society of Anesthetists, which six years later became the New York Society of Anaesthetists, composed of twenty-three members from around the New York area. At about the same time a group which called themselves the "American Association of Anesthetists" met sporadically and on June 12, 1912 became organized as a formal society During the ensuing decade or so, several "sectional societies of anesthetists" were formed in various parts of the United States and Canada. In 1919, Frances McMechan, one of the greatest pioneers of American anesthesiology, formed the "National Anesthesia Research Society" with the objective to develop closer liaisons between the basic sciences and clinical anesthesia. Six years later this became "The International Anesthesia Research Society", which included anesthetists from all over the world, with the objective of encouraging anesthesia research. In 1923 the "American Society of Regional Anesthesia" was started by a group of anesthetists and neurosurgeons who were interested in regional anesthesia. By 1926 the various sectional groups got together to form the "Association of Anesthetists of the United States and Canada". Meanwhile, the New York Society of Anesthetists, under the leadership of Gwathmey, Buchanan and others, grew in size and accepted members from various parts of the United States, culminating in 1936 in the formation of the American Society of Anesthetists, which was renamed the American Society of Anesthesiologists in 1945.

It is obvious that in the first four decades of the present century, growth of physician anesthetists in the United States was steady but very slow. I will give figures to indicate the pattern of growth, because I know it best and because, except for differences in the time sequence, the growth of American anesthesia reflects the pattern of the development of anesthesiology in most other countries. Although exact figures for the first two decades are not available, it is estimated that by 1920 there were about 200 physician anesthetists, by 1930 there were 300, by 1935 400, and by 1940 about 900.

During this period there was a commensurate growth in the diffusion of scientific information about anesthesia, and specialty training programs in anesthesiology. In 1914 James Gwathmey published the first American book titled *Anesthesia*; a year later "American Yearbook of Anesthesia and Analgesia" began publication and in 1916 P. Flagg published *The Art of Anesthesia.* In 1920 Arthur Guedel published his monograph *Signs of Anesthesia* and two years later Gaston Labat published the classical treatise *Regional Anesthesia,* and the journal *"Current Researches in Anesthesia and Analgesia"* began publication. Some 15 years later, in 1937, Guedel published a more extensive book, *Inhalation Anesthesia,* and a year later Henry K. Beecher published the book *Physiology of Anesthesia.* In 1940 the journal "Anesthesiology" began publication.

By 1930 anesthesiology specialty training programs had been developed at the New York Medical College and New York Postgraduate Medical School by Buchanan (who later initiated a program at Columbia University), at Iowa by Harding, at Wisconsin by Waters, at the Mayo Clinic by Lundy and in Los Angeles by Guedel. These pioneers were referred to as the first generation of anesthesiologists, and produced a second generation which included Rovenstine, Dripps, McCuskey, Beecher, Tuohy, and Tovell. These, in turn produced the third generation of anesthesiologists, which included Cullen, Papper, Eckenhoff, Bonica, Foldes and Apgar. In 1937 the American Board of Anesthesiologists was organized and subsequently, the American College of Anesthesiologists.

Similar development occurred in Britain, only somewhat faster. Hewitt's book was repeatedly revised and several editions of Boyle's book were published. In 1923 the "British Journal of Anaesthesia" began publication, nine years later Langton Hewer's *Recent Advances in Anaesthesia* appeared.

During these formative years, a number of scientific and technical advances were made, including the introduction of such agents as ethylene by Luckhart in 1923, divinyl ether by Leake in 1930, cyclopropane by Waters and associates in 1933 and the ultra fast-acting barbiturates, sodium amytal by Zerfaes in 1928, hexobarbital (Evipal) by Weiss and associates in 1932 and thiopental (Pentothal) by Lundy in 1934. Marked improvement in equipment included the introduction of carbon dioxide absorption by the to and fro method in a clinical practice by Waters in 1923 and the circle method by Sward in 1930; more sophisticated anaesthetic machines by Boyle of England in 1917, by the former Austrian Ricci Foregger in New York a few years later, and by Minnit of London in 1933. In 1930 Magill and Rowbotham developed endotracheal anesthesia, which had been proposed previously by Trendelenburg and others in Germany and subsequently endobronchial anesthesia by Waters and others, which together with the introduction of "controlled ventilation" introduced by Guedel made possible development of thoracic surgery. Other important advances made during this period included the investigation of the pharmacokinetics and the pharmacology of anesthetics by Haggard and other basic scientists.

Unfortunately, many of these advances were not widely applied to improve the anesthetic care of surgical and obstetric patients. For one thing, the correct application of much of the new knowledge and improved techniques required a medical background as well as anesthesia training: and there were simply not enough anesthesiologists to supervise anesthesia services, let alone give direct patient care. Although nurse anesthetists in America had done a creditable job, they did not have the medical background essential to optimal application of the new knowledge. In addition, the chasm between basic scientists and clinicians retarded the application of the new knowledge to patient care. Finally, as previously mentioned, in many countries surgeons discouraged the development of medical

anesthesiology by their persistence to dominate all aspects of surgical care, and continuing
the administration of their own regional anesthesia and then relegating the intraanesthetic
care of patients to untrained personnel — a situation which not infrequently resulted in complications.

Although these deficiencies were recognized by a few pioneer anesthesiologists, it did
not become apparent to the rest of the medical profession until the early part of World War
II. The disastrous results with anesthetics at many installations during the early part of
World War II dramatically exposed the urgent need for better-trained anesthetic personnel.
Consequently, training programs for physicians and nurses were rapidly developed in both
military and civilian hospitals.

Period of Growth

With this war-time stimulus, anesthesiology in the United States, Britain, and many of the
developed countries underwent a period of phenomenal growth. Following the war, many
physicians whose interest in anesthesia had been stimulated by their military experience
sought formal training. This trend was encouraged by many surgeons who, having become
accustomed to physician anesthesia during the war, demanded the same for their civilian
patients. Consequently, the number of anesthesiologists in the United States increased four
fold during the years 1945—50, and since then it has continued to grow so that currently
the American Society of Anesthesiologists has a total membership of slightly more than
16,000 physicians, of which 12,000 are active practitioners. In Britain the pattern of growth
was similar.

After the war, in many countries on the European continent and in other parts of the
world, some prominent surgeons had the foresight to realize and appreciate the importance
of anesthesiology and selected a few outstanding surgical assistants for anesthesiology training in Britain and the United States. In Sweden this occurred even before World War II and
Torsten Gordh was sent to Wisconsin to train with Ralph Waters in the late 1930s, and upon
his return initiated medical anesthesiology in Scandinavia. Promptly after the war, Lassner
went to Montreal to train with Bourne and subsequently returned to Paris, where he continued his training with his mentor, Kern, who in turn had trained in Britain during the war.
Otto Mayrhofer was sent to Columbia to train with Prof. Papper, Rudolf Frey was sent to
the Mayo Clinic to train with Lundy and his associates, and Zindler went to Philadelphia to
train with Dripps and his colleagues. Moreover, as I will emphasize later, Bruno Haid went to
Iowa to train with Cullen. A number of other anesthesiologists on the European continent
received this kind of special training. Moreover, after the war a very important teaching center was developed in Copenhagen, where many of the first generation anesthesiologists in
continental Europe received their training. As a result of all of these activities, anesthesiology has grown rapidly in most of these countries.

Even more impressive than the growth in numbers has been the increase in breadth and
scope of the specialty. The traditional task of the anesthesiologist was limited to the administration of anesthesia, but as surgeons came to appreciate the specialized knowledge and unique skills of the anesthesiologist in maintaining ventilation, circulation, and other vital functions, they began to relegate more and more responsibility. The application of this specialized knowledge and skill was greatly enhanced by the introduction of curare and other muscle
relaxants in the 1940s and the technique of "deliberate" or induced hypotension and hypothermia. This trend to broaden the techniques and responsibilities first took place in the

operating room and then was extended to the preoperative and postoperative management of patients.

This type of total anesthetic care had a major impact on surgical practice and it has been critical to the success of open heart surgery, lung and brain operations, organ transplantations, radical operation for cancer, and surgery on the critically ill, the very old, and the very small infants. Moreover, in response to the surgeon's needs, some anesthesiologists began to concentrate in such special areas as pediatric anesthesia, cardiovascular anesthesia, and neurosurgical anesthesia. The critical role clinical anesthesia has played in the development of American surgery was recently acknowledged in the *Study on Surgical Services for the United States (SOSSUS) Report* which stated "Anesthesiology has made an outstanding contribution to the improvement of surgical care. It has made for greater safety, comfort and survival in the operating room and in the intensive care unit after the operation." I am confident that most enlightened surgeons in other countries feel the same about their anesthesiology programs.

The Maturity of the Specialty

It is obvious that during the past quarter century, the specialty has matured as a clinical and scientific discipline. Clinically, it followed logically that the same knowledge and skills acquired in the operating room could be used to great advantage in obstetric patients and in the management of patients with acute or chronic respiratory disease or those who are critically ill and require support of vital function with artificial ventilation in the medical ward. Since the early 1950s anesthesiologists have provided vigorous leadership in the development of modern respiratory therapy services, in the management of acute and chronic pain states and more recently, in the development of intensive care units and in the development of critical care medicine. As a result of specialized interest and activities, and because of the advent of large amounts of new information, there has been a recent trend to develop sub-specialities in anesthesiology. Consequently, today many anesthesiologists limit most of their professional efforts to such sub-specialties as pediatric anesthesia, obstetric anesthesia, neurosurgical anesthesia, cardiac anesthesia, pain diagnosis and therapy, intensive care and respiratory care.

Many anesthesiologists have done outstanding scientific investigations and contributed fundamental and clinically relevant information on the physiology and pathology of the brain and the nervous system, of respiration, of circulation, and the function of many other organs. Moreover, a number of anesthesiologists have contributed significantly to the studies of such pathologic states as myasthenia gravis: a disease to which Prof. Foldes, who is in the crowd today, has made significant contributions. Others have done important studies of tetanus on patients sent to their intensive care units, and still others have helped to elucidate various medical and surgical physiopathologic processes. The great progress in the science and art of anesthesiology is well summarized in the monograph by Professors E.M. Papper, S.H. Ngai and L.C. Mark, Anesthesiology: Progress Since 1940 (U. of Miami Press, 1973).

The contributions of medical science and practice made by numerous anesthesiologic colleagues in Austria, Germany and Switzerland are so many that it would require the entire day to just mention, let alone describe. These contributions are well known and appreciated by medical colleagues in other countries. Many are summarized in the outstanding textbook on anesthesiology in the German language edited by Professors Frey, Huegin, and

Mayrhofer and the excellent journal, "Der Anaesthesist." The very rapid growth of academic anesthesiology during the past two decades in these three countries and in the rest of continental Europe is reflected by the very recent founding of the European Academy of Anesthesiology. The basis of the new organization, spearheaded by Prof. Jean Lassner, have been summarized by Prof. Jan Crul in his inaugural address published in the June 1979 issue of ACTA Anaesthesiologica Belgica.

Current Status of Anaesthesiology

The objectives of modern surgical anesthesia are: a) to prevent pain and suffering in the patient and induce mental tranquility; b) to prevent or minimize abnormal reflex responses caused by the surgical stimulation, such as serious cardiac arhythmia and disturbance and respiratory cardiovascular functions; c) to avoid or minimize significant alterations of the patient's body functions that may be caused by the anesthetic; d) to effectively treat certain serious alterations in body functions caused by disease, such as increased intracranial pressure caused by a tumor or blood clot by using hyperventilation; e) to help the surgeon minimize the blood loss during radical operations by using controlled or "international hypotension;" and f) to provide the surgeon with optimal operating conditions which require among other things prevention of any movement on the part of the patients, to provide a quiet operating field, and to provide complete muscle relaxation for intra-abdominal and orthopedic operations.

To achieve these objectives, it is essential for the anesthesiologist to have thorough knowledge of normal and abnormal physiology; to help prepare the patient psychologically, physiologically and pharmacologically, to select and administer the best drug or combination of drugs and techniques; to continuously monitor the patient's body functions during the operation; to diagnose and promptly treat any and all serious alterations caused by the anesthesia or surgery, or both; to communicate, coordinate and cooperate with other members of the surgical team; and in all other ways to apply the anesthesiologist's specialized knowledge, skills and expertise to the care of the patient before, during and after the operation.

Currently most people in developed countries are provided with high quality anesthetic care by the more than 50,000 practicing physician anesthetists, and in some countries by a number of nurse anesthetists and anesthetist assistants. Scientific knowledge, skills and expertise of anesthesiologists, especially those in major medical centers, have permitted surgeons to continue to push the frontiers of surgery. Consequently, more and more operations are being done on the most critically ill, the very old, and the very young (premature) newborn infants and progressively; more radical operations have been performed for organ transplantation, cancer, heart disease and other conditions which in former years precluded surgical therapy.

Other important factors which have improved the quality and safety of anesthesia have been: a) the advent of vastly better inhalation, intravenous and local anesthetics, of muscle relaxants and other drugs used as part of anesthesia therapy; b) the refinement of older techniques and the introduction of new ones in general anesthesia (e.g., balanced anesthesia) and regional anesthesia (e.g., segmental analgesia — anesthesia), and the application of sophisticated technology that permits comprehensive monitoring of patients' vital functions before, during and after the operation. All of these factors — the knowledge of the administrator, better agents and techniques, better patient monitoring — have made anesthesia highly effective and safe. Moreover, the vast array of drugs with very specific action and the highly sophisticated instrumentation in current use permit the anesthesiologists to fulfill virtually all other objectives.

Role of W.F.S.A.

During the past quarter century, the World Federation of Societies of Anaesthesiologists has played and important role in the development of anesthesia in many parts of the world. The plan for an international organization of anesthesiologists to aid and encourage the practice of the specialty was first suggested by Prof. Robert Monod and Dr. Marcelle Thalheimer of Paris, France at the congresses held in London, England and Paris in 1951. As a result of this initial discussion, a committee was appointed to explore the possibility of forming a truly representative world organization of anesthesiologists. Subsequently, the committee met on several occassions and eventually developed plans for the First World Congress of Anesthesiologists, which was held in Scheveningen, the Netherlands, on September 5–10, 1955. The first officers of the Federation were: Professor Harold R. Griffith of Canada, President; Professors C.R. Ritsema von Eck of the Netherlands and R. Frey of Germany and Drs. A. Goldblatt of Belgium and M. Curbelo of Cuba, Vice Presidents; and Dr. Geoffrey Organe of England, Secretary-Treasurer. Professor Otto Mayrhofer was a member of the first Executive Committee. Moreover, it is of interest to note that the anesthesiology societies of Austria, Germany and Switzerland were three of the 26 countries which were represented at the First World Congress.

From the outset, the primary purpose of the Federation was to make available the highest standards of anesthetic care and resuscitation to all the people of the world. This is to be accomplished by: a) assisting and encouraging formation of national societies; b) promoting the education and training of anesthetists and dissemination of scientific information; c) sponsoring a quadrennial World Congress of Anesthesiologists and several regional anesthesiology congresses in various sections of the world; d) recommending training standards and providing information about postgraduate clinical and research training; e) encouraging anesthesia research in all areas; f) establishing safety measures; and g) providing advice to national and international agencies about any and all aspects of anesthetics. Despite the fiscal constraints imposed on the Federation by the very low subscription rates, it has been successful in achieving its objectives, especially the dissemination of scientific information through its various world congresses: the second congress was held in 1960 in Toronto, Canada, with Professor Ritsema van Eck as President; the third was held in 1964 in Sao Paulo, Brazil, where Professor Organe was elected President; the fourth was held in London, England, in 1968, when Professor Foldes became President; the fifth Congress was held in Kyoto, Japan, in 1972, when Professor Mayrhofer was elected President after serving as a member of the Executive Committee and as Secretary-General for eight years. The Seventh Congress is scheduled to be helf next September in Hamburg, Germany, where Prof. Karl Horatz has been heading the department of anaesthesia and resuscitation over more than a quarter of century. It has the promise of being an outstanding meeting.

In addition, the Federation has sponsored the European, Latin American and Asian Australasian Congresses which are held every four years midway between world congresses and through sponsorship and support of anesthesiology teaching centers first in Vienna, and subsequently Caracas, Venezuela, and Manila, the Philippines; through the publication of monographs on resuscitation and obstetric anesthesia; by sponsoring and supporting visiting professors to these teaching centers and other places; and through a new program called Visiting Education Teams (VET) which will be composed of a senior and junior anesthesiologist, who, upon the invitation of a host country, will visit and teach in that country through the sponsorship of the Federation. Hopefully, more innovative programs will be developed in the future.

Achievements of Professor Bruno Haid

It deserves reemphasis that, while the development of anesthesiology on the European continent has lagged behind that of American and British anesthesia for varying periods ranging from 5 to 15 years, many countries have caught up, and in some areas the specialty has acquired more prestige and greater status than in the United States and the United Kingdom. This is especially true in the recently developed area of intensive care and critical medicine. In a number of European countries, this important segment of modern medical care is controlled and provided by the department or institute of anesthesiology. In contrast, in the United States we are still struggling with surgeons and internists to have some role in intensive care, let alone control it. In this regard, you have come a very long way, and I want to congratulate you for this significant achievement.

One of the most impressive examples of what has happened to European anesthesiology is the development of anesthesiology here in Innsbruck. I wish to end my presentation by reciting some of the achievements that have already been mentioned. Indeed, one of the most important reasons for my participation in your congress is to focus on the development of anesthesiology in Innsbruck.

Of the many, many medical centers that I have visited during the past three decades, non have impressed me more by their progress than the program headed by Prof. Bruno Haid. As one who has followed its growth rather closely over the past twenty-five years, I am very pleased and somewhat amazed by what Prof. Haid has accomplished at this medical center. Although every leader needs the support of his colleagues, the achievements in Innsbruck are primarily and predominantly due to Bruno Haid. His bright mind, his perseverance, his willingness to work long and hard, his intense motivation and zeal and his loyalty to the program which has caused him to forgo going to attractive meetings (as many of us have done) and his exceptional human traits, have made it possible for him to make unsurpassed achievements during the past twenty-five years.

Through the foresight of Prof. Breitner, who was one of the few exceptions amon surgeons I mentioned earlier, in 1949 Dr. Haid, then Assistant Professor of Surgery, was sent to Iowa to train with the late Prof. Stuart Cullen. The aforementioned characteristics of Bruno not only made it possible for him to be awarded a Masters in Anesthesiology from the University of Iowa, but to become eligible to write the first part of the American College of Anesthesiologists. In 1951 Dr. Haid returned to Innsbruck to be Head of the Division of Anesthesia in the Department of Surgery. Again, with Prof. Breitner's help, the Ministry of Education of Austria was persuaded to approve a training program in Anesthesiology. In 1954 I had the pleasure and privilege of representing the American Board of Anesthesiology for the purpose of inspecting the program as part of the examination for certification by that body. Despite the very meager physical facilities which have been mentioned, and resources that consisted of a small room and three volunteer coworkers, Prof. Haid was providing high quality anesthetic care. In the course of that visit, I was impressed by the qualities of great leadership manifested by Haid, which have become more and more evident with the passage of time. Subsequently, Prof. Haid became certified by the American Board of

Anaesthesiology (ABA), and I am informed he is the only one in Europe with ABA certification.

In 1959 Prof. Haid achieved another "first." The anesthesiology program became an independent department of anesthesia and a chair was established — the first on the European continent. This was accomplished with the help of Sir Robert Macintosh, who in 1937 had been given the first endowed chair of anesthesiology in the world. In collaboration with the Departments of Surgery and Radiology, Anesthesiology began to plan the development of a new building, which was realized ten years later. By this time, Prof. Haid had acquired this important responsibility of directing and controlling general intensive care as part of the Department of Anesthesiology.

In 1975 the program was further advanced to the present title of "Clinic of Anesthesiology" consisting of the 3 main sections: Anesthesia, Reanimation-Resuscitation and Intensive-Therapy ("ARI"-Clinic). This program includes one of the largest intensive care units of Europe, with 16 beds. I am informed that last year the unit treated over 400 patients with only a 24% mortality, which is a remarkable achievement.

During these many years, Pof. Haid has done remarkable things for the people of Innsbruck, the people of Tirol and of course, indirectly for the people of Austria, Europe, and indeed for world anesthesiology. To make these impressive achievements, one has to have the outstanding leadership qualities which I have mentioned. Ladies and gentlemen, I hope you will join me by standing and paying tribute to Prof. Bruno Haid for the great achievements and impressive contributions he has made to anesthesiology.

I wish to end this discourse by again expressing my great pleasure and delight in the opportunity of being with you today, and in participating in this ceremony opening the Central European Congress of Anaesthesiology. From reading the program, I am confident that it will be a highly successful scientific meeting, during which there will be dissemination of new and important information that will help all of us take better care of our patients. Equally important will be the many social events which will permit all of us to meet and interact with colleagues from throughout Europe and other parts of the world. Finally, I wish to thank Prof. Haid and the Organizing Committee for affording me the privilege of giving this address.

Panel III
Die präoperative Anaesthesieambulanz

Vorsitz: W.F. List

Einführung

W.F. List

Unter einer präoperativen Ambulanz soll eine Organisationsform verstanden werden, die eine frühzeitige präoperative Befunderhebung zur Feststellung der Anästhesiefähigkeit und des Anästhesierisikos durch Anästhesiologen ermöglicht. Chirurgische Patienten mit elektiven Eingriffen sollen entweder noch vor ihrer Spitalsaufnahme oder aber unmittelbar nachher in einer derartigen Ambulanz gesehen werden. Die Untersuchungen werden in eigenen Räumlichkeiten der Anästhesieabteilung bzw. des Anästhesieinstitutes oder der Anästhesieklinik durchgeführt. Dadurch ist die Gewähr gegeben, daß der Anästhesiologe schon frühzeitig mit dem chirurgischen Patienten in Kontakt kommt und alle notwendigen Befunde zur Feststellung der Anästhesiefähigkeit (Narkosetauglichkeit) und des Anästhesierisikos erheben kann. Zwischen 25 und 40 % unserer Patienten zeigen neben der chirurgischen Erkrankung noch medizinische Befunde, die beachtet werden müssen (Kyei Mensah et al. 1974). Das operative Risiko und die Operationsletalität wird durch medizinische Begleiterkrankungen deutlich erhöht (Goldman et al. 1977).

Bisher war es doch so — jedenfalls in meiner Institution — daß präoperative Befunde vom chirurgischen Patienten selbst in mehreren Ambulanzen und Labors zusammengetragen werden mußten. Dann wurde sehr oft vom Chirurgen ein Internist angefordert, der die Operationstauglichkeit meist bei „schonender Narkose" feststellt. Der Anästhesiologe sah die Patienten erst am Vorabend der Operation. Eine oft sehr lange Liste von Patienten mußte in kürzester Zeit beurteilt und prämediziert werden. Nicht selten mußte die Anästhesiefähigkeit auch noch mit unzureichenden Befunden abgeklärt werden. Ein Absetzen der Operation führte zu Schwierigkeiten mit dem Patienten, mit dem Operationsprogramm und dem Chirurgen.

Aus den einleitenden Worten geht schon hervor, daß eine gewisse semantische Verwirrung bezüglich der Bedeutung der Worte Operationstauglichkeit und Anästhesiefähigkeit (Narkosetauglichkeit) besteht. Nachdem ich in keinem chirurgischen Lehrbuch die genaue Definition für Operationstauglichkeit finden konnte, möchte ich meine eigene Beschreibung zur Diskussion stellen.

Eine Operationstauglichkeit wurde meist bei Patienten angefordert, bei denen neben der chirurgischen Erkrankung noch Begleiterkrankungen vermutet wurden. Sie wurde von einem Internisten auf Grund der Anamnese und der von ihm erhobenen Befunde festgestellt. Die internistische Operationstauglichkeit ist keine Anästhesiefähigkeit und der Internist trägt auch keinerlei Mitverantwortung für das Wohlergehen des Patienten während und nach der Anästhesie. Er kann auch keine Mitverantwortung tragen, da er weder die Wahl der Anästhesie beeinflussen, noch das Wissen um die Vorgänge während und nach Operationen und den dabei auftretenden Problemen hat. Der Anästhesiologe kann sich also keineswegs auf die Operationstauglichkeit, die vom Internisten gestellt wurde, verlassen, sondern muß seinerseits durch entsprechende Untersuchungen die Anästhesiefähigkeit und das Anästhesierisiko feststellen.

Unter Anästhesiefähigkeit eines Patienten verstehen wir eine vom Anästhesiologen fest-
gestellte Tauglichkeit des Patienten, einen chirurgischen Eingriff mit einer gezielten Schmerzausschaltung (Blocks) bzw. Allgemeinanästhesie durchführen zu können. Neben der Anästhesiefähigkeit muß auch das Anästhesierisiko abgeschätzt werden. Maßgebend für die Anästhesiefähigkeit und Risiko sind nicht nur die Befunde des Herz-Kreislaufsystems, der Atmung,
des Labors, sondern auch das Wissen um die Pharmakodynamik der Anästhesiemittel, Beatmung und intra- bzw. postoperativ auftretenden Problemen wie Hypovolämie, Hypoxie,
Rhythmusstörungen usw.

Der Anästhesiologe übernimmt damit die volle Verantwortung, sowohl dem Patienten
gegenüber, als auch in forensicher Hinsicht. Die Feststellung der Anästhesiefähigkeit kann
nicht auf ein anderes Fachgebiet delegiert werden.

Um den bisher bei der präoperativen Befunderhebung durch Anästhesiologen aufgetretenen Schwierigkeiten aus dem Weg zu gehen, war es notwendig, die präoperative Befundung
auf neue Grundlagen zu stellen. Der erste Vorschlag für eine derartige Anästhesieambulanz
oder Anästhesieklinik wurde bereits 1949 von Alfred Lee (Anaesth. 1949) gemacht. Trotzdem hat sich dieses Konzept bis heute nur sehr zögernd durchgesetzt, wohl vor allem auf
Grund von Personalschwierigkeiten, die in fast allen Anästhesieabteilungen herrschen.

Mit dieser Paneldiskussion soll Ihnen, meine sehr geehrten Damen und Herren, die zur
Feststellung der Anästhesiefähigkeit notwendigen Screeninguntersuchungen dargelegt werden. Es wird eine Frage der Organisation und der örtlichen Gegebenheiten einer solchen Ambulanz sein, wie die noch nicht vorhandenen Befunde erhoben und in welcher Form die Zusammenarbeit mit anderen Fächern — vor allem der Internen Medizin — erfolgt. Die Erfahrungen, die mit derartigen präoperativen Ambulanzen in unseren Nachbarländern bestehen,
zeigen verschiedene Modelle auf, die wir zur Diskussion stellen. Die statistischen Beweise, die
die Notwendigkeit einer frühzeitigen und vollständigen Befunderhebung vor Operationen zeigen, sollen Sie auch überzeugen, eine derartige Anästhesieambulanz in Ihrer Institution ein-
zurichten. Schließlich wird Ihnen noch Ihre rechtliche Verantwortung dem Patienten und
Gesetzgeber gegenüber von einem Fachmann auf diesem Gebiet, Herrn Dr. Weissauer, dargestellt.

Folgende Vorteile konnten wir durch die Einführung der Präoperativen Ambulanz feststellen: Für den Patienten hat sich eine wesentliche Vereinfachung der präoperativen Abklärung und eine Verkürzung des Spitalsaufenthaltes um 1—2 Tage ergeben. Der Chirurg kann
seine Betten jetzt gezielter und mit weniger Leerlauf belegen. Das Krankenhaus hat durch die
Einsparung von Spitalstagen und Betten wegen einer zu geringen Bettenkapazität ebenfalls
Vorteile. Und schließlich hat der Anästhesiologe die Möglichkeit, den Patienten frühzeitig
kennenzulernen, mit ihm persönlichen Kontakt zu haben, eine gezielte Befunderhebung durchführen zu können, um auch zu einer richtigen Einschätzung und Einordnung des Patienten
in ein Anästhesierisikoschema zu kommen. Die Wahl des Anästhesieverfahrens und des An-
ästhesiemittels wird dadurch erleichtert.

Literatur

Goldman L, Caldera OL et mult. al. (1977) Multifactorial index of cardiac risk in noncardiac surgical pro-
    cedures. N Engl J Med 297:845—850
Kyei-Mensah K, Thornton JA (1974) The incidence of medical disease in surgical patients. Br J Anaesth
    46:570—574
Lee A (1949) The anaesthetic outpatient clinic. Anaesth 4:169

Präoperative Diagnostik und operatives Risiko

H. Lutz

Es gilt heute als gesichert, daß in der Vorbereitung des Patienten auf den operativen Eingriff viele Ansatzpunkte für eine Senkung des operativen Risikos zu sehen sind. Dies wird nicht zuletzt durch eine Reihe gutdokumentierter Studien (Tabelle 1) über die Letalität bei elekti-

Tabelle 1. Letalitätsquoten bei Notoperationen und bei elektiven Eingriffen. Zusammenstellung der Befunde verschiedener Autoren

Autor	Alter unters. Pat.	Letalität % Notoperation	Elektiver Eingriff
v. Bramann u. Herold	> 80	46,9	13,1
Lorhan	> 80	38,7	23
Aubry et al.	> 70	45	2
Cogbill	> 65	23,2	17,8
Cole	> 60	18,6	6,5
Haug u. Dale	> 60	21,9	5,7
Shelby u. Lorhan	–	10,0	0,6

ven Eingriffen und bei Notoperationen unterstrichen [4, 5, 11, 20, 27]. Auch die kürzlich abgeschlossene Auswertung der von uns registrierten Anästhesiekomplikationen aus mehr als 100 000 Anästhesieprotokollen der letzten 5 Jahre bestätigt diese seit langem bekannte Tatsache nachdrücklich (Tabelle 2). Darüber hinaus zeigt die Auflistung unserer Komplikationen, daß der Schwerpunkt der intraoperativen Komplikationen im kardiovaskulären Bereich liegt und daß hier Unterschiede zwischen der Gruppe der Allgemeinanästhesien und dem Kollektiv der Regionalanästhesien nicht bestehen. Gegenwärtig darf man davon ausgehen, daß zwar Einigkeit über die Notwendigkeit von Befunderhebungen und Diagnostik besteht, daß aber über den Umfang dieser Maßnahmen selbst unter namhaften Anästhesisten recht unterschiedliche Meinungen vorliegen [15]. Wir vertreten seit 1972 den Standpunkt, daß vor jedem operativen Eingriff mit einem orientierenden breit gefächerten Untersuchungsprogramm (screening) die wesentlichsten Informationen über die Organfunktionen des Patienten gewonnen werden sollten [20]. Dies gilt auch für kleine operative Eingriffe, da die Komplikationsquote der sogenannten „Kurznarkose" nicht niedriger ist, als die einer Narkose bis zu zwei Stunden Dauer (Tabelle 3). Eine Reduzierung des präoperativen Diagnostikprogrammes halten wir deshalb nur dann für vertretbar, wenn die Dringlichkeit des operativen Eingriffes dies gebietet.

Tabelle 2. Intraoperative Komplikationen bei mehr als 100 000 Anaesthesien, unterteilt in Allgemein- und Regionalanaesthesien bei Planoperationen und Noteingriffen, durchgeführt am Institut für Anaesthesiologie und Reanimation des Klinikums Mannheim im Zeitraum 1974–1978

Komplikation	110743 Anaesth.		96767 Allgemeinanesth. 84419 Planoperationen		12348 Notoperationen		13976 Regionalanaesth. 12193 Planoperationen		1783 Notoperationen	
	n	%	n	%	n	%	n	%	n	%
Injektionsschwierigkeiten	241	0,21	197	0,23	44	0,35	–	–	–	–
Erschwerte Intubation	997	0,90	871	1,03	126	1,02	–	–	–	–
Zahnbeschädigung	155	0,13	141	0,16	14	0,11	–	–	–	–
Allergische Reaktion	261	0,23	185	0,22	11	0,09	63	0,51	2	0,11
Hypertonie	1238	1,11	993	1,17	156	1,26	78	0,63	11	0,61
Schwere Hypotension	1486	1,34	843	0,99	311	2,5	283	2,32	49	2,74
Herzrhythmusstörung	1812	1,63	1272	1,50	299	2,42	189	1,55	52	2,91
Kreislaufstillstand	72	0,06	28	0,03	34	0,27	6	0,05	4	0,22
Exitus in tabula	35	0,03	4	0,004	27	0,21	2	0,01	2	0,11
Singultus	82	0,07	58	0,07	22	0,18	2	0,01	–	–
Erbrechen	245	0,22	198	0,23	41	0,33	2	0,01	4	0,22
Aspiration	89	0,08	52	0,06	36	0,29	–	–	1	0,05
Atemwegsspasmus	344	0,31	284	0,33	29	0,23	31	0,25	–	–
Gerätetechnischer Fehler	152	0,14	137	0,16	15	0,12	–	–	–	–
Lagerungsschaden	18	0,01	14	0,01	3	0,02	1	0,008	–	–
Schwere Blutung	686	0,62	359	0,42	217	1,75	89	0,72	21	1,17
Total	7913	7,03	5636	6,61	1385	11,15	746	7,07	146	8,14

Tabelle 3. Komplikationsquoten und 4-Wochen-Letalität in Abhängigkeit von der Operationszeit

Operationszeit (min)	Komplikationsquote (%)	4-Wochen-Letalität (%)
0– 15	3,4	2,4
16– 60	2,3	1,9
61–120	3,2	3,3
121–180	7,4	5,9
181–240	8,7	7,7
241–300	9,4	8,8
> 300	14,0	17,9
Gesamt	3,6	3,2

In der täglichen Praxis erfolgt die Durchführung einer präoperativen Diagnostik und die Einschätzung des operativen Risikos am zweckmäßigsten und zuverlässigsten mit Patientenfragebögen, einem den wesentlichsten Forderungen gerecht werdenden Untersuchungsprogramm und einer Risiko-Checkliste. Der 1971 in unserem Institut entwickelte Patientenfragebogen (Ahlborn, Klose 1971) ist nach vielen Verbesserungen und Modifikationen inzwischen an vielen Anästhesieabteilungen im Routinegebrauch. Der Fragebogen erhöht zweifelsohne die Zuverlässigkeit der Befunderhebung, ohne eine wesentliche Mehrbelastung bei der

Prämedikationsvisite zu verursachen. Das 1972 von uns vorgeschlagene präoperative Untersuchungsprogramm [20] wurde in den zurückliegenden Jahren mehrfach verbessert und hat 1978 eine bemerkenswerte Unterstützung durch den Berufsverband Deutscher Internisten gefunden (Abb. 1). Die noch bestehenden geringen Unterschiede in den gewünschten Untersuchungen besitzen keinen Einfluß auf die Einschätzung des operativen Risikos. Sie betreffen lediglich Blutproben, wie Protein- und Natriumkonzentration, die Gamma-GT und orientierende Blutgerinnungsparameter, die als Entscheidungshilfen bei der Infusionstherapie und Auswahl des Anästhesieverfahrens von Wert sind. Im Jahre 1975 haben wir eine Anästhesie-Checkliste zur präoperativen Risikoeinschätzung (Abb. 2) vorgeschlagen (Lutz, Klose, Peter 1975), die inzwischen mehrfach überprüft und verbessert worden ist. Ausgangspunkt für die Entwicklung einer derartigen Liste war das unzureichende und nicht auf objektivierbare Kriterien beruhende Beurteilungsverfahren bei den ASA-Risikogruppen (Abb. 3). Auch bei der Aufschlüsselung der Anästhesietodesfälle nach der ASA-Nomenklatur wurde in vielen Studien gezeigt (Beecher a. Todd 1954; Edwards 1965; Boba 1961), daß keine Korrelation zwischen Risikogruppe und Letalität herzustellen ist. Die letzte Überprüfung der eigenen Risiko-Checkliste (Abb. 4) zeigt hingegen eine gute Korrelation verschiedener intra- und postoperativer Komplikationen mit den von uns errechneten Risikogruppen. Am auffälligsten ist dies bei den kardiovaskulären und bronchopulmonalen Komplikationen. Stoffwechselerkrankungen hingegen besitzen nur einen geringen Einfluß auf das operative Risiko. Auch der letzte Ausdruck der bei uns registrierten intraoperativen Komplikationen zeigt eine gute Korrelation zur verwendeten Risikogruppeneinteilung (Abb. 5).

Inzwischen liegt eine größere Zahl teilweise gut dokumentierter Untersuchungen zum operativen Risiko bei bestimmten Erkrankungen vor, so daß die Zuordnung der Einzelbefunde in eine Wertungstabelle mehr und mehr verbessert werden konnte. Dabei lassen sich 4 Schwerpunkte bilden: Cardiovaskuläre Erkrankungen, bronchopulmonale Erkrankungen, Stoffwechselkrankheiten und Allgemeinzustand, sowie Operationszeit und Operationsart.

Präoperative Untersuchungsprogramme	
Inst. f. Anästhesiologie Mannheim	Berufsverband Deutscher Internisten
–	BKS
Hämoglobin, Hämatokrit	Großes Blutbild
Serumprotein oder Serumalbumin	–
Blutzucker	Blutzucker
Elektrolyte Kalium	Elektrolyte Kalium
Natrium	–
Transamin. SGPT	Transamin. SGPT
–	*Gamma-GT*
Kreatinin	Kreatinin
Quickwert	Quickwert
–	*Thrombozytenzahl*
–	Urinanalyse
Blutgruppe	Blutgruppe
EKG (ohne Altersbegrenzung)	EKG (ohne Altersbegrenzung)
Lungen-Rö-Aufnahme	Lungen-Rö-Aufnahme

Abb. 1. Präoperatives Untersuchungsprogramm des Instituts für Anästhesiologie und Reanimation am Klinikum Mannheim und des Berufsverbandes Deutscher Internisten

Präoperative Risiko-Checkliste

0	1	2	4	8	16	Pkt
Geplante Operation, nicht dringlich	Geplante Operation, bedingt dringlich	Nicht geplante Op., dringlich	Soforteingriff			
Oberflächenchirurgie	Extremitäteneingriff	Operation m. Eröffnung der Bauchhöhle	Operation m. Eröffnung von Thorax o. Schädel	Zweihöhleneingriff	Polytrauma / Schock	
Alter 1 - 39 Jahre	0 - 1 Jahre 40 - 69 Jahre	70 - 79 Jahre	> 80 Jahre			
Voraussichtl. Op.zeit < 60 Min.	61 - 120 Min.	121 - 180 Min.	> 180 Min.			
Normgewicht ± 10%	10 - 15% Untergew.	10 - 30% Übergew. 15 - 25% Untergew.	> 30% Übergew.			
Normotonie < 160, < 95 mm Hg	Behandelte Hypertonie (kontrolliert)	Unbeh. od. kurzfristig beh. Hypertonie	Behandelte Hypertonie (unkontrolliert)			
Herzleistung normal	Rekomp. Herzinsuff.	Angina pectoris			Dekomp. Herzinsuff.	
EKG normal	Mäßige EKG-Veränd.	Schrittmacher-EKG	Fehlend. Sinusrhythmus > 5 ventrik. Extrasyst./Min			
Kein Herzinfarkt	Herzinfarkt > 2 Jahre	Herzinfarkt > 1 Jahr	Herzinfarkt > 6 Mon.	Herzinfarkt < 6 Mon.	Herzinfarkt < 3 Mon.	
Atmung normal	Obstruktion beh.	Obstruktion unbeh.	Bronchopulmonater Infekt-Pneumonie	Restriktion	Manifeste Ateminsuffizienz; Cyanose	
Laborwerte Leber normal	Laborwerte Leber leichte Veränderungen	Laborwerte Leber schwere Veränderungen				
Laborwerte Niere normal	Laborwerte Niere leichte Veränderungen	Laborwerte Niere schwere Veränderungen				
Laborw. SBH u. Elektr. normal	Laborw. SBH u. Elektr. leichte Veränderungen	Laborw. SBH u. Elektr. schwere Veränderungen				
Hb > 12.5 g %	Hb 12.5 - 10.0 g %	Hb < 10.0 g %				
Verbrennungsindex (% Verbr. Fläche x Alter)	bis 20	bis 40	bis 60	bis 80	> 80	
					Anzahl Punkte	

Abb. 2. Präoperative Risiko-Checkliste des Instituts für Anästhesiologie und Reanimation am Klinikum Mannheim

ASA-Risikogruppen		% Todesfälle					
I	Gesunder Patient	56	17	0	32	33	5
II	Pat. mit leichter Allgemeinerkrankung	56	21	15			19
III	Pat. mit schwerer Allgemeinerkrankung	44	46	31			44
IV	Pat. mit inaktivierender Allgemeinerkrankung	44	46	41	68	67	23
V	Moribunder Patient		16	10			9
Untersucher		BEECHER/TODD	EDWARDS	DRIPPS	BOBA/LANDMESSER	CLIFTON/HOTTEN	MEMERY

Abb. 3. ASA-Risikogruppen und Zusammenstellung von Nachuntersuchungsergebnissen verschiedener Untersucher. Zwischen der Höhe des Risikos und der Letalitätsquote besteht keine Korrelation

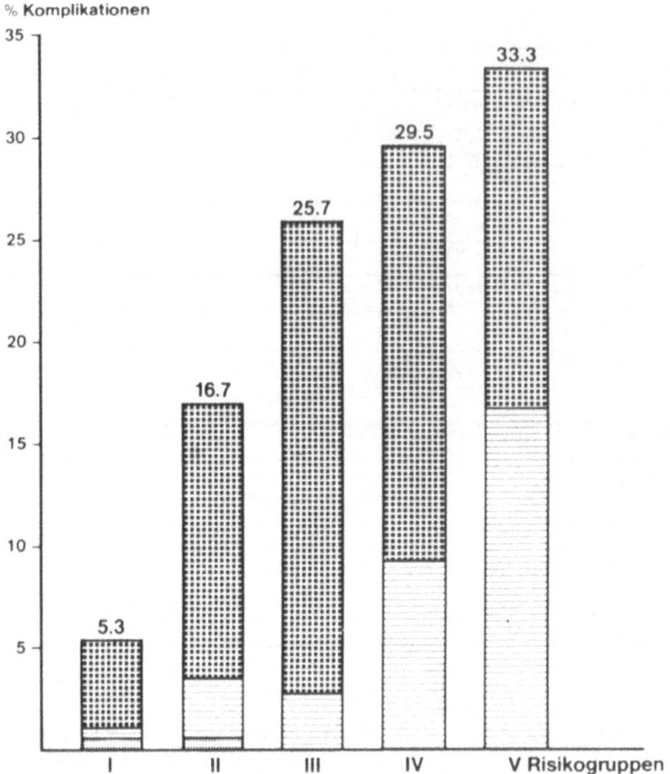

Abb. 4. Graphische Darstellung der Überprüfung der einen Risiko-Checkliste. Die Häufigkeit der Komplikationen steigt mit der Höhe des ermittelten Risikos an. Kardiovaskuläre (dunkles Karo) und bronchopulmonale (schraffiert) Komplikationen stehen im Vordergrund

1. Kardiovaskuläre Erkrankungen

Goldman et al. [9] haben den Einfluß kardiovaskulärer Erkrankungen auf das operative Risiko sehr eingehend untersucht. Danach sind folgende Erkrankungen in abnehmender Signifikanz mit dem operativen Risiko korreliert (Tabelle 4): Manifeste Herzinsuffizienz — Myokardinfarkt innerhalb der letzten 6 Monate — fehlender Sinusrhythmus oder Vorhofextrasystolen — mehr als 5 ventrikuläre Extrasystolen pro Minute — Aortenklappenstenose.

Aus vielen anderen Untersuchungen ([1, 8, 17, 22, 28] Topkins a. Artusio 1964) wird deutlich (Tabelle 5), daß der überstandene Herzinfarkt während der ersten drei Monate als absolute Kontraindikation für eine Allgemeinanästhesie gelten muß und daß erst 3 Jahre nach dem Infarkt das operative Risiko dieser Kranken dem eines gesunden Patienten entspricht.

Die Hypertonie — behandelt oder unbehandelt — ist Ursache einer Reihe nicht vorhersehbarer und schwer zu beeinflussender kardiovaskulärer Komplikationen. Dies sind insbesondere ausgeprägte Hypotensionen, Hypertensionen und Arrhythmien (Tabelle 6). Alle Komplikationen wurden häufiger beobachtet, wenn die Hypertonie unbehandelt war.

KOMPLIKATIONEN	ANZAHL DER PAT					
	I 6909	I 6305	I 4145	I 1291	I 256	I 18906
	RISIKO I	RISIKO II	RISIKO III	RISIKO IV	RISIKO V	GESAMT
INJEKTIONSSCHWIER	16 0.23	15 0.23	13 0.31	5 0.38	0 0.00	49 0.25
ALLERG.REAKTION	20 0.28	25 0.39	25 0.60	2 0.15	0 0.00	72 0.38
SCHWERE HYPOTENS	19 0.27	49 0.77	102 2.46	41 3.17	16 6.25	227 1.20
HYPERTONIE	18 0.26	56 0.88	103 2.48	47 3.64	4 1.56	229 1.20
HERZRHYTMUSSTRG.	57 0.82	61 0.96	107 2.58	52 4.02	9 3.51	286 1.51
ASYSTOLIE	2 0.02	2 0.03	3 0.07	3 0.23	3 1.17	13 0.06
ERSCHW.INTUBATION	43 0.62	114 1.80	71 1.71	11 0.85	4 1.56	243 1.28
ZAHNBESCHAEDIGUNG	6 0.08	13 0.20	5 0.12	2 0.15	0 0.00	26 0.13
ATEMWEGSSPASMUS	42 0.60	34 0.53	18 0.43	11 0.85	0 0.00	105 0.55
SINGULTUS	7 0.10	14 0.22	5 0.12	0 0.00	0 0.00	26 0.13
ERBRECHEN	43 0.62	31 0.49	21 0.50	5 0.38	3 1.17	103 0.54
ASPIRATION	9 0.13	12 0.19	5 0.12	1 0.07	1 0.39	28 0.14
SCHWERE BLUTUNG	2 0.02	23 0.36	44 1.06	25 1.93	8 3.12	102 0.53
EXITUS I.T.	2 0.02	1 0.01	1 0.02	1 0.07	17 6.64	22 0.11
LAGERUNGSSCHAEDEN	0 0.00	1 0.01	1 0.02	0 0.00	0 0.00	2 0.01
GERAETETEC.FEHLER	7 0.10	12 0.19	4 0.09	0 0.00	3 1.17	26 0.13
GESAMT(1327)	293 4.24	463 7.34	528 12.73	206 15.95	69 26.56	1558 8.24

```
ANAESTHESIEN MIT 1 KOMPLIKATIONEN   1133
ANAESTHESIEN MIT 2 KOMPLIKATIONEN    162
ANAESTHESIEN MIT 3 KOMPLIKATIONEN     28
ANAESTHESIEN MIT 4 KOMPLIKATIONEN      3
ANAESTHESIEN MIT 5 KOMPLIKATIONEN      1
```

Abb. 5. Originalausdruck der Verteilung von Komplikationen in Abhängigkeit von der Risiko-Checkliste des Instituts für Anästhesiologie und Reanimation am Klinikum Mannheim bei rd. 19 000 fortlaufend registrierten Anästhesien des Jahres 1979. Die Brauchbarkeit der Risiko-Checkliste wird besonders deutlich durch die gute Korrelation der kardiovaskulären Komplikationen und der Gesamtkomplikationsquote in Abhängigkeit von den ermittelten Risikogruppen

Tabelle 4. Wertigkeit kardiovaskulärer Risikofaktoren (nach [9])

Befund	Multivar.-Diskrim. Funkt.-Koeffiz.
Dekompensierte Herzinsuffizienz	0,451
Myokardinfarkt < 6 Mon. vor Operation	0,384
Fehlender Sinusrhytmus	
Vorhofextrasystolie	0,283
> 5 ventrikuläre Extrasyst./Min.	0,278
Aortenklappenstenose	0,119

Tabelle 5. Häufigkeit eines Reinfarktes in Abhängigkeit vom Intervall Primärinfarkt – Operation (nach Knapp et al. 1966)

Zeitinvervall Infarkt-Operation	Patienten mit präoperativem Myokardinfarkt	Patienten mit postoperativem Reinfarkt
unter 6 Monaten	7	7 (100%)
6 Mon. – 1 Jahr	21	7 (33%)
1 Jahr –2 Jahre	22	9 (41%)
2 Jahre – 3 Jahre	25	3 (12%)
über 3 Jahre	352	0
Total	427	26 (6%)

Tabelle 6. Kardiovaskuläre Komplikationen in Abhängigkeit von vorbestehender Hypertonie

Komplikation	10 827 Pat. mit Hypertonie		8 423 Pat. behandelt		2 404 Pat. unbehandelt	
	n	%	n	%	n	%
Hypotension	1124	10,38	768	9,11	356	14,81
Hypertension	917	8,46	619	7,34	298	12,43
Arrhythmie	1276	11,78	962	11,42	314	13,07
Gesamt	3317	30,62	2349	27,87	968	40,31

2. Bronchopulmonale Erkrankungen

Erkrankungen der Atemwege und der Lunge sind für das präoperative Risiko nur von untergeordneter Bedeutung; sie bestimmen aber in erheblichem Maße den postoperativen Verlauf, so daß sie in der präoperativen Diagnostik besondere Aufmerksamkeit erfordern. In einer Studie konnten wir zeigen (Lutz, Klose, Peter 1976), daß sie zwar nur mit 4,9% am Gesamtkrankengut (Tabelle 7), jedoch mit 15% an den postoperativen Komplikationen und sogar mit 30% an der 4-Wochen-Sterblichkeit beteiligt sind. Diese Zahlen stimmen gut mit Unter-

Tabelle 7. Komplikationsquoten und 4-Wochen-Letalität in Abhängigkeit von kardiovaskulären und bronchopulmonalen Komplikationen

| Erkrankung | 30 126 Patienten | | Komplikationen | 4-Wochen-Letalität |
	n	%	(%)	(%)
Kardiovaskuläre Erkrankungen	2802	9,3	28,3	20,2
Bronchopulmonale	1476	4,9	15,3	29,8

suchungen von Collins [6], Palmer [23] und Wightman [30] überein, die die Komplikationsrate bei akuten oder chronischen Lungenerkrankungen auf das 3- bis 4fache erhöht sehen. Für Patienten mit deutlich eingeschränkter Lungenfunktion haben Collins [6], Stein ([29], 1970) und Bryant [3] eine Risikosteigerung auf mehr als das zwanzigfache gefunden.

3. Stoffwechselerkrankungen

Unter den Stoffwechselerkrankungen ist der Diabetes mellitus am stärksten im operativen Krankengut verbreitet. Störungen anderer Hormonsysteme sind vergleichsweise selten.

Bei rechtzeitiger Erkennung und zuverlässiger Korrektur der gestörten Funktionen ist das operative Risiko nicht nachweisbar erhöht; es sei denn durch Folgeerkrankungen, wie durch diabetesbedingte Gefäßveränderungen. In gleicher Weise haben Leber- und Nierenerkrankungen keinen wesentlich höheren Einfluß auf das operative Risiko.

4. Allgemeinzustand, Operationszeit, Operationsart

Da Lebensalter und Leistungsabnahme der Organe im allgemeinen parallel laufen, läßt sich eine altersabhängige Zunahme des operativen Risikos nachweisen (Tabelle 8). Ein deutlicher Anstieg findet sich nach dem 70. Lebensjahr; eine Beobachtung, die auch von Goldman [9] bestätigt wurde.

Auch die extreme Mangelernährung und das Übergewicht sollten in einer Risikobeurteilung berücksichtigt werden. Bei Patienten mit einem Übergewicht von mehr als 30% des Sollgewichtes ist die postoperative Sterblichkeit — vor allem durch postoperative Lungenkomplikationen bedingt — um das zwei- bis dreifache erhöht [10, 18].

Tabelle 8. Komplikationsquoten und 4-Wochen-Letalität in Abhängigkeit vom Lebensalter

Altersgruppen	Komplikationen %	4-Wochen-Letalität %
0–39 Jahre	1,8	1,4
40–69 Jahre	5,0	4,6
70–89 Jahre	8,7	8,4
> 90 Jahre	18,1	29,5

Ebenso kann die Dauer des operativen Eingriffes gut mit der Komplikations- und Letalitätsquote korreliert werden (Tabelle 3). Hier ist auffällig, daß eine Erhöhung des operativen Risikos nach mehr als 2 Stunden Operationszeit resultiert. Erneut soll darauf hingewiesen werden, daß die sogenannten „Kurzeingriffe" keinesfalls ein geringeres Risiko zeigen, als Operationen bis zu 2 Stunden Dauer.

Einfluß auf das Risiko hat auch die Art des operativen Eingriffs. Wir fanden einen Anstieg der Komplikations- und Letalitätsquoten in der Reihenfolge Oberflächen-, Extremitäten-, Abdominal-, Thoraxchirurgie zu den Zweihöhlenoperationen. Auch in der Studie von Goldman [9] ist die Abhängigkeit des operativen Risikos von der Art der Operation — hier allerdings nur für die intraperitonealen und intrathorakalen Eingriffe geprüft — gut dokumentiert.

Auf der Grundlage der in letzter Zeit mitgeteilten Untersuchungsbefunde über den Einfluß bestimmter Vorerkrankungen auf das operative Risiko, sowie unter Berücksichtigung der Ergebnisse der letzten Überprüfung unserer Risikotabelle haben wir die Checkliste überarbeitet (Abb. 2). Sie enthält jetzt Angaben über die Dringlichkeit des Eingriffs, die Art und Dauer der Operation, den Allgemeinzustand des Patienten, sowie Informationen über seine kardiozirkulatorische-, bronchopulmonale- und Stoffwechselsituation. Da die kardiozirkulatorischen Informationen den größten Stellenwert für die Einschätzung des operativen Risikos besitzen, sind die dafür vorgesehenen Spalten drucktechnisch besonders hervorgehoben.

Wir sind uns bewußt, daß auch mit Hilfe einer derartigen Checkliste das Risiko des operativen Eingriffes im Einzelfall nicht absolut zuverlässig erfaßt werden kann. Zu viele Faktoren besitzen mitunter nicht voraussehbare schwerwiegende Einflüsse, so daß es immer wieder Bereiche geben wird, die nicht voll ausgelotet und abgewogen werden können. Für die tägliche Routine steht jedoch ein System zur Verfügung, das seine Bewährungsprobe bestanden hat, mehrfach mit guten Ergebnissen überprüft worden ist und vor allem die Einschätzung des operativen Risikos nicht mehr allein dem Zufall überläßt.

Zusammenfassung

Das Schicksal eines operierten Patienten wird entscheidend von seinen Vorerkrankungen und der sorgfältigen Vorbereitung auf den operativen Eingriff bestimmt. Kardiovaskuläre und bronchopulmonale Erkrankungen bilden die wesentlichsten Risikofaktoren. Lebensalter, Operationszeit und Operationsart können das Risiko des operativen Eingriffs zusätzlich erhöhen. Die bisher in vielen Untersuchungen analysierten Risikofaktoren werden hinsichtlich intra- und postoperativer Komplikationen gewertet und einer neuentwickelten Risiko-Checkliste zugeordnet. Die Überprüfung dieser Risiko-Checkliste zeigt, daß eine gute Korrelation der eingetretenen Komplikationen in Abhängigkeit vom vorberechneten Risikograd resultiert.

Literatur

1. Arkins R, Smessaert AA, Hicks RG (1964) Mortality and morbidity in surgical patients with coronary artery disease. J Amer med Ass 190:485
2. Brigden W (1971) Disease of the Myocardium. In: Beeson PB, Dermott WMc (eds) Textbook of Medicine. W.B. Saunders Comp, Philadelphia
3. Bryant LR, Rams JJ, Trinkle JK, Malette WG (1970) Present-day risk of thoracotomy in patients with compromised pulmonary function. Arch Surg 101:140

4. Cogbill ChL (1967) Operation in the aged. Arch Surg 94:202
5. Cole WH (1953) Operability in the young and aged. Ann Surg 138:145
6. Collins CD, Drake CS, Knowelden J (1968) Chest complications after upper abdominal surgery. Their anticipation and prevention. Brit Med J 1:401
7. Diament ML, Palmer KNV (1967) Spirometry for preoperative assessment of airways resistance. Lancet 1:1251
8. Fraser JG, Ramachandran PR, Davis HS (1967) Anesthesia and recent myocardial infarction. J Amer med Ass 199:318
9. Goldman L, Caldera DL, Nussbaum SR, Southwick FS, Krogstad D, Murray B, Burke DD, O'Malley TA, Goroll AH, Caplan CH, Nolan J, Carabello B, Slater EE (1977) Multifactorial Index of cardiac risk in noncardiac surgical procedures. N Engl J Med 297:845
10. Gould AD Jr (1962) Effect of obesity on respiratory complications following general anesthesia. Anesth Analg (Cleve) 41:448
11. Haug CA, Dale WA (1952) Major Surgery in old people. Arch Surg 64:421
12. Hedley-Whyte J, Burgess GW, Feeley ThW, Miller MG (1976) Applied physiology of respiratory care. Little, Brown a. Comp, Boston
13. Holdmann M (1965) Klinische Elektrokardiographie. Thieme, Stuttgart
14. Hunter PR, Endry-Wal P, Bauer PGE, Stephens FO (1968) Myocardial infarction following surgical operations. Brit med J 4:725
15. Hutschenreuther K (1979) Diskussion zu Sorgfalt bei der Voruntersuchung und Vorbehandlung. Anästhesiologie und Intensivmedizin 36
16. Keep KR (1962) The value of anesthesia outpatient clinics. Lancet 2:446
17. Knapp RB, Topkins MJ, Artusio JT (1962) The cerebral accident and coronary occlusion in anesthesia. JAMA 182:332
18. Latimer RG, Dickmann M, Day WC, Gunn ML, Schmidt CD (1971) Ventilatory patterns and pulmonary complications after upper abdominal surgery determined by preoperative and postoperative computerized spirometry and blood gas analysis. Am J Surg 112:622
19. Lundsgaard-Hansen P, Pappova E (1973/74) Respiratorische Insuffizienz, kolloidosmotischer Druck und Albumintherapie. Infusionstherapie 1:624
20. Lutz H, Klose R, Peter K (1972) Untersuchungen zum Risiko der Allgemeinanästhesie unter operativen Bedingungen. Dtsch med Wschr 97:1816
21. Lutz H (1979) Sorgfalt bei der Voruntersuchung und Vorbehandlung. Anästhesiologie und Intensivmedizin 2:31
22. Mattingly ThW (1963) Patients with coronary artery disease as a surgical risk. Amer J Cardiol 12:279
23. Palmer KNV, Diament ML (1968) Relative contributions of obstructive and restrictive ventilatory impairment in the production of hypoxaemia and hypercapnia in chronic bronchitis. Lancet 1:1233
24. Palmer KNV, Gardner AJS (1964) Effect of partial gastrectomy on pulmonary physiology. Brit Med J 1:347
25. Rovenstein EA, Taylor IB (1936) Postoperative respiratory complications: Occurance following 7 874 anesthesias. Am J Med Sci 191:807
26. Schlenker JD, Hubay CA (1973) The pathogenesis of postoperative atelectasis. A clinical study. Arch Surg 107:846
27. Shelby EA, Lorhan PH (1968) Age as factor in mortality after cholecystectomie. Anaesth Analg Curr Res 47:733
28. Skinner JF, Pearce ML (1964) Surgical risk in the cardiac patient. J chron Dis 17:57
29. Stein M, Koota GM, Simon M, Frank HA (1962) Pulmonary evaluation of surgical patients. JAMA 181:765
30. Wightman JAK (1968) A prospective survey of the incidence of postoperative pulmonary complications. Brit J Surg 55:85

Ausmaß und Wert präoperativer Voruntersuchungen zur Abklärung der Anaesthesietauglichkeit

H. Bergmann

Jeder kennt wohl die Realität langjähriger klinischer Praxis: ein gar nicht oder nur ungenügend voruntersuchter Patient wird präoperativ gar nicht oder nur ungenügend vom Anaesthesisten gesehen oder beurteilt und entweder aus einem freundschaftlichen Kompromiß oder aus einem nicht freundschaftlichen Zwang des Chirurgen heraus — womöglich noch als eben aufgenommener und unter Zeitdruck stehender „Straßenfall" — für eine elektive Operation akut anaesthesiert. Dem Zwischenfall sind damit Tür und Tor geöffnet, das anzustrebende Ideal einer, dem Dringlichkeitsgrad des Eingriffes entsprechend ausreichenden Voruntersuchung zum Zwecke der Senkung des Operationsrisikos, worunter wir die Summe aus Anaesthesierisiko und operativem Risiko verstehen wollen, wird damit klar mißachtet.

Die *Problematik* präoperativer Voruntersuchungen liegt nun im *Zeitfaktor* einer häufig umständlichen stationären Organisationsform, in der *Aussagekraft* der ausgewählten Befunde, die sich oft als verkehrt proportional zu ihrer praktischen Durchführbarkeit erweist, in der *Invasivität*, also dem Untersuchungsrisiko der Befundung, das dem daraus entspringenden Nutzen entsprechen muß, und nicht zuletzt auch im *Kostenaufwand*, der ebenfalls in Relation zum „benefit" gesetzt werden sollte.

Ein gefordertes *präoperatives Untersuchungsprogramm* (Tabelle 1) muß daher standardisiert sein, um als Routinevorgang „gewohnheitsmäßig und ohne besonderen Anlaß vorgenommen" ablaufen zu können, rationell den Zeitfaktor und den Aufwand zu optimieren und Informationslücken ebenso wie Exzesse zu vermeiden. Es wird im wesentlichen aus *Suchtesten* bestehen, die einfach und rasch auch in großer Menge — im Laborbereich durch die Automation begünstigt — durchgeführt werden können und bisher nicht bekannte Krankheiten aufzudecken imstande sind und es wird dann durch *Abklärungsteste* und Aussagen über Detailfunktionen von Organen ergänzt werden müssen, wenn der Suchtest positiv oder eine Krankheit bereits bekannt ist.

Tabelle 1. Umfang der Voruntersuchung

Ist-Bestand (kleiner bis mittlerer Eingriff, „gesunder" Patient, unter 40 Jahre)
Klinische Untersuchung, Körpergewicht und -größe, RR, Puls (Frequenz, Regularität), Harn Sacch., Alb.
→ grobklinischer Einblick, Adipositas, Hochdruck, Rhythmusstörungen

Soll-Umfang (gilt auch für über 40 Jahre und großen Eingriff)
EKG, Thorax-Rö., kleine Spirometrie
Hkrit, Gesamteiweiß, Blutgruppe, Rh, Antikörper
SGPT, HB_SAG BUN, Kreatinin
Elektrolyte, K, Na Blutzucker

Als *Ergebnis* der Voruntersuchung erwarten wir uns eine Abklärung der „Anaesthesie-tauglichkeit", die eine etwa notwendige Vorbehandlung und die Auswahl der Anaesthesie-mittel und -methode mit einschließt.

Als *Ist-Bestand* wird nun nicht selten, weil es sich „ohnehin" nur um einen kleinen oder mittleren Eingriff bei einem „gesunden" Patienten unter 40 Jahren handelt, neben einer kli-nischen Untersuchung das Körpergewicht, die Körpergröße, eine Blutdruck- und Pulsmes-sung mit Beurteilung von Frequenz und Regularität und etwa noch eine Harnuntersuchung auf Zucker und Eiweiß vorgelegt.

Als *Soll-Umfang*, für Patienten jeden Alters und jeder Eingriffsgröße zu fordern, möch-ten wir dem entgegenstellen: EKG, Thorax-Röntgen und kleine Spirometrie, Haematokrit, Gesamteiweiß, Blutgruppe/Rh und Antikörpersuchtest, SGPT, HB_sAG, BUN, Kreatinin, die Elektrolyte K und Na im Serum und den Blutzucker (siehe auch [3]).
In Form einer *organspezifischen Aufschlüsselung* soll nun auf diese Forderung etwas näher eingegangen werden.

1. Untersuchungsprogramm Herz [5, 6, 9, 11, 17] (Tabelle 2)

Abgesehen von der klinischen und physikalischen Beurteilung wird also das Untersuchungs-programm „Herz" neben der Blutdruck- und Pulsmessung das *Elektrokardiogramm* in Ruhe, nicht unbedingt aber in Belastung, mit allen Ableitungen umfassen, womit Reizbildungs- und -leitungsstörungen, eine Myokardischaemie und auch ein etwa einmal abgelaufener Infarkt aufgedeckt werden können. Es wird sodann das *Thorax-Röntgen* die Herzgröße, Vitien, eine Stauung und schließlich auch angeborene Herz- und Gefäßanomalien aufzudecken imstande sein. Beim pathologischen Ausfall dieses Screenings werden weitere spezielle Untersuchungen einzusetzen sein.

Tabelle 2. Untersuchungsprogramm Herz

Klinisch	Dyspnoe, Schmerz (A.P.), Herzklopfen, Synkope, Halsvenen
Perkussion — Auskultation	
RR, Puls	Frequenz, Rhythmus
Elektrokardiogramm	
Ruhe/Belastung, alle Ableitungen	
	Reizbildungs-, Reizleitungsstörungen, Ischämie, St. p. Infarkt
Thorax-Röntgen	
	Herzgröße, Vitien, Stauung, angeborene Herz- und Gefäßanomalien
→	Spezielle Untersuchungen

2. Untersuchungsprogramm Lunge [1, 8, 11, 13, 17, 19] (Tabelle 3)

Auch das Untersuchungsprogramm „Lunge" wird naturgemäß neben dem klinischen und physikalischen Befund das *Thorax-Röntgen* enthalten, seine Leistungsgrenzen muß man aber kennen: Eine bisher nicht bekannte Tuberkulose läßt sich mit einer Frequenz von 0,2 bis 4,4% erwarten, ein Malignom in einer Häufigkeit von etwa 1/4⁰/oo aufdecken. Gutartige Tu-

Tabelle 3. Untersuchungsprogramm Lunge

Klinisch   Dyspnoe, Sputum
Inspektion – Perkussion – Auskultation
Thorax-Röntgen
                    Tbc (0,2–4,4°/oo/Neumann [20])
                    Malignom (0,27 °/oo/Brett [3])
                    Sarkoidose, Pneumokoniose, Pneumothorax, Bronchiektasien, Emphysem (++),
                    Komporession der Luftwege (Tu, Cy, Ly)
Lungenfunktionsprüfung
VK/insp., Sekundenkapazität, Atemgrenzwert
                    Größe und Verteilung der Ventilation,
                    Hinweise auf Atemmechanik und Atemreserven, grob: Restriktion/Obstruktion
Resistance   (FD 5, Oszillationsmethode), BGA/kap
→   Spezielle Untersuchungen (auch bei Resektion)

---

more, eine Sarkoidose oder Pneumokoniose, ein Pneumothorax, Bronchiektasien, ein höhergradiges Emphysem und auch eine Kompression der Luftwege durch einen Tumor, eine Cyste oder Lymphknoten können ebenfalls nachgewiesen werden.

Funktionelle Aussagen sind jedoch erst durch eine *Lungenfunktionsprüfung* möglich. Aufgrund der heute verfügbaren Meßmethoden sollte diese die als „kleine Spirometrie" bezeichnete Parameter Vitalkapazität, Sekundenkapazität und Atemgrenzwert umfassen, womit Aussagen zur Größe der Ventilation, Hinweise auf Atemmechanik und Atemreserven und eine grobe Einschätzung einer etwaigen Restriktion oder Obstruktion gemacht werden können. Sie sollte aber auch einen oszillatorisch gemessenen Resistance-Wert und eine kapilläre Blutgasanalyse enthalten, die eine Obstruktion besser darzustellen bzw. eine respiratorische Insuffizienz nachzuweisen imstande ist.

Für Lungenresektionen und bei pathologischem Ausfall des Screenings tritt ein spezielles Untersuchungsprogramm in Kraft.

3. Untersuchungsprogramm Leber [23] (Tabelle 4)

Tabelle 4. Untersuchungsprogramm Leber

Klinisch   Palpation
SGPT   Leberzelldestruktion, gut leberspezifisch
Hepatitis B Antigen (HB$_S$AG)
(RIA, EIA, Haemagglutination – 3. Generation-Tests)
                    Hepatitis B, Infektiosität
                    gesunde Virusträger 0,2%
(Vorsichtsmaßnahmen im Operationssaal!?)
→   Spezielle Untersuchungen
Weitere Enzyme der *Leberzelldestruktion*
                    GOT, LDH
Verschluß (Cholestase)
                    alk, Phosphatase, LAP, Gamma GT
Elektrophorese

Zur Beurteilung der Leberfunktion ist das gut leberspezifische Enzym *SGPT* als Ausdruck einer Leberzelldestruktion als Suchtest allgemein anerkannt. Die Einbeziehung eines *HB$_S$AG*-Screenings ist zu diskutieren. Eine Meßmethode der 3. Generation (RIA, EIA oder Haemagglutination) ist imstande, noch 2 ng/ml Hepatitis B Antigen nachzuweisen, als *ein* Hepatitis B Marker ist der Test zu akzeptieren, die Frequenz gesunder Virusträger liegt bei 0,2%. Wie weit bei genereller Einführung dieser Untersuchung zusätzlich Vorsichtsmaßnahmen im Operationssaal praktikabel und sinnvoll sein werden, kann im Augenblick wohl noch nicht eindeutig entschieden werden.

Weitere Enzymuntersuchungen (Leberzelldestruktion: GOT, LDH; Verschluß/Cholestase: alkalische Phosphatase, LAP, Gamma GT) und eine Elektrophorese geben zusätzlich Auskunft über eine pathologische Leberfunktion, brauchen u.E. jedoch im Primärscreening nicht enthalten zu sein.

4. Untersuchungsprogramm Blut-Niere-Stoffwechsel [23] (Tabelle 5)

Und nun noch zum Untersuchungsprogramm Blut-Niere-Stoffwechsel: Um den Hydrierungszustand bzw. eine Anaemie und die daraus resultierende Notwendigkeit von Infusion und Transfusion einschätzen zu können, halten wir einen *Haematokrit*- bzw. *Haemoglobin*-Befund für ausreichend. Der Forderung des Berufsverbandes Deutscher Internisten nach dem großen Blutbild können wir uns nicht anschließen. Ebenfalls zur Vorbereitung auf eine Transfusion und zur Vermeidung pseudoakuter Transfusionssituationen gehört die grundsätzliche Vorbestimmung der *ABO-Blutgruppe*, des *Rh-Faktors* und ein *Antikörperscreening*, auf dem dann auch die Kreuzprobe aufbaut. Mit der Bestimmung des *Gesamteiweiß* sind schließlich Hypalbuminaemien aufzudecken und wird ebenfalls Einfluß auf Ausmaß und Art einer Infusionsvorbehandlung zu nehmen sein.

Tabelle 5. Untersuchungsprogramm Blut – Niere – Stoffwechsel

Haematokrit/Hb Hydrierung, Anaemie, Trf.	
Blutgruppe/Rh/AK (Ausgangspunkt für KP)	
Gesamteiweiß (Hypalbuminaemie, Infusion)	
BUN (RN = 10 + 1,07 x BUN)	grob
Kreatinin (100 : Kr = GFR ml/min)	empfindlicher
Elektrolyte K (Hypokaliaemie), *Na* (Hydrierung)	
Blutzucker (Diabetesaufdeckung)	
Säure-Basen pH, BE	
→	Spezielle Untersuchungen

Der *Harnstoff-Stickstoff,* formelhaft mit dem Reststickstoff verknüpft, ist ein grober, die Bestimmung des *Serum-Kreatinins* ein empfindlicherer Parameter der Nierenfunktion bzw. des Glomerulumfiltrates, und sollte bei keiner Voruntersuchung fehlen. Ebenso sind Elektrolytbestimmungen von *Kalium* und *Natrium* zum Ausschluß von Hypokaliaemien und zur Aussage über den Hydrierungszustand wertvoll, sollte bei der großen Zahl nicht bekannter Diabetiker auf einen *Blutzucker* nicht vergessen werden und im Rahmen der Blutgasanalyse mit dem *pH* und *Basenüberschuß* auch der Säure-Basen-Haushalt einer Bestimmung unterzogen werden. Der Berufsverband Deutscher Internisten fordert schließlich noch die *Thrombozytenzahl* und den *Quickwert*. Wir nehmen dies zur Kenntnis, sind der Meinung, daß bei Machbarkeit dem auch entsprochen werden sollte, glauben aber, daß der de facto Einfluß dieser Werte auf die Beurteilung der Anaesthesietauglichkeit zumindest nicht von globalem Interesse sein dürfte.

Die *präoperative Risikobeurteilung* [2, 7, 12, 16, 18] bedient sich nun verschiedener Klassifikationen: Die *ASA-Methode*, von Saklad 1941 [22] eingeführt, kann als grobe, aber augenscheinlich doch klinisch praktikable Vorgangsweise, die immerhin seit 38 Jahren geübt wird, angesehen werden [10]. Owens et al. [21] haben ihr erst kürzlich einen Mangel an wissenschaftlicher Präzision vorgeworfen und eine Art Modernisierung verlangt. Die *Lutz'sche Checkliste* [15, 16] zwingt zur Befundung und kann schon aus diesem Grund als wertvolle Bereicherung angesehen werden. Die Suche nach einer Organisationsform zur präoperativen Voruntersuchung als Routinemaßnahme führt schließlich zur Anaesthesieambulanz als mögliches Optimum [4].

Literatur

1. Anderson WG (1974) Respiratory aspects of the preoperative examination. Brit J Anaesth 46:549–554
2. Anderton JM (1972) The value of joint anaesthetic and surgical preoperative assessment. Brit J Anaesth 44:183–190
3. Brett GZ (1959) Bronchial carcinoma in men detected by selective and unselective miniature radiography: a review of 228 cases. Tubercle 40:192
4. Dick W, Ahnefeld FW, Fricke M, Knoche E, Milewski P, Traub E (1978) Die Anaesthesieambulanz. Erfahrungen mit einer neuen Organisationsform der pränarkotischen Untersuchung und Beratung. Anaesthesist 27:450–458
5. Fleming PR (1974) Cardiological aspects of the preoperative examination. Brit J Anaesth 46:555–557
6. Goldman L, Caldera DL, Nussbaum SR, Southwick FS, Krogstad D, Murray B, Burke DS, O'Malley TA, Goroll AH, Caplan ChH, Nolan J, Carabello B, Slater EE (1977) Multifactorial index of cardiac risk in noncardiac surgical procedures. New Engl J Med 297:845–850
7. Goldstein A, Keats AS (1970) The Risk of Anesthesia. Anesthesiology 33:130–143
8. Herzog H, Keller R (1974) Die präoperative Diagnostik bei Lungenfunktionsstörungen. In: Lawin P Morr-Strathmann U (Hrsg) Kongreßbericht DGAW, Jahrestagung 23.–26.11.1972 Hamburg. Springer, Berlin Heidelberg New York pp 452–466
9. Huth K, Sirbulesch R, Knorpp K, Lasch HG (1976) Myokardiale und koronare Risikofaktoren. Klin Anaesthesiol Intensivther 11:61–68
10. Keats AS (1978) The ASA Classification of Physical Status – A Recapitulation. Editorial Views. Anesthesiology 49:233–236
11. Kerr IH (1974) The preoperative chest X-ray. Brit J Anaesth 46:558–563
12. Kyei-Mensah K, Thornton JA (1974) The incidence of medical disease in surgical patients. Brit J Anaesth 46:570–574
13. Lichtenauer I (1975) Lungenfunktionsprüfung am Krankenbett. Anästh Inform 16:323–327
14. Lutz H (1979) Sorgfalt bei der Voruntersuchung und Vorbehandlung. Anästh Intensivmed 20:31–35
15. Lutz H, Klose R, Peter K (1972) Untersuchungen zum Risiko der Allgemeinanästhesie unter operativen Bedingungen. Dtsch med Wschr 97:1816–1820
16. Lutz H, Klose R, Peter K (1976) Die Problematik der präoperativen Risikoeinstufung. Anästh Inform 17:342–351
17. Maigaard S, Elksaer P, Stefansson T (1979) Value of routine preoperative radiographic examination of the thorax and ECG (Abstr.). Anesthesiology Excerpta Medica 14:5
18. Marx GF, Matheo CV, Orkin LR (1973) Computer analysis of postanesthetic deaths. Anesthesiology 39:54–58

19. Matthys H, Rühle KH (1976) Lungenfunktionsdiagnostik zur Erfassung des Risikopatienten in der Anästhesiologie. Klin Anästh Intensivther 12:8–13
20. Neumann G (1972) Die Bedeutung der Röntgenreihenuntersuchung für die Tuberkulosebekämpfung. Adv Tuberc Res 18:103
21. Owens WD, Felts JA, Spitznagel EL jr (1978) ASA Physical Status Classifications: A Study of Consistency of Ratings. Anesthesiology 49:239–243
22. Saklad M (1941) Grading of patients for surgical procedures. Anesthesiology 2:281–284
23. Whitby LG (1974) Biochemical screening tests for the anaesthetist. Brit J Anaesth 46:564–569

Kleine Spirometrie, Ruhe- und Belastungsblutgase als präoperative Kriterien für die respiratorische Funktion

K. Harnoncourt und W. Ragossnig

Im folgenden Referat sollen zunächst die Überlegungen des Internisten vorgestellt werden, die nach jahrelanger Erfahrung mit der früher allgemein üblichen konsiliarischen „Feststellung der Operationstauglichkeit" zu einer engen Zusammenarbeit mit den Anästhesiologen im Rahmen einer präoperativen Ambulanz geführt haben. Die vom Internisten üblicherweise geforderte Stellungnahme bei Patienten, welche einer Operation zugeführt werden sollen, betrifft zwei Gesichtspunkte, die für unsere Überlegungen voneinander getrennt werden müssen.

1. Die Stellungnahme zur Operationsindikation:
In allen jenen Fällen, bei welchen diese Entscheidung nicht vom Anästhesierisiko abhängt, wird sie wie bisher auf konsiliarischem Weg zwischen dem Internisten und dem Chirurgen zu treffen sein.

2. Die Stellungnahme zur Narkosetauglichkeit:
Was diese Stellungnahme anbelangt, ist die enge Zusammenarbeit zwischen dem Internisten und dem Anästhesiologen erforderlich. Der Internist hat dabei die Aufgabe, nach Risikofaktoren zu suchen und gegebenenfalls vorbeugende und therapeutische Maßnahmen zu verordnen. Der Anästhesist, der die Verantwortung für die Beherrschung dieser Risiken rund um die Operation zu tragen hat, muß so früh wie möglich genau informiert sein, um das für den jeweiligen Fall günstigste Vorgehen rechtzeitig planen und mit dem Chirurgen koordinieren zu können.

Die präoperative Anästhesieambulanz befaßt sich ausschließlich mit der in Punkt 2. angegebenen Problematik. Zur Vermeidung zeitraubender und aufwendiger Doppelgleisigkeiten wurde in Graz daher vor bald 2 Jahren vom Institut für Anästhesiologie, gemeinsam mit der II. Med. Abteilung, ein präoperatives Untersuchungsprogramm erstellt, welches den Anforderungen beider Disziplinen entspricht. Dieses Programm fußt auf Erfahrungen, welche mit einem Gesunden-Screening-Test (AKL-Test) zur Aufdeckung von kardiorespiratorischen Risikofällen, bei damals fast 10000 Untersuchungen gemacht worden waren [3]. In der im Institut für Anästhesiologie eingerichteten Ambulanz werden die Untersuchungen von eigens dafür geschulten Teams durchgeführt und interdisziplinär gemeinsam befundet. Durch diese Organisation ist gewährleistet, daß das Gros der problemlosen Fälle auf raschestem Weg zur Operation gelangt. Die Risikofälle werden entweder nach einem gemeinsam erstellten und mit dem Chirurgen abgesprochenen Konzept vorbehandelt und rund um die Operation überwacht, oder, wenn nötig, einer internistischen Station zur Operationsvorbereitung bzw. zur Weiterbehandlung zugewiesen.

Diese Organisationsform hat sich zunächst als besonders ökonomisch erwiesen. Entgegen den Befürchtungen mancher Kritiker, hat sie darüberhinaus durch die bessere interdisziplinäre Zusammenarbeit und Kommunikation auch die diagnostische Effektivität verbessert.

Es ist anzunehmen, daß es durch Berücksichtigung der laufend hinzukommenden Erfahrungen in Zukunft möglich sein wird, eine weitere Steigerung zu erreichen.

Nun zu den konkreten Ergebnissen dieser präoperativen Ambulanz, von welchen wir in diesem Referat jene vorzustellen haben, welche zur Erfassung von respiratorischen Risikofällen erhoben werden. Respiratorische Störungen nehmen bekanntlich in der Skala der intraoperativen Komplikationen den zweiten Platz ein und stehen bei den postoperativen Komplikationen bei weitem an erster Stelle. Die hohe Morbidität an Erkrankungen der Atmungsorgane, die je nach Altersgruppe zwischen 5 und 50% liegt [1], ist dafür verantwortlich. Eine effiziente präoperative Diagnostik hat die Aufgabe, diese respiratorischen Risikofälle zu erfassen und einer gezielten Prophylaxe, Überwachung und atemgymnastischen Betreuung [2] zuzuführen.

Das Untersuchungsprogramm der präoperativen Anästhesieambulanz in Graz enthält neben den allgemein üblichen Kriterien wie Anamnese, Untersuchungsbefund, Thoraxröntgen usw. routinemäßig atemphysiologische Parameter. Es sind dies die „Kleine Spirometrie", die nach den Richtlinien der Österreichischen Standardisierung vorgenommen und bewertet wird [4], sowie die Blutgasanalyse aus dem arteriellen Kapillarblut. In speziellen Fällen (Verdacht auf Diffusionsstörung oder Verteilungsstörung) bringen die Belastungsblutgase eine weitere Klärung. Es stehen somit folgende Funktionswerte zur Beurteilung zur Verfügung:
1. VC exsp. und VC exsp. in % des unteren Grenzwertes,
2. FEV_1 und FEV_1 in % der VC exsp.,
3. $FEV_1 \times 30$ und $FEV_1 \times 30$ in % des unteren Grenzwertes,
4. PO_2, PCO_2, pH, BA in Ruhe,
5. PO_2, PCO_2, BA nach Belastung.

Durch die modernen und einfach zu handhabenden Geräte, die heute überall zur Verfügung stehen, fällt das Argument, welches früher gegen eine routinemäßige Anwendung vorgebracht wurde, nämlich, daß der Aufwand in Relation zum Nutzen zu groß wäre, weg. Wir meinen, daß aus diesem Grund auch das individuelle Vorgehen nach einem Flußschema, wie es von Matthys und Rühle empfohlen wird [5], keinen Vorteil bringt, denn dabei kann der jeweils nächste Untersuchungsschritt immer erst dann erfolgen, wenn die Vorbefunde ausgewertet und beurteilt sind.

Für die Befundung verwenden wir die in Tabelle 1 angegebenen Grenzwerte, welche sich bei der oben erwähnten Screening-Gesundenuntersuchung (AKL-Test) bewährt haben. Was

Tabelle 1. Grenzwerte der atemphysiologischen Parameter

Vitalkapazität	
VC zwischen 110 und 80% des unteren Grenzwertes	= verdächtig
VC unter 80% des unteren Grenzwertes	= eingeschränkt
Einsekundenkapazität	
FEV_1 zwischen 75 und 65% der VC	= verdächtig
FEV_1 unter 65% der VC	= eingeschränkt
Atemgrenzwerte	
FEV_1 x 30 zwischen 100 und 80% des unteren Grenzwertes	= verdächtig
FEV_1 x 30 unter 80% des unteren Grenzwertes	= eingeschränkt
Blutgasanalyse	
PO_2 unter 60 mm Hg	= vermindert
PCO_2 über 45 mm Hg	= erhöht

die Kleine Spirometrie anlangt, beziehen sie sich auf die „unteren Grenzwerte" des Standardisierungsprogrammes für die Lungenfunktionsdiagnostik [4] der Österreichischen Arbeitsgemeinschaft für klinische Atemphysiologie.

Von den bisher untersuchten 4562 Fällen konnten 2007 bereits statistisch ausgewertet werden. Im Gegensatz zur „Kleinen Spirometrie", die nur in 4/5 der Fälle ein brauchbares Ergebnis lieferte, konnte in jedem Fall eine relevante Blutgasanalyse erzielt werden. Dies wohl deshalb, weil sie vom Zustand und der Kooperationsfähigkeit der Probanden nicht beeinflußt wird. Der hohe Ausfall spirometrischer Werte ist zum Teil aber auch darauf zurückzuführen, daß zahlreiche Unfälle und Akutpatienten in die Statistik mit einbezogen sind. Es war zu erwarten und hat sich auch gezeigt, daß die Blutgasanalyse gerade bei diesen, nicht spirometrierbaren Patienten ein besonders wichtiges Beurteilungskriterium darstellte.

Die Tabelle 2 zeigt eine Zusammenfassung der statistischen Auswertung der Ergebnisse. Bei 2/3 der Fälle sind keine pathologischen Befunde erhoben worden. Jeder 3. von diesen hatte allerdings einen Verdachtsbefund, auf den die nachbehandelnden Ärzte hingewiesen werden. Unter den 104 Fällen mit pathologischen Belastungsblutgaswerten fanden sich fast ausschließlich inadäquate Belastungsazidosen mit normalem Gasaustausch. Es bestätigte sich damit, daß die Ergometrie zur Feststellung respiratorischer Risikofälle weniger beiträgt als zur Diagnose von kardiozirkulatorischen Risikofällen. In Einzelfällen liefert sie freilich Informationen, die sonst einen größeren funktionsdiagnostischen Aufwand erfordern würden. So fanden sich, wie aus der Tabelle 3 hervorgeht, immerhin 5 Fälle mit ausgeprägter Diffusionsbehinderung (Emphysem, Zustand nach Lungenembolismus usw.), die noch einen normalen Ruhegasaustausch aufwiesen, bei geringer Belastung aber bereits respiratorisch dekompensierten. Durch das völlige Fehlen einer respiratorischen Reserve gehören diese, unter Ruhebedingungen oft wenig auffälligen Patienten in eine hohe Risikogruppe für postoperative Komplikationen. In 5 Fällen mit pathologischen Ruheblutgasen wurde andererseits die vermutete Gasaustauschstörung durch die guten Belastungswerte ausgeschlossen.

Tabelle 2. Die pathologischen Blutgaswerte von 2007 Untersuchungen

pathologische Blutgaswerte insgesamt	86	100 %
(ohne Bel. Azidose)		
bei normaler Spirometrie	8	9,5%
davon nach Bel. normal	5	0,2%
bei pathologischer Spirometrie	32	39,5%
bei fehlender Spirometrie	41	47,6%
erst nach Belastung	5	0,2%

Aus der Tabelle 3 geht weiters hervor, daß die Blutgasanalyse gerade in jenen Fällen, wo eine Kleine Spirometrie nicht vorgenommen werden konnte, einen besonders hohen Anteil von respiratorischen Störungen aufdecken konnte.

Ich glaube, daß wir aus diesen bisher erhobenen Befunden den Schluß ziehen dürfen, daß sich der screeningmäßige Einsatz der Kleinen Spirometrie und der arteriellen Blutgasanalyse zur Erfassung von respiratorischen Risikofällen gut bewährt hat. Die Ergometrie bringt für diese Indikation wesentlich weniger, da sie aber für kardiozirkulatorische Fragestellungen eingesetzt wird, steht sie auch für die seltenen respiratorischen Indikationen routinemäßig zur Verfügung.

Tabelle 3. Die bei 2007 statistisch ausgewerteten Fällen erhobenen Befunde zur Erfassung von resp. Risikofällen

Blutgasanalyse in Ruhe PO_2, PCO_2, pH, BA (Ohr)	2007	100 %
Kleine Spirometrie VC_{exsp}, FEV_1, FEV_1 x 30	1713	85,5%
davon nicht beurteilbar	95	4,5%
keine Kleine Spirometrie	294	14,5%
Ergometrie BGA, EKG, RR, HR	446	22,0%

Da diese Untersuchungen heute einfach und rasch durchgeführt werden können und die dazu erforderlichen Einrichtungen überall zur Verfügung stehen, ist das Grazer Programm auch so ökonomisch, daß es für eine allgemeine Anwendung empfohlen werden kann.

Literatur

1. Ahnefeld FW, et al. (1976) Der Risikopatient in der Anästhesie. Vorwort Klinische Anästhesiologie und Intensivtherapie, Band 12. Springer, Berlin Heidelberg New York
2. Benzer H, Fitzal S, et al. (1973) Prae- und postoperative Atemtherapie. Anästh Inform 8:303
3. Harnoncourt K (1976) Leistungsbeurteilung der cardiorespiratorischen Funktionen in Form eines Suchtests. Wien Med Wschr 126:274–276
4. Harnoncourt K, et al. (1976) Die Standardisierung der Lungenfunktionsdiagnostik in Österreich. Öst Ärzteztg 31/18:1019–1057
5. Matthys H, Rühle RH (1976) Lungenfunktionsdiagnostik zur Erfassung des Risikopatienten in der Anästhesiologie. Klinische Anästhesiologie und Intensivtherapie Band 12:8–13. Springer, Berlin Heidelberg New York

Die Anästhesieambulanz – Konzept, Organisation, Realisierung

W. Dick

Die psychologische Legitimation für eine Verbesserung der Beziehungen zwischen Anästhesist und Patient wurde erst jüngst wieder nachdrücklich dokumentiert. Das Institut für Demoskopie in Allensbach brachte zutage, daß 90% der befragten Personen als ersten einer Liste verschiedener Wünsche äußerten, „daß bei einer Operation die Narkose durch einen Facharzt gemacht wird" [1].

Daß die psychologische Tätigkeit des Anästhesisten nicht erst mit der Anästhesie selbst beginnen soll, vielmehr ein Schwergewicht der präoperativen Phase gebührt, ist geläufig und wird auch durch Untersuchungen von Leigh et al. aus dem Jahre 1977 belegt [4], wonach die präoperative Visite des Anästhesisten als einzige unter den verschiedenen Maßnahmen geeignet war, Angst und Furcht des Patienten vor dem Eingriff und der Narkose zu mildern.

In optimaler Weise kann der Anästhesist einer derartigen Vertrauensstellung gerecht werden, wenn er – wie alle anderen Fachgebiete auch – Zeit, Ruhe, eine geeignete Atmosphäre und adäquate räumliche Möglichkeiten bereithält. Diesem Ideal käme wohl eine Organisationsform am nächsten, bei der ein Patient, sobald er vom Operateur einen Operationstermin erhalten hat, in die Sprechstunde des Anästhesisten geht mit der Fragestellung, ob er über seine Operationsfähigkeit hinaus (die ja letztlich der Operateur feststellt) auch anästhesierbar sei. Wird er für nicht anästhesierbar gehalten, so muß er anästhesierbar *gemacht* werden. Dazu sollten eigene und konsiliarische Einrichtungen zur Verfügung stehen.

Die Realisierung einer derartigen gedanklichen Konzeption ist in verschiedener Weise vorstellbar [2]:

1. Der Patient wird so früh stationär einbestellt, daß genügend Zeit zur präoperativen Untersuchung und gegebenenfalls Vorbehandlung besteht, ein prinzipiell begrüßenswerter, aber volkswirtschaftlich teurer Weg und nur für solche Krankenhäuser geeignet, deren Betten zu allenfalls 50% ausgelastet sind.

2. Die Einrichtung einer Sprechstunde bzw. einer Ambulanz des Anästhesisten, in der die Patienten noch in der vorstationären Phase voruntersucht und gegebenenfalls vorbehandelt werden.

3. Eine Kombination beider Möglichkeiten.

Dem Department für Anästhesiologie der Universität Ulm wurde nach einem internen Probelauf zum 1.10.1976 die offizielle Einrichtung einer Anästhesieambulanz konzidiert, deren Tätigkeitsbereich sich zunächst auf die Urologische Klinik, die Frauenklinik, die Hals-, Nasen-, Ohren- und Augenklinik sowie die Dermatologie und die Kinderklinik erstreckte.

Für die letzten drei Monate des Jahres 1976 wurden DM 40 000,– für Investitionen und DM 3 000,– für den laufenden Bedarf bewilligt, im Jahre 1977 dann DM 50 000,– an Investitionen und DM 30 000,– für den laufenden Bedarf, in den Jahren 1978 und 1979 schließlich je DM 25 000,– für restliche Investitionen und je DM 30 000,– für den laufenden Be-

<table>
<tr><td colspan="3" align="center">Finanzierung</td></tr>
<tr><td></td><td align="center"><u>Investitionen</u></td><td align="center"><u>laufender Betrieb</u></td></tr>
<tr><td>1.10. - 31.12.
1976</td><td align="center">40 000 DM</td><td align="center">3 000 DM</td></tr>
<tr><td>1977</td><td align="center">50 000 DM</td><td align="center">30 000 DM</td></tr>
<tr><td>1978</td><td align="center">23 000 DM</td><td align="center">30 000 DM</td></tr>
<tr><td>1979</td><td align="center">25 000 DM</td><td align="center">30 000 DM</td></tr>
<tr><td colspan="3" align="center">= 0,50 DM/poliklinisch behandelter
Patient der Univers. Kliniken</td></tr>
</table>

Abb. 1. Abschätzung des Finanzbedarfes einer Anästhesieambulanz

trieb (Abb. 1). Damit bestritten wurde die Einrichtung der Warteräume, des Sekretariats, der Untersuchungsräume, spezieller Geräte wie Belastungsergometer, EKG, Defibrillator, Lungenfunktionsmeßplatz, Möglichkeiten zur ambulanten Inhalations- und Möglichkeiten zur ambulanten Schmerztherapie.

Die Patienten, die uns ambulant direkt vom Hausarzt oder der Fachsprechstunde zugewiesen werden, erreichen die Anästhesieambulanz mit einem Überweisungsbogen, der Angaben darüber enthält, welcher operative Eingriff für welchen Termin geplant ist, welche fachspezifische Diagnostik noch vor der Operation erforderlich ist und welche Unterlagen bereits mitgegeben werden können (Abb. 2).

In der Anästhesie-Ambulanz erfolgt die fachanästhesiologische Untersuchung inklusive aller Zusatzuntersuchungen [3]. Werden Leistungen benötigt, die nicht im Spektrum der Anästhesie-Ambulanz enthalten sind, wird der Patient direkt etwa zur Internistischen Ambulanz überwiesen.

Wiederum mit Hilfe eines speziellen Mitteilungsbogens erhalten überweisender Hausarzt und Fachambulanz eine Information, aus der die Gesamtbeurteilung der Situation des Patienten hervorgeht; die Mitteilung enthält aber auch — wo nötig — definierte Vorschläge und Empfehlungen zur Vorbehandlung bestehender Funktionsstörungen aus anästhesiologischer Sicht. An Einleitung und Einhaltung dieser Vorbehandlung wird die termingerechte Durchführung der Anästhesie und damit des operativen Wahleingriffs geknüpft (Abb. 3).

Im letzten 3 Monatszeitraum des Jahres 1976, also mit offizieller Einrichtung der Anästhesieambulanz, wurden 7% aller anästhesierten Patienten ambulant voruntersucht, 22% suchten die Ambulanz als schon stationäre Patienten auf, noch 71% wurden überhaupt nicht in der Ambulanz vorgestellt. Um realistische Zahlen zu erhalten, muß jedoch die Gesamtzahl der Anästhesien um Geburten und Notfälle reduziert werden, da derartige Patienten niemals die Chance erhalten, in der Anästhesieambulanz vorgestellt zu werden. Nach dieser Korrekturberechnung wurden 11% der Patienten ambulant, 36% schon stationär untersucht und nur etwas über 50% überhaupt nicht der Anästhesieambulanz zugeführt (Abb. 4).

7900 Ulm, den

Überweisende Klinik Tel.	Adressette

An die
Anästhesieambulanz

Klinikbereich Michelsberg

Bei unserem Patienten ....
ist ein operativer Eingriff geplant.

Vorgesehene Operation: ....

Vorgesehener Aufnahmetermin: ....

Unsererseits ist eine <u>stationäre</u> <u>Fach</u>diagnostik vor der ersten erforderlichen Narkose von .... Tagen
notwendig.

Der Patient erhält folgende Unterlagen zu Ihrer Kenntnis:
Arztbrief
Krankenblatt, evtl. frühere Krankenblätter
Röntgenaufnahmen
EKG
Laborwerte
etc.

Wir bitten, den Patienten nach der Untersuchung zu uns zurückzuschicken   Ja/Nein

Besondere Bemerkungen: ....
....
....

Überweisender Arzt

Abb. 2. Beispiel eines Überweisungsformularbogens von der Fachambulanz in die Anästhesieambulanz

Anästhesieambulanz

Department für Anästhesiologie
der Universität Ulm
Klinikbereich Michelsberg

7900 Ulm, den
Prittwitzstraße 43
Tel. 07 31 / 1 79 41 18

Frau/Herrn

Sehr geehrte(r) Frau /Herr Kollegin (Kollege)!

Nach Überweisung aus der Ambulanz der _______________________________
Klinik ist heute Ihr Patient

____

im Hinblick auf die geplante Allgemeinnarkose/Lokalanästhesie anästhesiologisch voruntersucht
worden. Wir haben die folgenden Befunde/Diagnosen erhoben:

a) Gegen die Anästhesie bestehen keine Bedenken.

b) Eine Anästhesie ist erst nach Vorbehandlung möglich.

c) Eine Anästhesie ist erst nach Vorbehandlung und erneuter Vorstellung des Patienten
   möglich.

Folgende Behandlung halten wir im Hinblick auf den geplanten Eingriff in Narkose für
angezeigt:

____

____

____

____

Wir bitten um erneute Vorstellung des Patienten am _______________________________

Besondere Bemerkungen: ____

____

____

Mit freundlichen Grüßen

Abb. 3. Beispiel eines Mitteilungsbogens der Anästhesieambulanz an die Fachambulanz

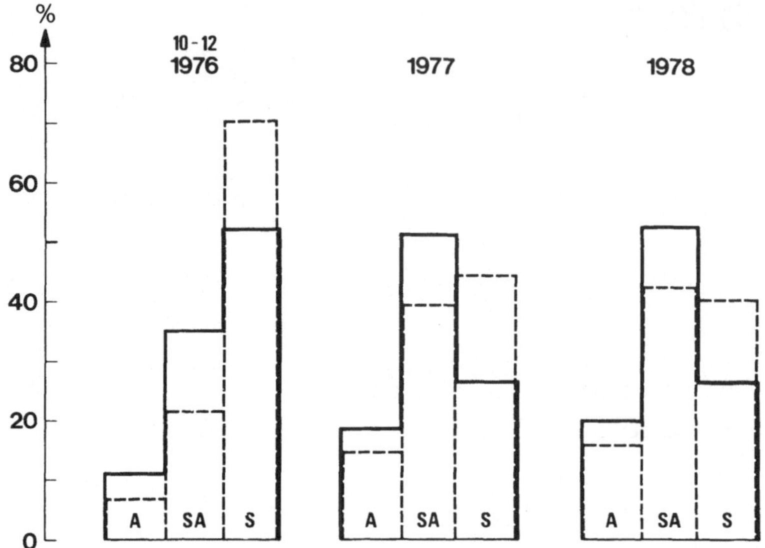

Abb. 4. Übersicht über die Verteilung der anästhesierten Patienten aus den Jahren 1976 bis 1978 auf ambulant untersuchte (A), stationär in der Ambulanz untersuchte (SA) und stationär untersuchte (S) Patienten

In den Jahren 1977 und 1978 hat sich das Bild grundlegend gewandelt. Nach Bereinigung des Zahlenmaterials um Geburten und Notfälle wurden annähernd 20% der Patienten ambulant untersucht und 52% bzw. 53% als schon stationäre Patienten in der Ambulanz. Zusammengenommen ergibt sich daraus ein prozentualer Anteil von 73% aller anästhesierten Patienten; in Absolutzahlen bedeutet dies etwas mehr als 3500 Patienten pro Jahr oder im Durchschnitt 14 Untersuchungen pro Tag. Tatsächlich müssen an manchen Tagen bis zu 50 Patienten allein zur Voruntersuchung und Verordnung der präoperativen Vorbereitung und Prämedikation die Ambulanz durchlaufen. Daneben werden ambulante Inhalationstherapie und Schmerzbehandlung durchgeführt.

Werfen wir einen Blick auf die Einzelleistungen der Anästhesie-Ambulanz im Rahmen der Voruntersuchungen und der Verordnungsmaßnahmen, so zeigt sich, daß alle 3 650 Patienten einer eingehenden klinischen Untersuchung unterzogen wurden, bei den ambulant untersuchten Patienten wurde zusätzlich zur Bestimmung der Laborwerte Blut entnommen. Eine EKG-Untersuchung war bei 30% der ambulanten und bei 54% der stationär voruntersuchten Patienten erforderlich. Für die Lungenfunktionsuntersuchungen lauten die entsprechenden Zahlen 8 beziehungsweise 16%. Verordnungen an den Hausarzt oder die Fachambulanz erwiesen sich bei 8% der ambulanten Patienten als notwendig, Verordnungen an die Station bei 60% der stationär voruntersuchten Patienten (Abb. 5).

Versucht man einen Überblick darüber zu gewinnen, ob und wie die präoperative Verweildauer der Patienten durch die Anästhesie-Ambulanz beeinflußt wird, so ergeben sich folgende Zahlen, die aus einer separaten Auswertung des ersten Halbjahres 1978 ermittelt wurden. Von den ambulanten Patienten konnten nahezu 30% am Aufnahmetag operiert werden, von den stationären Patienten jedoch nur 1%. Auch in der weiteren Häufigkeitsverteilung lagen die stationären Patienten immer leicht über den ambulanten (Abb. 6).

Leistungen der Anästhesieambulanz 1978			
	Ambulante Patienten	Stationäre Patienten	Zusammen
Klinische Untersuchungen	1003	2653	3656
Blutentnahmen	964	—	964
EKG	298 (30%)	1421 (54%)	1719 (47%)
Lungenfunktion	77 (8%)	415 (16%)	492 (13%)
Sonstiges	2	—	2
Verordnungen an Hausarzt oder Fachambulanz	83 (8%)	1601 (60%)	1684 (46%)

Abb. 5. Übersicht über die Leistungen der Anästhesieambulanz im Rahmen der Voruntersuchung und Prämedikation, unterteilt nach ambulant und stationär in der Ambulanz untersuchten Patienten

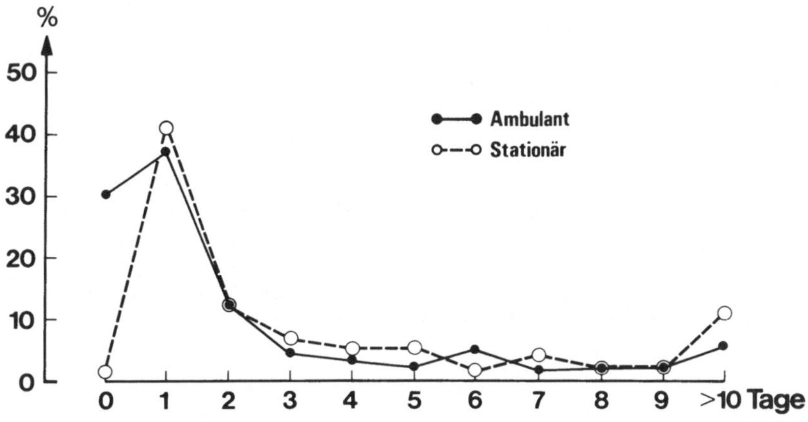

Abb. 6. Aufschlüsselung der präoperativen Verweildauer ambulant bzw. stationär in der Ambulanz untersuchter Patienten (durchgezogene Linie: ambulant untersuchte Patienten, gestrichelte Linie: stationär in der Ambulanz untersuchte Patienten)

Aus den Intervallaufzeichnungen erkennt man weiter, daß alle stationär in der Ambulanz untersuchten Patienten letztlich direkt am Aufnahmetag der Anästhesie-Ambulanz zugeführt worden waren. Trotzdem ergibt sich bei diesen Patienten eine um im Mittel 1,3 Tage höhere präoperative Verweildauer, die — in Zahlen ausgedrückt — einen Mehraufwand von nahezu einer halben Million DM ausmacht. Der wirtschaftliche Gesichtspunkt ist jedoch insofern problematisch, als Einsparungen, die zugunsten der Krankenkassen erfolgen, zu Lasten des Krankenhausträgers gehen und umgekehrt.

Wenn im vergangenen Jahr „nur" 20% aller anästhesierten Patienten ambulant voruntersucht worden sind, so erscheint dies auf den ersten Blick zu wenig. Tatsächlich muß jedoch in die Kalkulation der ursprünglichen Zielsetzung der Anästhesie-Ambulanz auch die Zahl derjenigen Patienten mit aufgenommen werden, die zwar schon stationär aufgenommen worden waren, die aber dennoch der Anästhesie-Ambulanz zugeführt wurden. Diese Patienten werden, der Auswertung zufolge, alle am Tage der stationären Aufnahme der Anästhesie-Ambulanz überwiesen. Ambulante und dieser Teil der stationär aufgenommenen Patienten zusammen ergeben eine Frequenz von über 70% aller anästhesierten Patienten, die heute in der Anästhesie-Ambulanz untersucht werden.

Unsere Auswertung hat auch gezeigt, daß bei den nur stationär in der Ambulanz untersuchten Patienten zwischen 58 und 84% vom Hausarzt oder auswärtigen Facharzt nach telefonischer Terminabstimmung mit der jeweiligen Fachklinik direkt dorthin überwiesen und dort stationär aufgenommen wurden. Derartige Patienten sind zwar zu irgendeinem Zeitpunkt einmal in der zuständigen Fachambulanz erschienen, haben sich jedoch zunächst nicht für einen erforderlichen operativen Eingriff entscheiden können, sondern haben diese Entscheidung später getroffen und ihrem Hausarzt mitgeteilt.

Wenn heute über 70% aller anästhesierten Patienten die Anästhesie-Ambulanz durchlaufen, so kommt dieser Prozentsatz dem ursprünglich gesteckten Ziel sehr nahe. Auch wenn nur 20% dieser Patienten in der vorstationären Phase vorgestellt wurden, so bedeutet die Vorstellung der schon stationären Patienten am Aufnahmetag einen erheblichen qualitativen Fortschritt, der darüber hinaus zur Vereinfachung organisatorischer Probleme beiträgt, suchen doch jetzt zahlreiche Patienten *einen* Anästhesisten in dessen Sprechstunde auf, nicht hingegen zahlreiche Anästhesisten zahllose, auf unterschiedliche Stationen verteilte Patienten.

Literatur

1. N.N. (1979) Bedürfnisse und Wünsche der Patienten im Krankenhaus. Der Deutsche Arzt 9:28
2. Dick W, Ahnefeld FW, Fricke M, Knoche E, Milewski P, Traub E (1978) Die Anästhesieambulanz. Erfahrungen mit einer neuen Organisationsform der pränarkotischen Untersuchung und Beratung. Anaesthesist 27:450
3. Lutz H, Klose R (1979) Operationsvorbereitung aus anästhesiologischer Sicht. Med Welt 30:639
4. Leigh JM, Walker J, Janaganathan P (1977) Effect of preoperative anaesthetic visit on anxiety. Brit Med J 2:987

Die anaesthesiologische Ambulanz

St. Jeretin und J. Voncina

Die anaesthesiologische Ambulanz besteht in Slowenien seit 1971, als die Zentrale Abteilung für Anaesthesie des Klinischen Zentrums gegründet wurde. Die ersten Erfahrungen mit solchen Ambulanzen gehen bei uns auf das Jahr 1962 zurück, als in Maribor und etwas später auf der Gynäkologischen Klinik in Ljubljana versuchsweise anaesthesiologische Ambulanzen eröffnet wurden.

Zur Zeit sind im Rahmen des C.A.R.S. (Zentraler Dienst für Anaesthesiologie und Reanimation) vier Ambulanzen tätig.

Tabelle 1. Übersicht der Anaesthesieambulanzen im Klinischen Zentrum Ljubljana

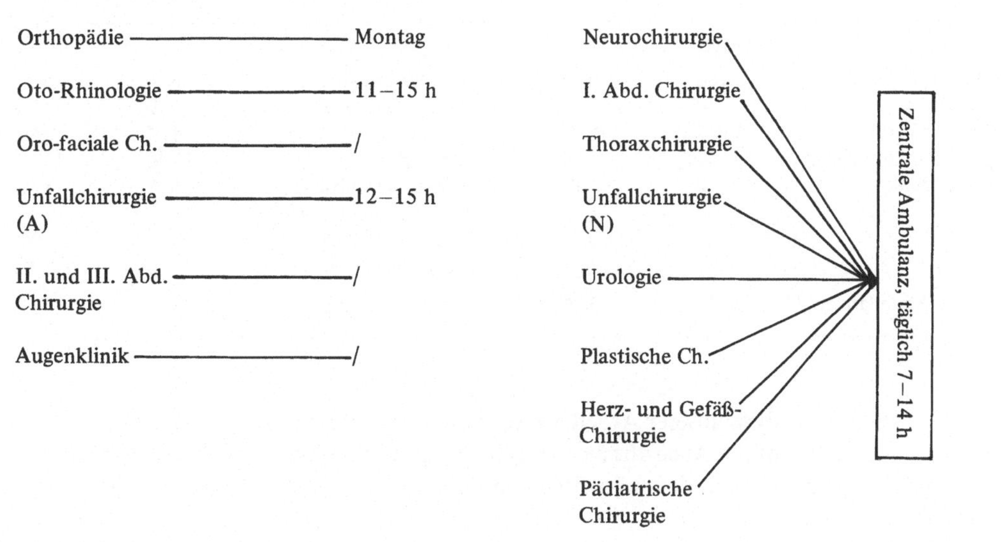

Die Aufgabe dieser ist, den Patienten vor Anaesthesie und Operation zu untersuchen und die Befunde verschiedener Labors und Fachärzte zu prüfen. Dann soll Anaesthesiefähigkeit und das Risiko festgestellt werden. Außerdem soll eine eventuell notwendige präoperative, medikamentöse Therapie bereits in der Ambulanz begonnen werden.

Tabelle 2. Die Funktionen der Anaesthesieambulanz

Anamnese (spezifisch)
Physischer Status
Laborstatus (Elektrolyte, Urea . . .)
EKG
Lungenfunktions-Screening
Funktionsdiagnostik: Leber, Niere
Diagnostik von genetischen u. metabolischen Erkrankungen
Konsultation
Therapie: Vorbereitung und Planen der Anaesthesie

Damit entspricht die Ambulanz dem bei uns üblichen Arbeitsschema: Facharztambulanz –
Hospitalisation – Behandlung.

Die Übersicht der tatsächlich geleisteten Arbeit der Ambulanzen zeigt, daß in den sogenannten lokalen Ambulanzen der verschiedenen operativen Kliniken nur 33% aller program-
miert operierten Patienten vorbereitet wurde. In der Zentralambulanz, die alle operativen
Kliniken im neuen Gebäude versorgt, ist die Situation ähnlich; 35% der Patienten wurden gesehen.

Tabelle 3. Anzahl und Prozentsatz der in den Anaesthesiologischen Ambulanzen untersuchten Patienten
im Zeitraum 1978/79

Orthopädie	1201	66%	Neurochirurgie	0	0%
Otorhinologie	464	64%	I. Abdominalchirurgie	624	54%
Oro-faciale Ch.	0	0%	Thoraxchirurgie	0	0%
Unfallchirurgie (A)	1125	97%	Unfallchirurgie (N)	424	55%
II./III. Abdominal-Ch.	0	0%	Urologie	1790	125%
Augenklinik	0	0%	Plastische Chirurgie (mit Verbrennungen)	595	47%
			Herz- und Gefäß-Ch.	0	0%
			Pädiatrische Chirurgie	0	0%
Lokale Ambulanzen	Σ 2820	36%	Zentrale Ambulanzen	Σ 3433	35%

Eine weitere Analyse unserer Arbeitsweise an den Ambulanzen zeigt, daß meistens nur
eine Anamnese, die auf die Anaesthesie bezogen ist, sowie ein physischer Status gemacht
werden. Sie dienen dann mit den mitgebrachten Befunden zur Feststellung der Anaesthesiefähigkeit.

Das EKG wird in allen 4 Ambulanzen geschrieben, jedoch nur in 3 ausgewertet. Lungenfunktionsprüfungen werden nur an der Zentralambulanz durchgeführt.

Aus Tabelle 4 kann man ersehen, daß eine Blutentnahme für laborchemische Untersuchungen nicht notwendig war. In allen 4 Ambulanzen wurde für jeden Patienten eine Zusammenfassung geschrieben und somit die Narkosefähigkeit dokumentiert. Am Tag vor der geplanten Anaesthesie wird der Patient nach seiner Untersuchung und Behandlung nochmals
vom Anaesthesisten besucht.

Tabelle 4. Untersuchungen, die in den Ambulanzen durchgeführt werden

	Orthopädie	Oto-Rhinologie	Oro-Faciale Chirurgie	Unfallchirurgie (A)	II./III. Abdominalchirurgie	Augenklinik	Neurochirurgie	I. Abdominalchirurgie	Thoraxchirurgie	Unfallchirurgie (N)	Urologie	Plastische Chirurgie	Herz- u. Gefäßchirurgie	Pädiatrische Chirurgie
Anamnese	+	+	/	+	/	/	/	+	/	+	+	+	/	/
Phys. Status	+	+	/	+	/	/	/	+	/	+	+	+	/	/
EKG	+	+	/	+	/	/	/	+	/	+	+	+	/	/
EKG Befundung	+	+	/	/	/	/	/	+	/	+	+	/	/	/
Lungenfunktion	/	/	/	/	/	/	/	+	/	+	+	/	/	/
Laboruntersuchungen	/	/	/	/	/	/	/	/	/	/	/	/	/	/
Zusammenfassung Narkosefähigkeit	+	+	/	+	/	/	/	+	/	+	+	+	/	/

Tabelle 5. Übersicht über die Frequenz der präoperativen Visiten am Krankenbett in % der Anaesthesien

Orthopädie	40%		Neurochirurgie	100%
Oto-Rhinologie	95%		I. Abdominalchirurgie	100%
Oro-Faciale Chirurgie	100%		Thoraxchirurgie	100%
Unfallchirurgie (A)	10%		Unfallchirurgie (N)	80%
II./III. Abd. Ch.	50%		Urologie	90%
Augenklinik	50%		Plastische Chirurgie	
			mit Verbrennungen	10%
			Herz- u. Gefäßchirurgie	50%
			Pädiatrische Chirurgie	40%
Lokale Ambulanzen	Σ 58%		Zentrale Ambulanz	Σ 71%

71% der Patienten vom Klinischen Zentrum werden am Krankenbett besucht, jedoch 58% der Patienten an den außenliegenden Kliniken.

Der Aufgabenbereich der anaesthesiologischen Ambulanz ist klar umrissen. Der untersuchende Facharzt für Anaesthesiologie kennt den Einfluß verschiedener Pharmaca und deren Interaktionen, des operativen Eingriffs, der Lagerung etc. auf die wichtigsten Organfunktionen und verringert damit Narkose- bzw. Operationsrisiko. Damit werden auch Narkosemorbidität und -mortalität herabgesetzt. Die Zusammenarbeit mit Operateur und Konsiliarärzten anderer Fächer werden verbessert.

Erstaunlich ist, daß nach achtjährigem Betrieb der Anaesthesieambulanz, nur 30—35% aller Patienten dort untersucht werden. Analysieren wir diesen niederen Prozentsatz, so kommen wir zur Feststellung, daß vor allem die jüngeren Chirurgen und Operateure anderer Fächer die Arbeit der Anaesthesieambulanz sehr begrüßen und schätzen.

Die Zusammenarbeit mit Konsiliarärzten anderer Fächer, vor allem den Internisten gestaltete sich schwieriger, da sich letztere nicht abgewöhnen konnten „Anaesthesie mit mög-

Tabelle 6. Die Stellung der Anaesthesieambulanz im Rahmen der operativen Kliniken

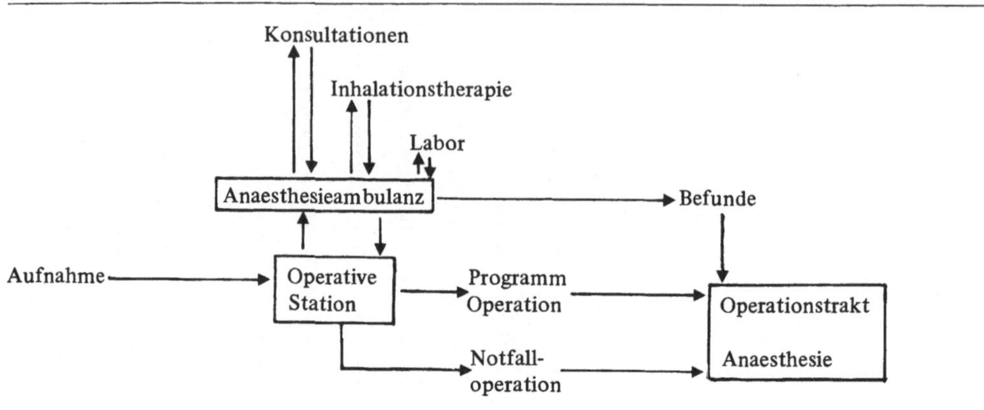

lichst viel Sauerstoff" im Befund zu schreiben. Folgende für den Anaesthesiologen nützliche und wichtige Fragen sollen vom Internisten beantwortet werden:

1. Genaue Diagnose internistischer Begleiterkrankungen.
2. Ist der Patient in bestmöglichem Zustand (Frage 1 betreffend) für Anaesthesie und Operation?
3. Welche Therapie zur Besserung des präoperativen Zustands soll eingeleitet werden?
4. Wie lange wird die präoperative Therapie dauern?
5. Welche Komplikationen sind zu erwarten?

So gezielte Konsultationen ergeben bessere Resultate als die routinemäßig ausgeführte fachärztliche Untersuchung. Auf Grund unserer Erfahrung kamen wir zur Meinung, diese teilen auch führende Internisten, daß die routinemäßige Untersuchung aller Patienten durch den Internisten präoperativ nicht notwendig ist.

Aufgabe des Anaesthesiologen ist es, den Kranken hinsichtlich der Narkosefähigkeit zu untersuchen, die erhobenen Befunde schriftlich zu erfassen und das Anaesthesieverfahren auszuwählen. Gezielte Konsultationen mit Fachärzten anderer Disziplinen sind von großem Nutzen.

Nach sorgfältiger Analyse aller Daten kamen wir ähnlich wie unsere Kollegen aus England zum Schluß, daß Ambulanzen nur erfahrene Anaesthesiologen betreuen sollen. Sie sollen eine ausreichende klinische Ausbildung haben, da die Anaesthesieambulanz ein Grenzgebiet zu anderen Fachambulanzen darstellt. Schließlich muß der Anaesthesiologe prüfen und beurteilen, ob der Patient den spezifischen Risiken und Belastungen gewachsen ist. Leider ergaben sich bei uns in Slowenien hier bei der Ausbildung zum Anaesthesiologen deutliche Mängel.

Es war nicht leicht, die Ambulanz einzuführen und mit anderen medizinischen Disziplinen in Einklang zu bringen, schwieriger war, den im Operationssaal durch die tägliche Routinearbeit überlasteten Anaesthesiologen dafür zu begeistern. Zuviele unserer Kollegen sahen nur eine Mehrbelastung des Personals und einen zu hohen finanziellen Aufwand. Sie waren der Meinung, daß die präoperative Visite am Krankenbett vollkommen genügt, diese wegen des besseren Kontaktes mit dem Patienten günstiger ist. *Allgöwer's* Satz: „Ein guter präoperativer Besuch ist schon die halbe Anaesthesie" wurde vielfach zitiert.

Tabelle 7. Vergleich der Prozentzahlen aller operierten Patienten zwischen anaesthesiologischer Ambulanz und Visite am Krankenbett

Orthopädie	66%	40%	Neurochirurgie	0%	100%
Oto-Rhinologie	64%	95%	I. Abdominalchirurgie	54%	100%
Oro-Faciale Chirurgie	0%	100%	Thoraxchirurgie	0%	100%
Unfallchirurgie (A)	97%	10%	Unfallchirurgie (N)	55%	80%
II./III. Abdominal-Chr.	0%	50%	Urologie	125%	90%
Augenklinik	0%	50%	Plastische Chirurgie		
			mit Verbrennungen	47%	10%
			Herz- u. Gefäßchirurgie	0%	50%
			Pädiatrische Chirurgie	0%	40%
Lokale Ambulanzen	Σ 36%	58%	Zentralambulanz	Σ 42%	71%

Tabelle 8. Begleiterkrankungen (aus der Zentralambulanz über 6 Monate 1979)

Herzerkrankungen	82	5,8%
Hypertonie	117	8,2%
Lungenerkrankungen	133	9,4%
Lebererkrankungen	41	2,9%
Diabetes mellitus	32	2,3%
Neurologische Erkrankungen	24	1,7%
Allergien	5	0,4%
Sonstige Begleiterkrankungen	123	8,7%
Summe	557	39,3%

Was sollte nun geschehen, um die Anaesthesiemorbidität und -mortalität zu senken, ohne den Patienten der seelenlosen Präzisionsmaschinerie eines modernen Großbetriebes auszusetzen? Vor einem geplanten operativen Eingriff soll der Patient in der Anaesthesieambulanz untersucht werden. Jeder Patient soll seinen Anaesthesisten am Tage vor der Operation und nach der Operation bzw. Anaesthesie sehen und sprechen. Damit haben wir alle Vorteile der Ambulanz und den psychologischen Effekt eines warmen persönlichen Kontaktes erreicht.

Tabelle 9. Vorteile der Anaesthesieambulanz

Psychologischer Effekt auf Patienten
Bessere Vorbereitung des Kranken
Kleineres Narkoserisiko
Kleinere Narkosemorbidität und -mortalität
Entlastung der Operativen Fächer
Bessere Ausnützung der Konsiliarärzte
Bessere Zusammenarbeit mit dem Operateur
Verkürzung der Liegedauer (Hospitalisation)
Genaue operative Terminplanung

Um dieses Ziel zu erreichen, braucht man mehr Anaesthesisten und ärztliches Hilfspersonal sowie mehr Räume und mehr technische Ausrüstung. Die angeführten Forderungen sind, weil sie eine größere finanzielle Belastung darstellen, schwer zu erfüllen; das Hauptproblem jedoch wird die Ausbildung des jungen Anaesthesisten sein. Er soll die Bedeutung, Vorteile und Sicherheit der Anaesthesieambulanz für den Patienten erkennen. Eine Ausweitung und Ergänzung der Ausbildungsprogramme oder des Lehrzielkatalogs wird nötig sein.

Die präoperative Ambulanz in Graz

K. Hudabiunigg

Seit November 1977 besteht am Institut für Anaesthesiologie der Universität Graz in Zusammenarbeit mit der II. Medizinischen Abteilung des Landeskrankenhauses Graz (Vorstand: Doz. Dr. K. Harnoncourt) eine Anaesthesieambulanz für ambulante und stationäre Patienten mit verschiedenen, aus dieser Einrichtung gestellten Forderungen. Die Hauptgründe für die Errichtung dieser Ambulanz waren das Verlangen nach einer Verkürzung des präoperativen Aufenthaltes durch Konzentration des Untersuchungsablaufes und daraus resultierend eine Einsparung an Patiententagen sowie die Verbesserung des individuellen Kontaktes mit den Patienten. Während des Jahres 1978 kam es zu einem Rückgang der durchschnittlichen Liegedauer aller chirurgischen Patienten von 14,3 Tagen (1977) auf 13,7 Tage, welcher natürlich multifaktoriell begründet ist, aber durch einen stichprobeartigen Vergleich gleicher Patientenkollektive aus den Vorjahren zum Großteil auf diese Institution zurückgeführt werden muß. Unter Nichtberücksichtigung der thorax- und cardiochirurgischen Patienten, der Jugendlichen und der Voruntersuchten, durchlaufen 51% aller Patienten, deren Operationen geplant sind, diese Untersuchungsstelle. Bei Überweisungen von anderen Krankenhäusern bzw. von medizinischen Kliniken und praktizierenden Ärzten werden alle auswärts durchgeführten Untersuchungen berücksichtigt, um Doppelbefundungen zu vermeiden. Diese Patienten scheinen in der Statistik nicht auf.

Die Patienten werden von den einzelnen Stationen nach Blutentnahmen mit Anfertigung eines Thoraxbildes in den ersten Tagen des stationären Aufenthaltes oder aber ambulant zugewiesen. Die präoperative Untersuchungsstelle ist mit einem Anästhesisten und einer Schwester besetzt und erstellt den in Tabelle 1 zu sehenden Untersuchungsbefund zur Klärung der Anästhesiefähigkeit und des Anästhesierisikos.

Das Hauptaugenmerk zielt dabei neben der Anamnese und der Klärung der bisherigen Medikation auf die Beurteilung der erhobenen Laborwerte (BB + SMA) des Thoraxbildes, die Erstellung einer kleinen Spirometrie, die Schreibung eines EKG's, der Blutgasanalyse und bei gegebener Notwendigkeit eine Belastungsuntersuchung. In Zusammenarbeit mit den Internisten wird abschließend ein präoperativer Therapieplan erstellt und der Patient in das Risikoschema der ASA eingereiht.

Wir hatten bei den bisher Untersuchten über 4500 Patienten, die der Abb. 1 zu entnehmende Altersverteilung.

Die Pyramide ist weit nach rechts verschoben, da auf Grund der angespannten personellen Situation und der Unmöglichkeit, mehr als 20–25 Personen pro Tag zu untersuchen, die ohnehin geringe Anzahl an Jugendlichen noch dadurch verringert wird, daß sie nicht den gesamten Untersuchungsablauf durchlaufen und daher nicht in dieser Studie aufscheinen.

Die Abb. 2 zeigt die Verteilung der einzelnen Risikogruppen in den verschiedenen Altersdekaden.

Tabelle 1

Institut für Anaesthesiologie	Station 6 B
der Universität Graz	Unt. Nr.: 3655
Vorstand: Univ. Prof. Dr. W. List	Graz, am 6.3.1979

Präoperative Untersuchung

Name	X.X., weibl.	geb. 4.12.1913 cm 163 kg 72
Adresse	Schillerstraße 6	Beruf
Diagnose	Cholelith	Operation
Anamnese:	Persumbran 1 x 1, Brinerdin mite 1 x 1 dzt. keines.	
	zeitweise subj. Gefühl von Rhythmusstörung.	
	Klin. kein Hinweis auf Dekompensation, leichte Bronchitis	
Medikation	Cedilanid seit Montag	Alk Nik
Blutchemie	path.: o.B.	
Thoraxröntgen	unauffällig	
Kleine Spirometrie	(nach AKL)	
exspir. Vitalkapazität (VC)	2400 l (u. Gr. 2500 l)	96% u. Gr.
1-Sek.-Kapazität (FEV$_1$)	2100 l (u. Gr. = 75% VC)	88% VC
indir. Atemgrenzwert		
(FEV$_1$ x 30)	63 l (u. Gr. 48 l)	131% u. Gr.
Belastungstest		

Fahrradergometer	U/min	70 Watt	5 Min.				
	pO$_2$	pCO$_2$	pH	BE	BE	RR	Puls
Ruhe vor Belastung	76	40	7,42	1		145/85	59
nach Belastung	91	36	7,40	−2	3	160/75	120
5 Min. nach Bel.	86	38	7,39	−1,5	2,5		

EKG in Ruhe	SR Mitteltyp	
nach Belastung	deutliche Zunahme der ST Streckensenkung	
Empfohlene Therapie	wie eingeleitet, bei Stenocardien Myocardon	
Weitere Befunde	keine	
Prämedikation		
am Vorabend	Temesta 1	Narkoserisiko 1
präoperativ	Thalamonal 1,5 ml	2
	Atropin 0,6 mg	3
		4
		5

Beurteilung: Op-tauglich.
Bei der gewählten Belastungsstufe Hinweis auf coronare Herzerkrankung.
Ausreichende körperliche Leistungsreserve.

                                   Beurteiler: OA Ragossnig,
                                                      OA Hudabiunigg

---

Nach Durchführung dieses Untersuchungsablaufes konnten 86% aller Patienten für sofort anästhesiefähig erklärt werden (Tabelle 2). Diese bekamen eine Prämedikation verordnet und wurden am Vorabend der Operation von ihren Anästhesisten besucht und über das zu erwartende Anästhesieverfahren informiert.

Bei 14% der Untersuchten lagen Ausschluß- bzw. Aufschubgründe für eine sofortige Operation vor. Diese verteilten sich entsprechend der Tabelle 3.

Neben den objektiven Kriterien aus diesem Untersuchungsablauf bestand bei 23% der Untersuchten auf Grund unklarer Angaben aus der Anamnese bezüglich vorhergegangener Erkrankungen des cardiovasculären Systems eine Unsicherheit über die entsprechende Ein-

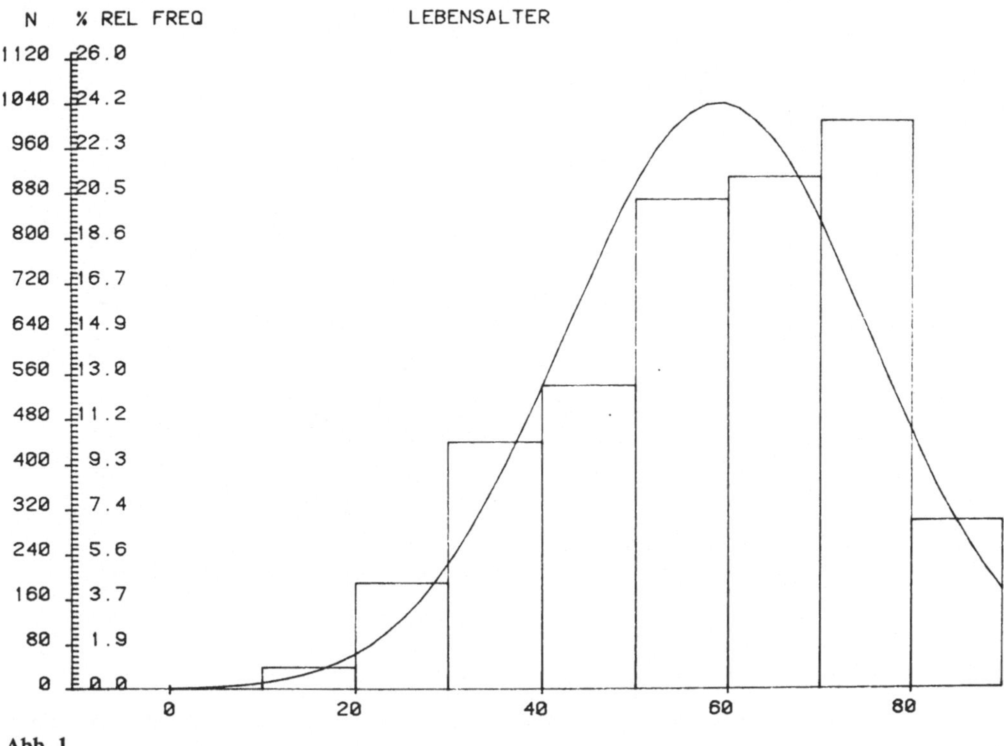

Abb. 1

ordnung in die verschiedenen Risikogruppen (Tabelle 4). Teilweise lagen nur Verdachtsmomente wie Adipositas oder ein Grenzwerthypertonus vor.

Bei diesen Patienten entschlossen wir uns zu einer Belastungsuntersuchung am Fahrradergometer mit einer Belastungsblutgasanalyse. Es wird dabei eine individuell vorgegebene Wattstufe (50–120) im Sinne einer submaximalen Belastung rektangulär für 5 Minuten geleistet.

Während der Belastung traten in 13% pathologische EKG-Befunde, in 8,3% pathologische RR-Werte und in 1% pathologische Blutgaswerte auf (Tabelle 5).

Nach den Ergebnissen dieser Ergometrie konnten wir 88% der Belastungsuntersuchten in eine günstigere Risikogruppe einordnen, als es allein auf Grund der anderen Befunde möglich gewesen wäre. Bei 12% erhöhte sich das Risiko nach den Erkenntnissen aus der Ergometrie.

Zusammenfassend darf nach 2 1/2jähriger Erfahrung mit der Anästhesieambulanz und unserer Feldstudie gesagt werden, daß die während dieser Zeit gewonnenen Erkenntnisse die Notwendigkeit einer genauen präoperativen Untersuchung bei über 20jährigen unterstrei-

Tabelle 2. Narkosetauglichkeit

86%	14%
Sofort	Aufschub
	+
	Ausschluß

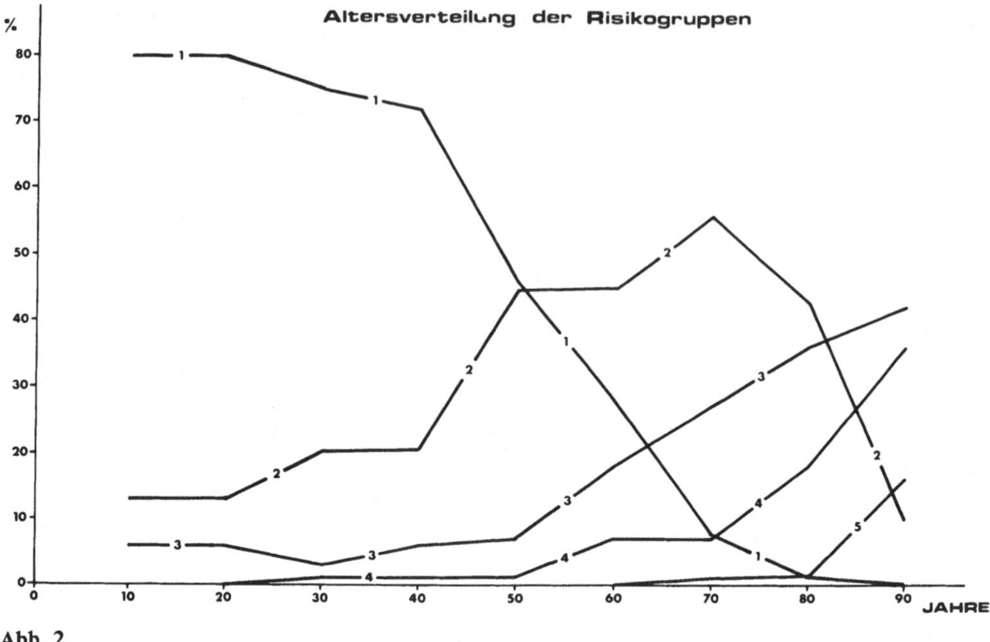

Abb. 2

chen. Unser Verfahren gewährleistet eine weitgehende, speziell auf die Anästhesie bezogenen Information für den die Narkose durchführenden Kollegen, und gibt dem Operateur die Möglichkeit, die Durch- oder auch Undurchführbarkeit des notwendigen chirurgischen Eingriffes zu erkennen.

Neben diesen, der Reduktion des Operations- und Anästhesierisikos dienenden Faktoren sollen aber die Vorteile, die speziell unserem Fachgebiet zugute kommen, nicht übersehen werden. Dies sind vor allem die Entwicklung eines individuellen Kontaktes mit dem Patienten und die Möglichkeit der Weiterbildung und Verbesserung der klinischen Erfahrung des Anästhesisten.

Tabelle 3. Ursachen

A:	Cardiale	
	3,5%	Hypertonus
	3,2%	latente Dekompensation
	3,0%	manifeste Dekompensation
	2,5%	schwere Rhythmusstörung
B:	Andere	
	1,5%	pulmonale Erkrankungen
	1 %	ungesicherte Euthyreose
	0,8%	Hämoglobin unter 100
	0,6%	Diabetes schlecht oder nicht eingestellt
	0,5%	Nierenerkrankungen
	1,8%	andere (Thrombophlebitis, Hepar, Gerinnung, Cerebrum)

Tabelle 4. Risikoklärung

	Ergometrie	
	n = 923	23%

Veranlassung

78%	„Kreislauf"
	Adipositas
	Grenzwerthypertonus
	„Kollaps"
16%	Herz
	angeb. Stenocardie
	„Myocardschaden"
	„Coronarinsuffizienz"
6%	Lunge
	post Resektion
	TBC
	Skoliose
	Diffusionsstörung

Tabelle 5. Ergebnisse Ergometrie

EKG pathol.	13 %
Belastungshypertonus	8,3%
Blutgase pathol.	0,1%

12%	**Risikoerhöhung**
88%	**Risikominderung**

Die präoperative Diagnose des cardiovasculären Risikos

W.F. List

Goldman et al. (1977) haben mit ihrem multifaktoriellen Index des cardialen Risikos bei chirurgischen Eingriffen die einzelnen Risikofaktoren, die für lebensgefährliche oder tödliche Zwischenfälle während und nach Operationen in Frage kommen, genannt und bewertet.

1. Präoperativ 3. Herzton oder Jugularvenenerweiterung	11
2. Myocardinfarkt vor weniger als 6 Monaten	10
3. Kein Sinusrhythmus oder Auftreten von supraventrikulären Extrasystolen	7
4. Mehr als 5 ventrikuläre Extrasystolen zu irgendeiner Zeit vor der Operation	7
5. Alter über 70 Jahre	5
6. Intraperitoneale, intrathorakale oder Aortenoperation	4
7. Deutliche Aortenklappenstenose	3
8. Notfallsoperationen	4
9. Schlechter Allgemeinzustand (RN, Kr, Blutgase, Leber)	3

Den höchsten Stellenwert bei dieser Risikoeinstufung nehmen neben der cardialen Insuffizienz und dem frischen Myocardinfarkt die ventrikulären und supraventrikulären Rhythmusstörungen ein.

Ähnliche Ergebnisse konnte auch Vormittag (1979) in seiner Untersuchung zum cardialen Risiko beim chirurgischen Patienten aufzeigen. Viele der cardialen Risikofaktoren können schon mit relativ einfachen Mitteln, nämlich der Anamnese, Inspektion, EKG und Blutdruckmessung während einer Ruheuntersuchung abgeklärt werden.

In einer derzeit noch laufenden Feldstudie der II. Medizinischen Abteilung des Landeskrankenhauses Graz zusammen mit dem Institut für Anästhesiologie der Universität Graz und der Steirischen Gesellschaft für Gesundheitsschutz konnte bei mehr als 14 000 Probanden ein Untersuchungsprogramm mit EKG, Puls und Blutdruck, Lungenfunktion und Blutgasen in Ruhe unter submaximaler Belastung gemacht werden. Aus einer Studie mit 3558 Feuerwehrmännern zwischen 20 und 60 Jahren, die als Atemschutzträger schweren Belastungen ausgesetzt sind und sich gesund fühlten, möchten wir die statistischen Ergebnisse, die das cardiovasculäre Risiko vor allem in den jüngeren Altersgruppen aufzeigen, bringen.

Unter Hypertonus wird ein Blutdruck von > 150/90 unter dem 40. Lebensjahr, von > 170/100 über dem 40. Lebensjahr entsprechend der Definition der WHO verstanden. Als Grenzwerthypertonus bis zum 40. Lebensjahr 150/90, über dem 40. Lebensjahr 170/100. Unter Belastungshypertonus verstanden wir einen Blutdruckanstieg von > 60 mm Hg unter submaximaler Belastung oder einem Blutdruck von > 200 mm Hg systolisch.

Belastungsuntersuchungen mit dem Fahrradergometer submaximale Belastung zwischen 125 und 200 Watt. 3446 Feuerwehrmänner wurden auf diese Weise belastet.

Aus der Goldman'schen Studie über das cardiale Risiko bei operativen Eingriffen und aus unserer eigenen Untersuchung geht eindeutig hervor, daß sowohl das EKG als auch der

Tabelle 1a. Aufschlüsselung des Untersuchungsgutes

3.558 (100   %) Feuerwehrmänner
 372 (10,6%) Auffällige Ruhebefunde
 260   trotzdem belastet
 112 (3,2%) pathologische Ruhebefunde

Tabelle 1b. Gewichtsverteilung

Normalgewicht	2.092 (58,8%)
Übergewicht von 20%	882 (24,7%)
Übergewicht von 40%	90 (2,6%)
Übergewicht > 40%	6 (0,2%)
10–20% über dem Normalgewicht	448 (13,7%)

Tabelle 1c. Auffällige Ruhebefunde: 372 von 3.558 (10,6%)

1. Pathologischer EKG-Befund	176 (4,9%)
2. Hypertonus	166 (4,6%)
3. Ruhetachykardie	8 (0,2%)
4. PO_2-Wert > 60 mm Hg	24 (0,7%)
5. PO_2-Wert > 45 mm Hg	3 (0,1%)
6. BA-Wert > − 5 mVal	15 (0,4%)
7. VC% unterer GRW.	5 (0,1%)
8. FEV_1 % VC < 65	15 (0,4%)

Tabelle 1d. EKG-Befunde in Ruhe (4,9%)

1. Rhythmusstörungen		3. Erregungsausbr. Störungen	
Sinustachycardie	8	Linkshypertrophie	106
Supraventr. ES	43	Rechtshypertrophie	6
Ventr. ES	33	Linksschenkelblock	4
AV-Knotenrhyth.	4	Rechtsschenkelblock	15
AV-Dissoziation	1		
VH-Flimmern	2		
2. Überleitungsstörung		4. Erregungsrückbildg. Stör.	
AV-Block 1. Grad	8	HW-Infarktnarbe	1
W-P-W-Syndrom	1	Außenschichtläs.	1
		ischäm. ST-Senkung	2

Tabelle 1e. Blutdruckverhalten

Normoton	2.872 (80,6%)
Grenzwerthypertonus	530 (14,8%)
Hypertonus	166 (4,6%)

Tabelle 1f. Pathologische Ruhebefunde n = 112 (3,1%)

EKG-Veränderungen	44 (1,2%)
Hypertonus	53 (1,5%)
Spirom. und Blutgase	15 (0,4%)

Tabelle 1g. Altersverteilung

Alter	Ges. Zahl Probanden	Auffällige Ruhebefunde	Patholog. Ruhebefunde
bis 20 J.	497 (13,9%)	28 (5,64%)	3 (0,6%)
21–30 J	1328 (37,4%)	122 (9, 1%)	48 (3,6%)
31–40 J.	1035 (29,1%)	114 (11, 0%)	32 (3,0%)
41–50 J.	572 (16,1%)	68 (11, 8%)	16 (2,7%)
51–60 J.	121 (3,4%)	35 (28, 9%)	11 (9,0%)
über 60 J.	5 (0,1%)	5 (100, 0%)	2 (40,0%)
	3558 (100,0%)	372 (10, 5%)	112 (3,1%)

Tabelle 1h. Mittlere Belastung   147 Watt

bis 20 Jahre	158 Watt
21–30 Jahre	157 Watt
31–40 Jahre	152 Watt
41–50 Jahre	148 Watt
51–60 Jahre	140 Watt

Tabelle 1i. Ergometriebefund (n = 3.3446)

1. Belastg. Hochdruck	133 (3,8%)	
2. Patholog. EKG	176 (5,1%)	
Rhythmusstörungen	145	
Überleitungsstörungen		2
Erregungsausbreitg. Störg.	2	
Erregungsrückbildg. Störg.	27	
3. Verdacht v. Coronarinsuffizienz	37 (1,1%)	

Blutdruck bei allen Altersklassen über 20 Jahren festgestellt werden sollte. Aus unserer Feldstudie geht darüberhinaus ein gesicherter statistischer Zusammenhang zwischen dem Auftreten von metabolischen Acidosen und Herzrhythmusstörungen hervor. Metabolische Acidosen, verursacht durch Hypoxie, Streß, lokale Ischämie und Hypovolämie bzw. auch Depression des Kreislaufes sind während der operativen und postoperativen Phase häufig. Dabei auftretende Rhythmusstörungen können zu einer akuten Gefährdung des Patienten führen. Eine verläßliche Prognose des cardialen Risikos auf Grund präoperativ erhebbarer Befunde ist derzeit noch nicht möglich (Vormittag 1979). Durch eine kontrollierte Arbeitsbelastung

(Ergometrie) können jedoch metabolische Acidosen ausgelöst werden und damit eine operative oder postoperative Streßsituation simuliert werden. Die Risikoeinschätzung des operativen Eingriffes kann damit verbessert werden.

So haben wir bei entsprechender Fragestellung in unserer Präoperativen Ambulanz auch Belastungsuntersuchungen zur Erkennung derartig gefährdeter Patienten durchgeführt. Die Belastungen werden submaximal zwischen 50 und 150 Watt über 5 Minuten mit dem Fahrradergometer durchgeführt. Untersucht wurden vor allem Patienten, bei denen präcordiale Herzbeschwerden ohne Zeichen im Ruhe-EKG auftraten und Patienten mit guter körperlicher Mobilität auch im höheren Alter und vor großen Eingriffen (z.B. Neorecti 70 Jahre).

Tabelle 2. Ausnahmen für präoperative Ergometerbelastung

1. Bekannte Erkrankungen des Herzens
2. Pathologisches Ruhe-EKG
3. Hypertonus
4. Manifeste Organ- und Stoffwechselerkrankungen
5. Ansteckende Erkrankungen
6. Ischämie oder orthopädische Störungen der Füße
7. Alter über 70 Jahre

Von den über 4500 Patienten unserer Präoperativen Ambulanz wurden 23% einer ergometrischen Belastungsuntersuchung zugeführt. Bei 13% dieser belasteten Patienten konnten wir Rhythmusstörungen mit ventrikulären Extrasystolen, ST-Senkungen, Schenkelblocks feststellen, bei 8% wurde ein Belastungshypertonus gefunden. Die Ergometerbelastung führte bei einigen unserer Patienten zu einer Veränderung der Risikoeinschätzung.

Eine eindeutige statistische Korrelation präoperativ erhobener pathologischer Befunde und intraoperativer Zwischenfälle konnten wir auf Grund zu geringer Zahlen noch nicht feststellen. Eine Schwierigkeit liegt auch darin, daß das System der Rückantworten über intraoperative Zwischenfälle und unseren präoperativen Befunden noch nicht vollständig ist. Wir haben ein Rückantwortblatt, das sowohl den Anästhesieverlauf als auch die postoperative Phase einschließt, seit kurzer Zeit in Austestung.

Abschließend sei festgestellt, daß wir für Ruheuntersuchungen des EKG, Puls und des Blutdruckes möglichst ab dem 20. Lebensjahr plädieren. Bei entsprechender Fragestellung sollten auch Belastungsuntersuchungen in einer präoperativen Ambulanz durchgeführt werden. Ein Screening der Myocardfunktion z.B. mit Hilfe der Systolischen Zeitintervalle (List 1973) ab dem 50. Lebensjahr sollte ebenfalls in Erwägung gezogen werden. Diese Untersuchungen können uns zusätzliche Erkenntnisse bringen und nach deren Therapierung dem Patienten eine noch größere Sicherheit während und nach dem chirurgischen Eingriff geben.

Literatur

Goldman L, Caldera DL, et al. (1977) Multifactorial index of cardiac risk in noncardiac surgical procedures. New England J Med 845−850
List WF, Rigler B, Kraft-Kinz J (1973) Verbesserung der Myocardfunktion von chirurg. Alterspatienten durch Einzeldosen von Beta-Methyldigoxin. Med Klin 68:1082−1086
Vormittag E (1979) Kardiale Komplikationen in der Chirurgie. Springer, Wien New York

Rechtliche Aspekte der präoperativen Untersuchung

W. Weissauer

Bei der Erörterung der rechtlichen Aspekte der präoperativen Untersuchung stellt sich zunächst die Frage: Wer trägt die ärztliche und rechtliche Verantwortung für die Beurteilung der Narkose- oder richtiger der Anaesthesiefähigkeit des Patienten und für die Wahl des Anaesthesieverfahrens? Die Antwort auf diese, für die Arbeitsteilung und die Zusammenarbeit ärztlicher Spezialisten typische Frage kann nicht zweifelhaft sein. Wer immer als ärztlicher Spezialist ein diagnostisches oder therapeutisches Verfahren anwendet, trägt auch die volle straf- und zivilrechtliche Verantwortung dafür, daß es unter Berücksichtigung der Umstände des konkreten Falles, also des Alters, etwaiger Begleiterkrankungen und sonstiger individueller Komponenten indiziert ist und lege artis ausgeführt wird. Der Arzt, der das Verfahren anwendet, muß deshalb die indizierenden gegen die kontraindizierenden Faktoren abwägen, er muß sich ein Bild über die bei diesem Verfahren drohenden Risiken machen und im Rahmen der spezifischen ärztlichen Sorgfaltspflichten seines Faches alle Vorkehrungen treffen, um die Eingriffsgefahren so gering wie möglich zu halten.

Umgemünzt auf die spezifischen Belange der Anästhesie besagt diese generalisierende Erkenntnis: Der Anästhesist trägt die Verantwortung für das Betäubungsverfahren und intraoperativ auch für die Überwachung, Aufrechterhaltung und Wiederherstellung der Vitalfunktionen. Seine ureigene Aufgabe ist es deshalb, zu prüfen und zu beurteilen, ob der Patient den spezifischen Risiken der Anästhesie und den Belastungen gewachsen ist, die sich für die Vitalfunktionen aus dem Betäubungsverfahren und dem speziellen Eingriff ergeben. Er kann diese Aufgabe und die mit ihr verbundene rechtliche Verantwortung nicht auf den Vertreter eines anderen Fachgebietes delegieren. Jeder Gedanke an eine solche Delegation muß schon deshalb a limine verworfen werden, weil sich untrennbar mit der Prüfung der Anästhesiefähigkeit die Frage nach der Wahl der optimalen Anästhesiemethode, nach der Art und Dosierung der Anästhetika und nach zahlreichen anästhesiologischen Details verbindet, die nur der schlüssig beantworten kann, der das Betäubungsverfahren durchzuführen hat und durch seine Methodenwahl auch selbst wieder entscheidenden Einfluß auf das anästhesiologische Risiko nehmen kann.

Ausführungen darüber, von welcher Bedeutung eine gründliche Anamnese und die Voruntersuchung des Patienten für die Beurteilung des Anästhesierisikos und für die Wahl des richtigen Anästhesieverfahrens sind, darf ich mir in Ihrem Kreise ersparen. Sorgfaltsmängel in diesem Bereich sind im Ergebnis wohl die primäre Ursache für die meisten Zwischenfälle, die zu forensischen Konsequenzen führen. Wenn noch Fortschritte bei der Senkung des Anaesthesierisikos zu erzielen sind, so liegen sie offenbar in der Verbesserung der anaesthesiologischen Voruntersuchung und der Vorbehandlung.

Gleichwohl meine ich, daß starre, zu Kunstregeln hochstilisierte Schemata über Art und Umfang anästhesiologischer Voruntersuchungen dem Fortschritt mehr schaden als nützen.

Man wird hier die individuellen Umstände nicht außer Betracht lassen dürfen und differenzieren müssen. Der erfahrene Anästhesist wird auf Grund einer sorgfältigen Anamnese dem Patienten manche Untersuchung ersparen können, die für einen weniger erfahrenen unerläßlich ist.

Mit dem vom Berufsverband Deutscher Anästhesisten empfohlenen Aufklärungs- und Anamnesebogen hoffen wir ein Hilfsmittel geschaffen zu haben, das eine sorgfältige Anamnese als Grundlage der Voruntersuchung erleichtert, ihre Ergebnisse dokumentiert und zugleich dem Patienten Hinweise für das Aufklärungsgespräch mit dem Arzt gibt.

Die rechtliche Verantwortung des Anästhesisten für die Beurteilung der Anästhesiefähigkeit, die heute außer jeder Diskussion stehen sollte, bedeutet selbstverständlich nicht, daß der Anästhesist die für diese Beurteilung erforderlichen Befunde stets selbst erheben müßte. Wie auch sonst im Rahmen der Arbeitsteilung in der Medizin, darf, ja muß er die Ergebnisse der von anderen Ärzten durchgeführten Voruntersuchungen zu Rate ziehen, zum einen um belastende und kostenträchtige Doppeluntersuchungen zu vermeiden, die schon unter dem Gesichtspunkt der Unwirtschaftlichkeit zu beanstanden wären, zum anderen aber auch, weil spezielle diagnostische Methoden weithin auch spezifische Fachkenntnisse erfordern. Der Anästhesist darf sich im Rahmen des Vertrauensgrundsatzes darauf verlassen, daß die ihm mitgeteilten Befunde und Untersuchungsergebnisse mit der gebotenen ärztlichen Sorgfalt erhoben sind. Er muß diese Untersuchungen um fehlende Glieder ergänzen und daraus das Schlußresümee ziehen.

Lautet es dahin, daß gegen die Anästhesiefähigkeit Bedenken bestehen, so ist damit noch nicht die abschließende Entscheidung getroffen. Ob die Operation gleichwohl durchgeführt werden soll, muß unter Abwägung der vom Anästhesisten mitgeteilten Bedenken gegen die Fakten getroffen werden, die aus der Sicht des Operateurs für den Eingriff hic et nunc sprechen. Diese Abwägung muß letztlich der Operateur treffen und verantworten. Der Anaesthesist darf sich — gleichfalls im Rahmen des Vertrauensgrundsatzes — darauf verlassen, daß diese Abwägung sachgerecht ist.

Das eine zentrale Problem dieses Panels scheint mir in der Frage zu liegen, welche der von ihm als erforderlich erachteten Voruntersuchungen der Anästhesie selbst vornehmen darf oder soll und bei welchen Untersuchungen er andere Fachgebiete einschalten muß. Vom Juristen erwarten Sie dazu gewiß keine konkrete Enumeration und keinen fachlichen Katalog, sondern allenfalls den Hinweis auf rechtliche Trennlinien. Auch insoweit muß ich mich freilich auf den Hinweis beschränken, wie diese Abgrenzung nach deutschem Recht zu sehen ist.

Der entscheidende Ansatzpunkt ist nach unserem Recht das in den Berufs- und Weiterbildungsordnungen der Landesärztekammern verankerte Gebot der Fachgebietsbeschränkung. Es zwingt den Arzt, der eine bestimmte Gebietsbezeichnung führt, sich grundsätzlich auf die ärztlichen Verrichtungen seines Gebietes zu beschränken. Die Berufs- und Weiterbildungsordnungen sind Satzungen autonomiebegabter öffentlicher Körperschaften; Verstöße gegen die Fachgebietsbeschränkung können im berufsgerichtlichen Verfahren geahndet werden. Eine weitere, im Ergebnis wohl noch wirksamere Sanktion liegt darin, daß die gesetzlichen Krankenkassen solche Leistungen nicht honorieren.

Für die Aufrechterhaltung des Prinzips der Fachgebietsbeschränkung lohnt es sich im Interesse des Leistungsstandards ärztlicher Spezialisten mit Entschiedenheit einzutreten. Ebenso entschieden muß aber auch der Standpunkt vertreten werden, daß die Fachgebiete keine mit starren Zäunen abgegrenzte Erbhöfe oder Schrebergärten sind, sondern daß sie sich in weiten Zonen überschneiden und überlappen. Die Definition der einzelnen Gebiete in unseren Weiterbildungsordnungen bezeichnet fachliche Aufgabenbereiche und nicht Monopole. Es ist deshalb nur konsequent, daß die deutschen Anästhesisten niemals ein Monopol für die Anästhesie gefordert und die fachliche Zuständigkeit der operativen Fächer für anästhesiologische Leistungen innerhalb ihrer jeweiligen operativen Aufgabenstellungen nicht in Zweifel gezogen haben.

Während im übrigen bisher keine Probleme erkennbar geworden sind, scheint sich das präoperative EKG in der Fachgebietsabgrenzung gegenüber dem Internisten zu einem neuralgischen Punkt zu entwickeln. Für mich ist freilich nur schwer nachvollziehbar, wie man dem Anästhesisten gerade in diesem Bereich die fachliche Zuständigkeit bestreiten will. Niemand zieht in Zweifel, daß er sich intraoperativ zur Überwachung der Herzfunktionen des EKG Monitorings bedienen darf, ja in Risikofällen bedienen muß, wenn ihm die dazu erforderlichen technischen Einrichtungen zur Verfügung stehen. Das gleiche gilt für die Zwischenfallstherapie und in weitem Umfang auch für die Intensivmedizin. Was der Anästhesist intraoperativ und in der Intensivmedizin darf, ja muß, dafür sollte ihm präoperativ die fachliche Kompetenz nicht abgesprochen werden können.

Dabei verkenne ich keinesweges, daß es eine Reihe von Fällen geben wird, in denen der Anästhesist den Spezialisten zur näheren Befundung des präoperativen EKG zu Rate ziehen muß. Es geht ja auch ersichtlich der Anästhesie nicht etwa darum, durch eigene diagnostische Leistungen andere Spezialisten aus der präoperativen Untersuchung zu verdrängen; Ziel aller Anstrengungen des Fachgebietes sollte es vielmehr sein, die präoperative Beurteilung der Anästhesierisiken auf breiter Basis zu intensivieren und dabei auch die Erkenntnisse zu gewinnen, die erforderlich sind, um andere Spezialisten rechtzeitig in diese Beurteilung einschalten zu können.

Die andere bedeutsame Frage scheint mir dahin zu gehen, *wann* die präoperative anaesthesiologische Untersuchung zur Prüfung der Anaesthesiefähigkeit durchgeführt werden soll. Die Antwort muß m.E. aus einer Vielzahl von Gründen lauten: Wenn irgend möglich so frühzeitig, daß eine nach der Beurteilung des Anästhesisten zweckmäßige Vorbehandlung durchgeführt werden kann, ohne zu einer Verschiebung des vom Operateur vorgesehenen Operationstermins zu zwingen. Dies erübrigt interkollegiale Auseinandersetzungen und die daraus resultierenden psychologischen Belastungen der Zusammenarbeit, erspart dem Patienten die mit Umdispositionen verbundenen Aufregungen und Zeitverluste und verringert das Gesamtrisiko, weil der Anästhesist dann bei der Entscheidung über die Vorbehandlung keine Konzessionen im Hinblick auf die bereits geplanten Operationstermine machen muß.

Bei nicht dringlichen Eingriffen spricht dies alles dafür, die präoperativen anästhesiologischen Untersuchungen und die Beurteilung der Anästhesiefähigkeit schon vor der stationären Aufnahme des Patienten durchzuführen. Im Bereich der sozialen Krankenversicherung wird dies bei uns freilich Widerständen begegnen, solange es nicht gelingt, den Nachweis zu führen, daß die gesonderte Berechnung der dabei anfallenden anästhesiologischen Leistungen durch die Ersparnisse bei der stationären Behandlung weit mehr als ausgeglichen wird. Erspart werden zum einen die Kosten für die stationäre Aufnahme des Patienten für die Dauer der Voruntersuchung. Zum anderen wird es in aller Regel möglich sein, auch die Vorbehandlung ambulant durchzuführen und damit die durchschnittliche Verweildauer deutlich zu senken. Und insgesamt kann wohl gelten: Was an präanästhesiologischen Voruntersuchungen finanziell eingespart wird, muß doppelt und dreifach bei der Therapie anästhesiologischer Komplikationen nachentrichtet werden.

Lassen Sie mich hoffen, daß die Referate und die Diskussion dieses Panels dazu beitragen, Schwierigkeiten und Hemmnisse, die einer angemessenen anästhesiologischen Voruntersuchung heute noch entgegenstehen, zu beseitigen.

Freie Themen
Präoperative Vorsorge

Vorsitz: W.F. List

Wertigkeiten verschiedener Parameter bei der präoperativen Beurteilung des Anaesthesie-Risikos

J.P. Striebel, R. Scherrer, I. Stähler-Hambrecht und H. Lutz

Die Einschätzung eines Patienten nach seinem Anästhesie- und Operationsrisiko stellt ein zentrales Problem in der operativen Medizin dar [1, 2, 13, 22]. Die optimale Nutzung aller präventiven Maßnahmen hat mit dazu beigetragen, daß es zu keinem wesentlichen Anstieg der intra- und postoperativen Letalität gekommen ist, und das, trotz erheblicher Ausweitung der Operationsindikationen, bezogen auf die Art des Eingriffes und das Alter des Patientengutes. Es besteht jedoch immer noch ein erhebliches Risiko, wenn man die möglichen hämodynamischen, respiratorischen und metabolischen Komplikationen ohne tödlichen Ausgang im Rahmen eines operativen Eingriffes in Betracht zieht [7, 18, 19, 32, 38]. Lutz und Peter [19] haben in einer Studie über das Risiko in der Anästhesie unter operativen Bedingungen eine Checkliste zur Erkennung und Reduzierung des Narkoserisikos erarbeitet. Damit soll für den Patienten der bestmögliche präoperative Zustand erreicht und vermeidbaren postoperativen Komplikationen vorgebeugt werden. In dieser Checkliste werden Angaben über Alter, Gewicht, Laborparameter, Operationsverfahren und Leistungsdaten der wichtigsten Organsysteme festgehalten. Während früher Risikoeinschätzungen nur anhand einzelner Kriterien vorgenommen wurden [25], soll mit Hilfe dieser Checkliste eine differenzierte Aussage über das zu erwartende Risiko gemacht werden. Ziel unserer Untersuchung war es, nachzuprüfen, inwieweit sich die anhand der Checkliste vorhergesagten Risiken auf den Anästhesieverlauf und die postoperative Phase auswirken.

Material und Methodik

Zur Untersuchung kamen innerhalb eines definierten Zeitraumes unausgewählt 331 Patienten aus dem chirurgischen, gynäkologischen und urologischen Operationsgut am Klinikum Mannheim. Bei allen Patienten wurde präoperativ anhand der Checkliste eine Risikoeinschätzung durchgeführt und über ein punktuelles Bewertungssystem (kein Risiko erhielt die Bewertungsziffer Null, maximales Risiko die Bewertungsziffer 16) die jeweilige Risikogruppe ermittelt. Die Anzahl der Patienten wurde auf mindestens 30 pro Operationsgebiet festgelegt. Alle Abweichungen vom Soll-Anästhesieverlauf wurden als Komplikationen definiert und gewertet. Der Beobachtungszeitraum umfaßte den gesamten Anästhesieverlauf und die Verweildauer im Aufwachraum. Aufgetretene Komplikationen wurden in hämodynamische, respiratorische und solche der Bewußtseinslage unterteilt.

Zu den hämodynamischen Komplikationen rechneten Hyper- und Hypotensionen mit mehr als 30% Abweichung vom Ausgangswert und Herzrhythmusstörungen, wie Kammerflimmern, Tachykardie ($>$ 100/min.), Bradykardie ($<$ 60/min.), Extrasystolen, Asystolien.

Die respiratorischen Komplikationen umfaßten sowohl Intubations- wie auch Beatmungsprobleme, Bronchospasmus, Singultus und Aspiration.

Als metabolische Komplikationen galten diabetische Stoffwechselentgleisungen und Allergien. Gesondert erfaßt wurden eine im Aufwachraum notwendige Atemhilfe, wie verlängerte O_2-Inhalation ($>$ als 20 Minuten postoperativ), eine weiterbestehende bzw. erneute Intubation + O_2 oder eine Nachbeatmung. Zusätzlich wurde die postnarkotische Bewußtseinslage nach den Kriterien kooperativ, bewußtseinsgetrübt, ohne Bewußtsein — festgehalten. Die als Komplikationen bezeichneten definierten Abweichungen vom Soll-Anästhesieverlauf wurden den Einzelkriterien der Checkliste, aus deren Summe sich die Riskiogruppe errechnet, gegenübergestellt (Tabelle 1).

Tabelle 1. Gegenüberstellung verschiedener Narkosekomplikationen und der Risikobeurteilung anhand von Parametern der Risiko-Checkliste

Narkose-Komplikation	Risikobeurteilung
Hämodynamik	Risikogruppe (1–5)
Art. Mitteldruck	Vorerkrankungen
Herzrhythmus	1 Herz-Kreislauf
Respiration	2 Atemwege
Technische Kompl.	3 Nieren, Elektrolyte
Beatmungs-Kompl.	4 Leber
	5 Diabetes mellitus
Metabolismus	6 Anämie
Glukoseverhalten	
Allergien	Alter
	Narkoseverfahren
Bewußtseinslage p. op.	Narkosedauer
kooperativ	Operationsart
bewußtlos	Geplante Operation
	Re-Operation
	Akut-Operation

Statistische Auswertung

Die Ergebnisse der Checkliste und die Abweichungen vom Soll-Anästhesieverlauf wurden in einem Erhebungsbogen protokolliert, mit Zahlen verschlüsselt und mittels Lochkarten auf einem Magnetband gespeichert. Es wurde eine statistische Häufigkeitsverteilung sämtlicher Daten erstellt und anschließend mit Hilfe des SPSS-Programm-Systems ein zwei- bis dreidimensionaler Vergleich der Einzeldaten bei gezielter Frage und Gegenüberstellung einzelner Parameter durchgeführt.

Ergebnisse und Diskussion

Die Risikogruppenverteilung des gesamten Patientengutes zeigt Abb. 1, der auch die Häufigkeit von Vorerkrankungen innerhalb der einzelnen Risikogruppen zu entnehmen ist. Die ho-

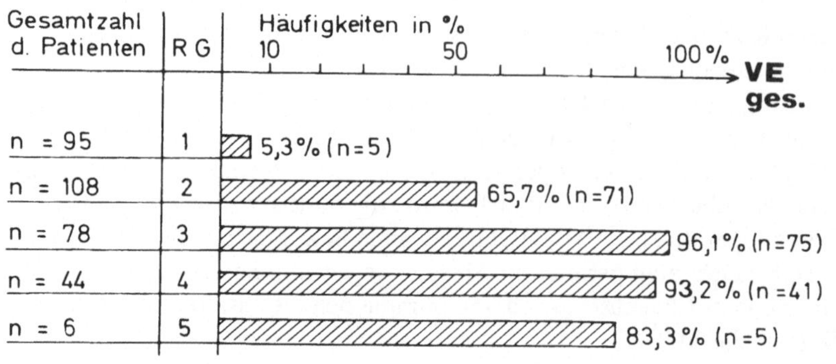

Abb. 1. Verteilung der Risikogruppen auf die Gesamtpatientenzahl und Anteil der Gesamtvorerkrankungen in den einzelnen Risikogruppen

he Anzahl von Patienten mit Vorerkrankungen in den Risikogruppen 2, 3, 4 und 5 bestätigt, daß die Vorerkrankungen auf die Risikoeinstufung einen wesentlichen Einfluß nehmen [11]. Im Gesamtkollektiv bestehen bei 59,5% Vorerkrankungen. Die Herz-Kreislauferkrankungen liegen mit 48,3% und die Atemwegserkrankungen mit 16,3% vorne.

Untersucht man die Abhängigkeit von Vorerkrankungen und Narkosekomplikationen (Abb. 2), so stellt man bei Patienten mit Herz-Kreislaufvorerkrankungen eine deutliche Häufung von hämodynamischen Komplikationen fest. Als Vergleich dienen Patienten, die keine Herz-Kreislaufvorerkrankungen aufweisen. Hämodynamische Komplikationen während der Narkose nehmen bei Patienten mit Herz-Kreislaufvorerkrankungen um mehr als das Doppelte zu [10]. Sie beinhalten im wesentlichen hypertone Kreislaufregulationen [29]. Es finden sich keine Unterschiede bezüglich Herzrhythmusstörungen, respiratorischen und metabolischen Komplikationen unter der Narkose und im Aufwachraum für Patienten mit und ohne Kreislaufvorerkrankungen.

Bei 54 Patienten war eine respiratorische Vorerkrankung bekannt. Im Vergleich mit Patienten ohne respiratorische Vorerkrankung steigt in erster Linie der Anteil respiratorischer, aber auch der hämodynamischer Komplikationen an. Dies gilt sowohl für die Narkoseeinleitung, als auch für die gesamte Narkosedauer. Im Aufwachraum benötigen diese Patienten vermehrt eine respiratorische Unterstützung [1, 12, 26, 30]. Memery [21] berichtet dazu, daß bei Todesfällen innerhalb der Anästhesie 3/4 aller Patienten in der präoperativen Phase schwere Lungenerkrankungen aufwiesen. Auf schmerzbedingte Verschlechterung der Ventilation bei respiratorischen Vorerkrankungen, hat Pooler schon 1949 hingewiesen [27]. Eine Beziehung zwischen Herzrhythmusstörungen und respiratorischen Vorerkrankungen ließ sich nicht zeigen.

Bei 32 Patienten war eine Nierenvorerkrankung bzw. eine Störung des Elektrolythaushaltes bekannt; in dieser Gruppe kommt es zu einer deutlichen Häufung von hämodynamischen Komplikationen während der Narkose. Die Analyse der hämodynamischen Komplikationen erbringt hypertone Kreislaufregulationsstörungen ebenso wie Herzrhythmusstörungen [23]. Obwohl bei beiden Kollektiven die respiratorischen Komplikationen gleich sind, ist die Zahl der Patienten, die im Aufwachraum einer respiratorischen Unterstützung mit Intubation und Sauerstoff bedurften, in der Gruppe mit Vorerkrankungen erhöht.

Bei Patienten mit vorangegangener Lebererkrankung (Abb. 3) kann in Anbetracht der kleinen Fallzahl nur sehr bedingt von einer Zunahme respiratorischer Komplikationen ge-

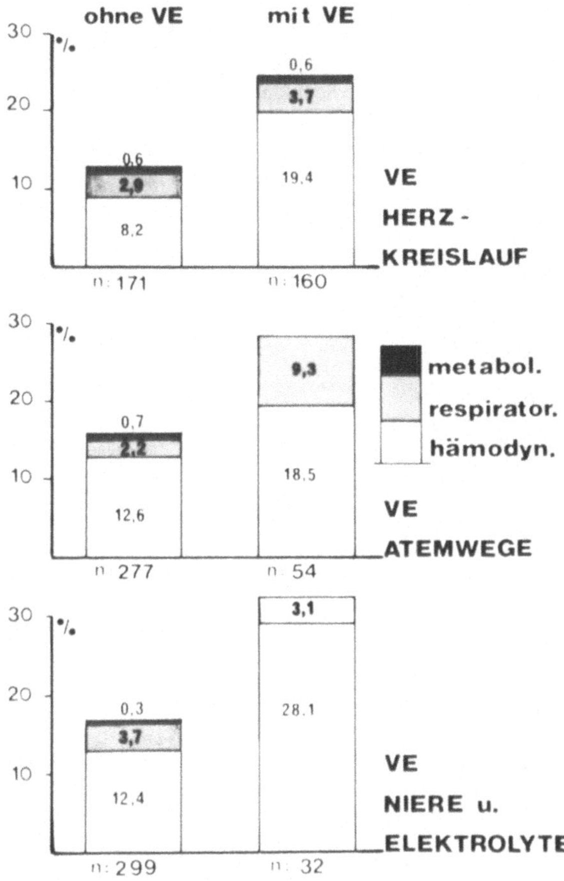

Abb. 2. Narkosekomplikationen bei verschiedenen Vorerkrankungen

sprochen werden. Zum Teil befinden wir uns hier im Gegensatz zu Ergebnissen anderer Untersucher [15], der Grund hierfür liegt aber möglicherweise in der Definition des Begriffes Lebererkrankung.

Patienten mit Diabetes mellitus zeigen eine Zunahme hämodynamischer Komplikationen während der Narkose. Diese sind fast ausschließlich hypertoner Natur und können bis in die Aufwachraumphase weiter verfolgt werden [24].

Das Lebensalter aller Diabetiker in diesem Kollektiv lag über 40. Bei 85,4% der Diabetes-Kranken waren zusätzlich Herz-Kreislaufvorerkrankungen bekannt [11], 41,2% litten an 3 und mehr Vorerkrankungen.

22 Patienten wiesen präoperativ einen erniedrigten Hb-Wert auf. Bei 40,9% dieser Patienten traten Komplikationen unter der Narkose auf. Es handelte sich dabei fast ausschließlich um hypotensive Kreislaufregulationen. Im Aufwachraum zeigten sich dagegen ausschließlich hypertensive Dysregulationen. Die Anzahl der Herzrhythmusstörungen ist in beiden Kollektiven, mit und ohne Anämie, nahezu gleich.

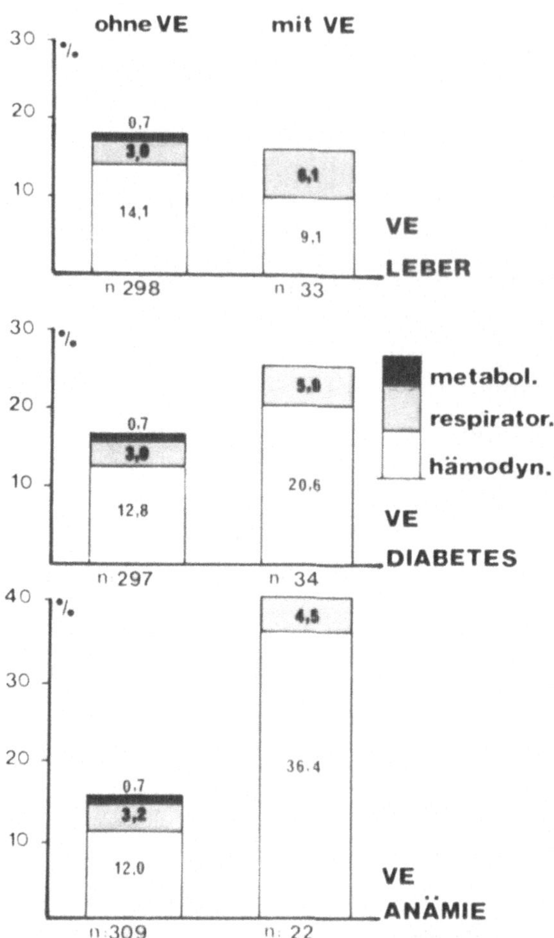

Abb. 3. Narkosekomplikationen bei verschiedenen Vorerkrankungen

Von Einfluß auf die Komplikationsrate ist auch die Narkosedauer [9, 18]. Bis zu 180 Minuten zeigen sich lediglich leichte Schwankungen, danach steigt die Komplikationsquote mit zunehmender Narkosedauer kontinuierlich an (Abb. 4). Es häufen sich sowohl hämodynamische wie auch respiratorische Komplikationen. Mit zunehmender Narkosedauer bedürfen diese Patienten auch im Aufwachraum vermehrter respiratorischer Unterstützung [38]. Dies entspricht Angaben von Mayrhofer [20], der eine deutliche Mortalitätszunahme in Abhängigkeit von der Narkosezeit beschreibt.

Vergleicht man die Art der Operation mit der Komplikationshäufigkeit, so haben operative Eingriffe im Oberbauch und in der Halsregion die größte Komplikationsrate (Abb. 5).

In Übereinstimmung mit anderen Literaturangaben [37] wird ein relativ hohes Operationsrisiko auch von Mayrhofer für gefäß- und abdominalchirurgische Eingriffe angegeben. Die Analyse der Komplikationen ergibt bevorzugt hämodynamische Komplikationen. Schädeloperationen weisen vermehrt hypotone, Ober- und Unterbaucheingriffe sowie Rücken-

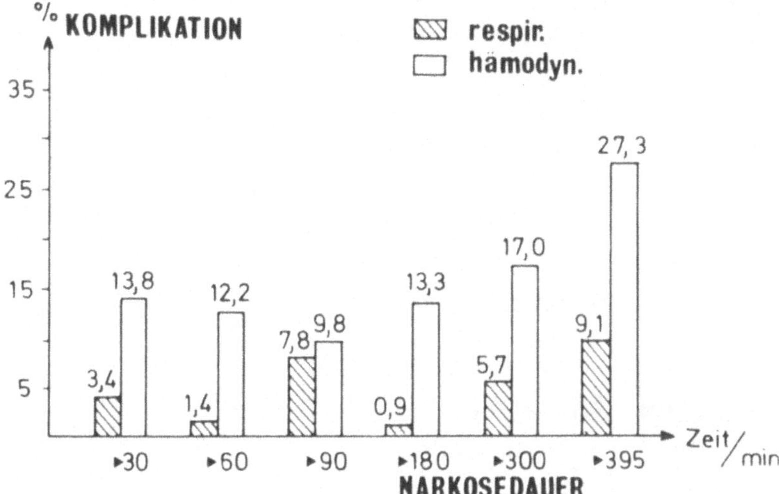

Abb. 4. Respiratorische und hämodynamische Komplikationen in Abhängigkeit von der Narkosedauer

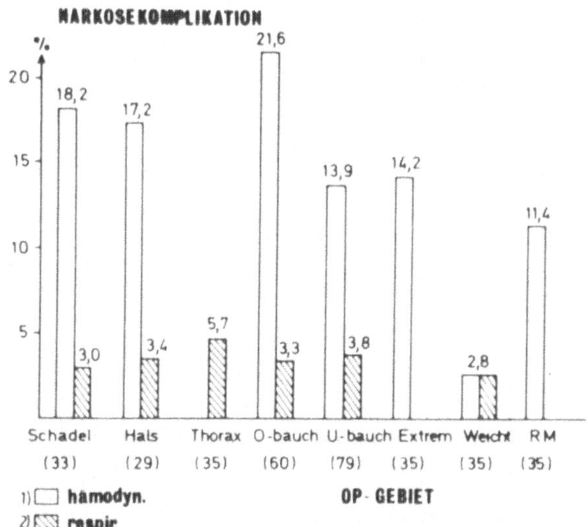

Abb. 5. Hämodynamische und respiratorische Narkosekomplikationen in Abhängigkeit vom Operationsgebiet

marksoperationen vermehrt hypertone Dysregulationen auf. Keine Unterschiede finden sich
bei Thorax-, Extremitäten- und Weichteiloperationen. Eine auffällige Häufung von Herzrhythmusstörungen unter Narkose tritt operationsbedingt bei Eingriffen im Carotisbereich
auf. Postoperativ finden sich jedoch weder für das Verhalten von Blutdruck, noch für das des
Herzrhythmus' Korrelationen zum operativen Eingriff.

Im Vergleich zu geplanten Operationen mit optimaler Vorbereitung ergibt sich bei akuten Eingriffen eine deutliche Zunahme der Komplikationsquote während der Narkose
(Abb. 6). Dies trifft sowohl für die hämodynamischen als auch die respiratorischen Kompli-

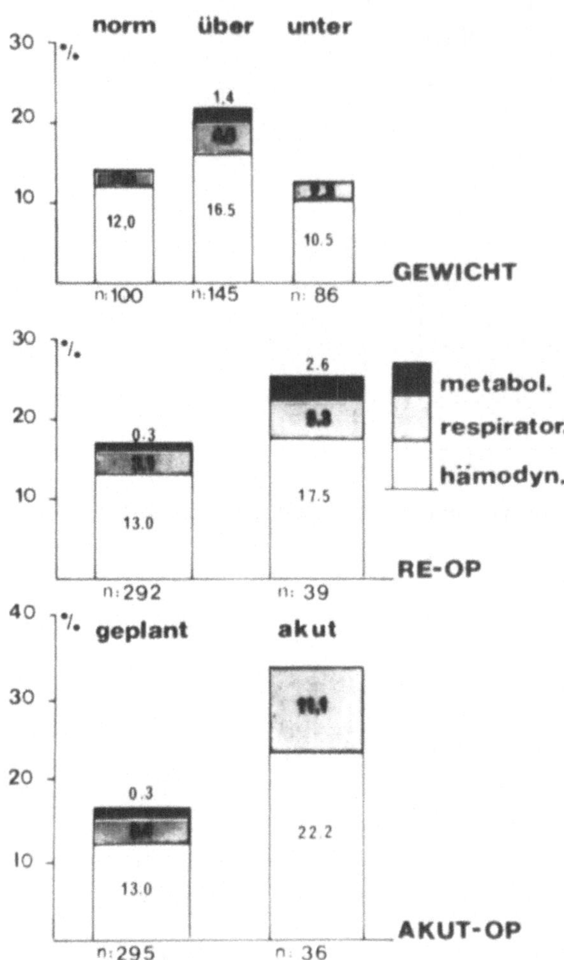

Abb. 6. Narkosekomplikationen in Abhängigkeit vom Körpergewicht, geplanten, Akut- und Reoperationen

kationen zu [3, 17, 31, 36]. Vergleicht man die unter Narkose aufgetretenen Blutdruckveränderungen, so finden sich bei notoperierten Patienten vermehrt hypo- wie auch hypertone Kreislaufregulationen. Der Prozentsatz der Patienten, bei denen postoperativ im Aufwachraum eine verlängerte O_2-Inhalation bzw. eine Nachbeatmung nötig war, ist bei Notoperationen höher. Das gleiche gilt für die Häufung von postoperativen Bewußtseinsstörungen. In Bezug auf Herzrhythmusstörungen ist zwischen elektiven Eingriffen und akuten Operationen sowohl unter Narkose wie auch im Aufwachraum kein Unterschied zu finden.

Stevens [33] beschreibt eine eindeutig höhere Mortalitätsrate nach Notoperationen. In unserer Studie lag die Mortalität bei Notoperationen bei 13,9% im Vergleich zu 2,7% bei elektiven Eingriffen. Weniger ausgeprägt ist der Unterschied in der Komplikationshäufigkeit bei Reoperationen.

Warner [35] beschreibt ein erhöhtes Narkoserisiko für den adipösen Patienten. Bei 43,8% unserer untersuchten Patienten lag eine Übergewichtigkeit von mehr als 10% des Soll-

Körpergewichtes vor. Hämodynamische Komplikationen während der Narkose treten bei Übergewichtigen häufiger und bei Untergewichtigen seltener auf als bei Normalgewichtigen. Die hämodynamischen Komplikationen werden vor allem durch hypertone Blutdruckregulationen verursacht. Respiratorische Komplikationen sind höher in der übergewichtigen Gruppe, Herzrhythmusstörungen wurden nicht beobachtet. Betrachtet man die Vorerkrankungen in Abhängigkeit vom Körpergewicht, so findet sich bei Übergewichtigkeit eine größere Häufigkeit für Herz-Kreislaufvorerkrankungen und für Diabetes mellitus. Die Ergebnisse dieser kleinen Studie spiegeln die von Postlethwait [28] beschriebene Konstellation von Diabetes mellitus und Hypertonie sowie Übergewicht wider.

Ab dem 50. Lebensjahr nehmen die in unserem Patientengut erfaßten Komplikationen gleichmäßig zu. Bei Differenzierung der Komplikationsart zeigt sich dies besonders in der Hämodynamik. Hypertone Dysregulationen nehmen ab dem 40. Lebensjahr stetig zu und erreichen einen Höchstwert im 7. Dezennium. Respiratorische Komplikationen haben in der Altersklasse der 50- bis 60jährigen den größten Anteil. Betrachtet man dazu die Verteilung der Risikogruppen auf die verschiedenen Altersklassen und die Vorerkrankungen, so wird dies verständlich (Abb. 7, Abb. 8). Mayrhofer und Mitthöfer finden, daß bei Patienten über 70 Jahren die Mortalität signifikant ansteigt. Sie führen dies auf die Folgen des physiologischen Alterungsprozesses und die darin kausal beinhaltete Polymorbidität zurück.

Bei kritischer Wertung der vorliegenden Daten kann man im Hinblick auf die Validität und Aussagekraft der verwendeten Risikocheckliste für den Anästhesieverlauf folgendes feststellen:

RISIKOGRUPPE

ALTER	1	2	3	4	5
−10 J.	19	●	●	●	●
−20 J.	12	5	●	●	●
−30 J.	14	5	1	1	●
−40 J.	20	21	1	1	●
−50 J.	20	32	10	6	●
−60 J.	10	30	19	14	●
−70 J.	●	8	32	12	●
−89 J.	●	7	15	10	6

Abb. 7. Die Verteilung der Risikogruppen auf die verschiedenen Altersstufen

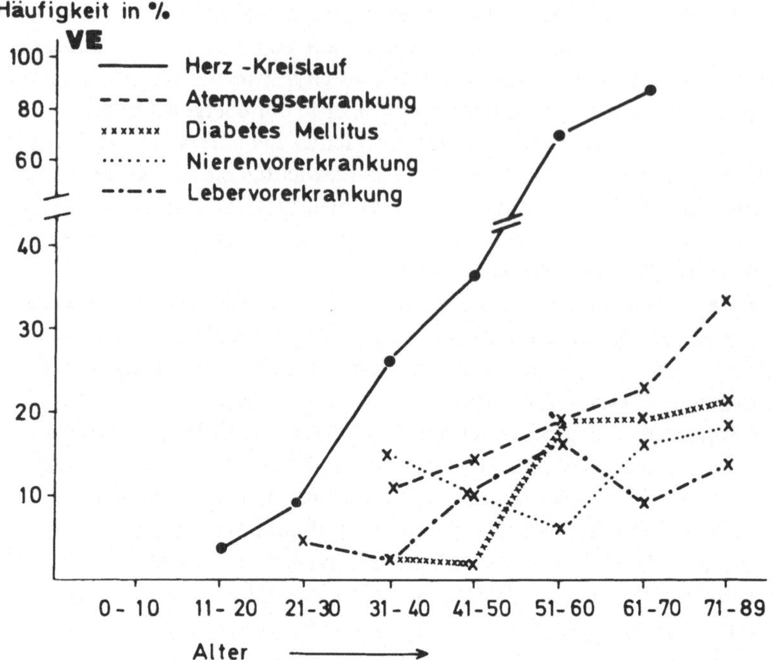

Abb. 8. Häufigkeiten verschiedener Vorerkrankungen auf die verschiedenen Altersstufen

1. Die Art und der Umfang der Vorerkrankungen beeinflußt wesentlich den Anästhesieverlauf.
2. Vorerkrankungen im Bereich des Herz-Kreislaufsystems und der Atemwege überwiegen und sollten bei der Beurteilung des Narkoserisikos Priorität haben.
3. Die Untersuchungsergebnisse bestätigen, daß bei höherem Alter, Übergewicht und zunehmender Narkosedauer das Anästhesierisiko zusätzlich steigt.
4. Notoperationen und Reoperationen zeigen häufiger Anästhesiekomplikationen als geplante Eingriffe.
5. Die präoperative Risikovorhersage trifft weitgehend zu, sowohl für die Anästhesie direkt, als auch für die unmittelbare postoperative Phase.
6. Die Zusammenhänge zwischen Vorerkrankungen, Risikoeinstufung und Anästhesieverlauf zeigen deutlich, daß für eine optimale Operationsvorbereitung in der Anästhesie die sachgerechte Anwendung einer Risikocheckliste unter besonderer Berücksichtigung der Kreislauf- und Atemfunktion unentbehrlich geworden ist (Abb. 9).

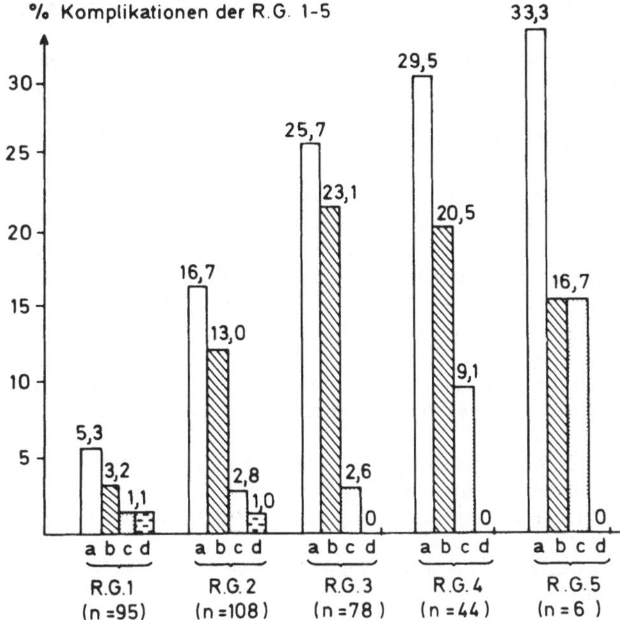

Abb. 9. Häufigkeit der Narkosekomplikationen in Abhängigkeit von der zugeordneten Risikogruppe

Literatur

1. Bergmann H (1969) Gestörte Atemfunktion als Anästhesierisiko. Wien Med Akad Wien 45
2. Brandesky G (1973) Prä- und postoperative Probleme. Langenbecks Arch Chir 334:755
3. Burn JMB (1974) Preoperative anaesthetic assessment clinic. Lancet 2:886
4. Clark RC, Jones GL, Greifenstein FE (1972) Anesthesia and hepatic necrosis. Amer J Obstet Gynec 113:1146
5. Cole F (1961) Anesthesia, surgery and death. Med Times 89:281
6. Cole WH (1953) Operability in the young and aged. Ann Surg 138:145
7. Cullen DJ, Cullen BL (1975) Postanesthetic complications. Surg Clin North Amer 55:987
8. Fisher A, Waterhouse TD, Adams AP (1975) Obesity: Its relation to anaesthesia. Anaesthesia 30:633
9. Fisk GC (1961) The time factor in surgery. Med J Aust 48:703
10. Goldman L, Caldera DL, Nussbaum SR, Southwick FS, Krogstad D, Murray B, Burke DS, O'Malley TA, Goroll AH, Caplan CH, Nolan J, Carabello B, Slater EE (1977) Multifactorial index of cardiac risk in non cardiac surgical procedures. N Engl J Med 297:845
11. Hallen B (1973) Computerized anesthetic record keeping. Acta Anesth Scand Suppl 52:5
12. Hedley-Whyte J, Burgess GE, Feeley ThW, Miller MG (1976) Applied physiology of respiratory care. Little, Brown a. Comp, Boston
13. Kaushik SP, Kaushik S (1972) A study of operative and anesthetic mortality. Indian J Med Res 60: 1361
14. Lamberth IE (1968) Obesity and anesthesia. Clin Anesth 3:56
15. Little DM jr, Wetstone HJ (1964) Anesthesia and the liver. Anesthesiology 25:815
16. Lutz H (1979) Sorgfalt bei der Voruntersuchung und Vorbehandlung. Anästhesiologie u. Intensivmedizin 2:31
17. Lutz H, Klose R (1979) Operationsvorbereitung aus anästhesiologischer Sicht. Med Welt 30:639
18. Lutz H, Klose R, Peter K (1972) Untersuchungen zum Risiko der Allgemeinanästhesie unter operativen Bedingungen. Dtsch Med Wschr 97:1816

19. Lutz H, Peter K (1973) Das Risiko der Anästhesie unter operativen Bedingungen. Langenbecks Arch Chir 334:671
20. Mayrhofer O (1970) Operationsrisiken alter Menschen unter besonderer Berücksichtigung der Arteriosklerose. Münchn Med Wschr 46:2071
21. Memery HN (1965) Anesthesia mortality in private practice. JAMA 194:1185
22. Moore DC, Bridenbaugh LD, Bagdi PA (1968) Tabulation of Anesthetic. Data: An Improved system. Anesthesiology 29:595
23. Pflüger H (1969) Anästhesieprobleme bei essentieller Hypertonie. Med Welt 35:1881
24. Pflüger H (1971) Anästhesieprobleme bei Diabetes mellitus. Med Klin 66:1225
25. Pitule H (1976) Zum Operations- und Narkoserisiko. Eine vergleichende Studie über die Aussagekraft zweier Op-Checklisten unter besonderer Berücksichtigung des postoperativen Verlaufs. Inaugural-Dissertation, Mannheim
26. Pontoppidan H, Laver MB, Geffin B (1970) Acute respiratory failure in the surgical patient. Advanc Surg 4:163
27. Pooler HE (1949) Relief of postoperative pain and its influence on vital capacity. Brit Med J 2:1200
28. Postlethwait RW, Johnson WD (1972) Complications following surgery for duodenal ulcer in obese patients. Arch Surg 105:438
29. Prys-Roberts C, Meloche R, Foex P (1971) Studies of anaesthesia in relation to hypertension. I. Cardiovascular responses of treated and untreated patients. Brit J Anaesth 43:122
30. Rügheimer E (1968) Prophylaxe und Therapie der respiratorischen Narkosekomplikationen. Langenbecks Arch Chir 322:1291
31. Rügheimer E (1970) Die akute Ateminsuffizienz in der prä- und postoperativen Phase von Noteingriffen. Langenbecks Arch Chir 327:896
32. Scheibe O, Dahm P (1970) Der Noteingriff in der Alterschirurgie unter besonderer Berücksichtigung der Begleiterkrankungen. Langenbecks Arch Chir 327:777
33. Stevens KM, Aldrete JA (1969) Anaesthesia factors affecting surgical morbidity and mortality in the elderly male. J Amer Geriatr Soc 17:659
34. Vormittag E (1975) Risikofaktoren und Pathogenese der postoperativen kardialen Dekompensation. Münchn Med Wachr 117:1929
35. Warner WA, Garrett LP (1968) The obese patient and anesthesia. JAMA 205:102
36. Wiemers K (1970) Wahl des optimalen Zeitpunkts bei Noteingriffen. Langenbecks Arch Chir 327:892
37. Wilkins LF, Knight CD (1958) Abdominal surgery in the aged. An analysis of 307 operations. Arch Surg 76:963
38. Wilson RD, Strother BF, Allen CR (1967) A study of the effects of a postanesthetic recovery room on mortality and morbidity in 9212 geriatric patients. Texas Rep Biol Med 25:35

Die Anamneseerhebung in der Anaesthesiologie –
ein Vergleich zwischen Fragebogen und Interview

D. Daub

Die Anamneseerhebung in der Anaesthesiologie ist, verglichen mit der Situation in den Fachrichtungen, die ihre Patienten stationär betreuen, behindert, weil der Anaesthesist seine Patienten einzeln aufsuchen — häufig dabei auch suchen muß. Deshalb werden in manchen Abteilungen Fragebögen zur Anamneseerhebung herangezogen, um ein screening der Patienten durchzuführen. In einem Versuch sollte nun überprüft werden, wie ein solcher Fragebogen aufgebaut sein sollte und wie effektiv er eingesetzt werden kann.

Vor fünf Jahren konnte die Qualität der anaesthesiologischen Anamneseerhebung im Klinikum der RWTH Aachen dadurch wesentlich verbessert werden, daß eine standardisierte Interviewtechnik eingeführt wurde. Anhand eines als check-list angelegten Anaesthesiedaten-Erfassungsbogens konnte die Objektivität durch die gute Strukturiertheit des Bogens verbessert werden. Die zu erfragenden Sachverhalte sind weitgehend vorgegeben; sie werden, wenn zutreffend, durch Unterstreichen markiert und, wenn notwendig, durch handschriftliche Eintragungen ergänzt. Soweit die Ausgangsposition.

In mehreren Vorversuchen wurde getestet, wie ein Fragebogen aufgebaut sein soll, um die größte Zahl von Informationen zu erfassen. Dieses Kriterium der maximalen Informationsmenge erschien das gegebene, weil davon ausgegangen werden mußte, daß die Anamnese nie vollständig erfaßt werden kann und deshalb mehr anamnestische Angaben auch zwangsläufig bessere Anamnese bedeuten mußten. Der endgültig für brauchbar befundene Fragebogen bestand fast ausschließlich aus sogenannten dichotomen, geschlossenen Fragen, auf die nur die Antworten „ja" und „nein" gegeben werden konnten. Ein weiteres Ergebnis der Vorversuche war, daß prinzipiell auch umfangreiche Fragebögen von den Patienten gerne und exakt ausgefüllt werden.

Im Zeitraum von November 1977 bis April 1978 wurden 150 Patienten der Abteilungen Chirurgie, Orthopädie, Hals-Nasen-Ohren und Gynäkologie am Vorabend eines größeren operativen Eingriffes sowohl nach der standardisierten Interviewtechnik als auch über den Fragebogen zu ihrer Anamnese befragt. Um Fremdeinflüsse auszuschalten, wurde die Hälfte der Patienten zuerst interviewt, dann wurde ihnen der Bogen vorgelegt, bei der anderen Hälfte wurde umgekehrt verfahren. Dem Interviewer war nicht bekannt, ob ein Fragebogen von dem betreffenden Patienten bereits ausgefüllt war oder ob er dafür vorgesehen war, einen solchen auszufüllen. Er war selbstverständlich nicht über eventuell vorliegende Befragungsergebnisse informiert.

Es soll hier nur ein Ergebnis des Versuches diskutiert werden: Die Anzahl der erfaßten Anamnesedaten liegt bei den Fragebögen wesentlich höher als bei den Interviews. Bei den 150 Patienten unseres Versuchskollektivs wurden insgesamt mit beiden Methoden 1820 anaesthesierelevante Fakten aus der Anamnese ermittelt, wobei über das Interview 615, über den Fragebogen jedoch 1684 Anamnesedaten dem behandelnden Anaesthesisten bekannt wurden.

Dieses Ergebnis ist überraschend, und es bedarf einer ausführlichen Erklärung. Zur Überprüfung von Befragungstests stehen im Wesentlichen drei Kriterien zur Verfügung, und zwar neben der bereits genannten Objektivität, die in beiden Verfahren etwa gleichermaßen erfüllt wird, die Reliabilität und die Validität. Die Reliabilität, in unserem Fall am besten durch die Reproduzierbarkeit des Testes überprüft, ist nicht gegeben, weil das Ergebnis der Befragung wesentlich von der präoperativen Situation beeinflußt wird. Die Validität des Testes ist ebenfalls nicht prüfbar, weil bei fast allen erfaßten Daten der Wahrheitsgehalt nicht bekannt und nicht erfaßbar ist.

Wie kann man sich — wenn schon nicht mit wissenschaftlichen Verfahren — dieses Ergebnis dennoch erklären? Denkbar sind die folgenden Erklärungsversuche:

1. Der Interviewer fragt nicht die gesamte „check-list" ab.

2. Der Patient hat bei Verwendung des Fragebogens mehr Zeit zu überlegen und erinnert sich so an mehr Einzelheiten.

3. Der Fragenbogen wurde nach den falschen Kriterien optimiert, das heißt, nicht die Anamnese mit den meisten positiven Antworten ist die beste; der Interviewer kommt mit gezielten Fragen der Wahrheit näher.

4. Der Patient kreuzt zweifelhafte Sachverhalte an oder aber aggraviert mit dem Ziel, mit dem Anaesthesisten persönlich zu sprechen. Dafür spricht, daß Patienten mit völlig leerer Anamnese die Frage bejahten, sie hätten dem Arzt etwas Wichtiges mitzuteilen; dagegen spricht die Tatsache, daß sich kein signifikant anderes Verhalten zeigt bei den Patienten, die zuerst interviewt worden sind zu denen, denen zuerst der Fragebogen vorgelegt wurde.

Als Fazit läßt sich zusammenfassen: Über den Fragebogen werden wahrscheinlich eher zu viele als zu wenige Anamnesedaten erfaßt; die Wahrheit, die keiner der Beteiligten kennt, liegt in der Mitte. Der Fragebogen kann die Prämedikationsvisite nicht ersetzen, weil in ihrem Verlauf auch eine Befunderhebung und Verordnungen notwendig sind. Der Fragebogen reduziert nicht einmal den Zeitbedarf der Visite, weil alle erfaßten Daten auf ihre Validität — soweit dies überhaupt möglich ist — überprüft werden müssen. Hinzu kommt, daß die Mehrzahl der Patienten der Methode des Fragebogens negativ gegenüberstehen, wenn sie befürchten müssen, daß das Ausfüllen der Bogen den Besuch eines Arztes ersetzen soll.

Aus diesen Gründen werden in unserer Abteilung Fragebögen für den Routinepatienten nicht eingesetzt. Wir haben lediglich, und das scheint eine sinnvolle Anwendung zu sein, die Bögen in die im Aachener Raum gesprochenen Sprachen und in die der dort beschäftigten Gastarbeiter übersetzt, um sie bei sprachlichen Verständigungsschwierigkeiten einzusetzen.

Untersuchungen zur präoperativen Angst

W. Tolksdorf, U. Gawol, R. Grund, J. Pfeifer, H. Lutz, J. Berlin, B. Berlin und D. Langrehr

Die Reduktion der präoperativen Angst gehört ebenso wie die Aufrechterhaltung der Funktionen von Kreislauf, Atmung und Stoffwechsel, sowie der Gewährleistung einer ausreichenden Analgesie zu den vornehmen Aufgaben des Anaesthesisten.

Wenn wir von Angst sprechen, so meinen wir jenen situationsabhängigen, unangenehmen, affektiven Zustand, welcher hervorgerufen ist durch einen aversiven Stimulus, hier Krankheit, Narkose und Operation.

Der Terminus Angst wird verwendet im Sinne des, im angloamerikanischen Sprachgebrauch verwendeten Begriffs der „state anxiety", als vorübergehendem Zustand, im Gegensatz zur „trait anxiety", die die Ängstlichkeit als relativ stabilen Charakterzug meint.

Der emotionale Zustand der Angst ist immer auch begleitet von somatischen Veränderungen, vorwiegend des vegetativen Nervensystems, weshalb die Angstreduktion nicht nur eine humane, sondern auch eine psychosomatische Notwendigkeit darstellt.

Neben der medikamentösen abendlichen und morgendlichen Prämedikation, mit anxiolytischer Komponente, muß dem Gespräch zwischen Patient und Anaesthesist eine erhebliche Bedeutung für die subjektive Befindlichkeit des Patienten und seiner psychosomatischen Reaktion beigemessen werden.

Es galt lange Zeit als selbstverständlich, durch beruhigende Worte und durch die Beschreibung des prä- und postoperativen Ablaufs, im Patienten eine Reduktion der Angst herbeizuführen. Die juristische Verpflichtung zur Risikoaufklärung jedoch beinhaltet unseres Erachtens eine Steigerung der Angst, was vielen Anaesthesisten Unbehagen und vielen Patienten schlaflose Nächte und eine risikoreichere Narkose und Operation bereitet. Da unseres Wissens bislang keine Studie existiert, in der dieses Problem bearbeitet wurde, untersuchten wir den Einfluß der Risikoaufklärung auf die Angst des Patienten vor Narkose und Operation, sowie ihr somatisches Korrelat anhand des Kreislaufverhaltens sowie des intraoperativen Narkosemittelverbrauchs.

In der Versuchsplanung mußten die Faktoren berücksichtigt werden, die wir als angstbeeinflussend anhand vorausgehender Pilotstudien isolieren konnten. Hierzu waren zu zählen: Das Alter der Patienten, das dem Ausmaß der Angst umgekehrt proportional ist, die zu erwartenden funktionellen und kosmetischen Operationsfolgen, sowie frühere Narkoseerfahrungen, die erheblich die präoperative Befindlichkeit beeinflussen. Wir wählten allgemein chirurgische und orthopädische Operationen, die anhand der Kriterie kosmetische und funktionelle Operationsfolgen einem mittleren Angstniveau zuzuordnen waren. Die Untersuchung wurde bei 44 Patienten durchgeführt, die nach einem zuvor festgelegten Randomisierungsplan in zwei Gruppen eingeteilt wurden.

Die Patienten der Gruppe I wurden während der präoperativen Visite am Abend vor der Operation in einem halbstandardisierten Gespräch über folgende individuelle und allgemeine Narkoserisiken aufgeklärt.

a) Individuelle Risiken:

Begleiterkrankungen von seiten des Herz-Kreislaufsystems, der Atemorgane und des Stoffwechsels.

b) Allgemeine Narkoserisiken:

die Möglichkeit unerwünschter Nebenwirkungen der Narkosemittel auf den Kreislauf, die Atmung sowie die Möglichkeit der allergischen Reaktion. Komplikationen, verursacht durch Intubation, wie Zahnschäden und postoperativer Heiserkeit. Die Möglichkeit technischer Fehler, die jedoch sehr selten vorkämen und in nahezu allen Fällen erkannt und behoben würden.

c) Nach der Aufklärung wurde den Patienten versichert, daß auch diese Risiken aufgrund unseres Fachwissens und der Erfahrung auf ein Minimum reduziert würden, und daß kein Grund bestünde, aufgeregt zu sein.

Auf die Patienten der Gruppe II wurde lediglich beruhigend eingegangen und weder auf das individuelle, noch das allgemeine Anaesthesierisiko hingewiesen. Es wurde ihnen versichert, daß sie die Narkose gut überstehen würden, und kein Grund zur Angst bestünde.

Alle Patienten hatten den Mannheimer Fragebogen zur Narkosevorbereitung ausgefüllt.

Die abendliche Prämedikation war mit 10 mg Valium p.o., die morgendliche mit Dolantin, Psyquil und Atropin, abhängig vom Körpergewicht, standardisiert.

Die Angst der Patienten wurde unmittelbar vor dem Gespräch, unmittelbar nach dem Gespräch und am Morgen der Operation mit dem, von der Arbeitsgruppe Mannheim/Groningen entwickelten Erhebungsbogen der subjektiven Befindlichkeit, kurz ESB genannt, gemessen. Zu denselben Zeitpunkten, sowie intraoperativ, postoperativ im Aufwachraum, sowie postoperativ auf Station, wurden der Blutdruck nach Riva-Rocci, als auch die Pulsfrequenz ausgewertet. Als statistisches Prüfverfahren verwendeten wir die Varianzanalyse.

Wir erhielten folgende Ergebnisse: Die Patienten beider Gruppen im Alter von 16 bis 65 Jahren unterschieden sich weder hinsichtlich der Alters- noch Geschlechtsverteilung voneinander. Auch im ESB-Wert als Angstparameter vor dem Gespräch, konnte mit 3,0 bzw. 3,3 kein Unterschied festgestellt werden.

2 Patienten, die über das Narkoserisiko aufgeklärt wurden, verweigerten nach dem Gespräch Narkose und Operation. Sie fielen aus der weiteren Auswertung heraus.

Während die aufgeklärten Patienten einen Anstieg des ESB-Wertes nach dem Interview und einen geringen Abfall unmittelbar präoperativ aufwiesen, der jedoch immer noch über dem Ausgangswert lag, kam es in der beruhigten Patientengruppe zu einem stetigen Abfall des Angstwertes. Der Unterschied zwischen beiden Gruppen zu den beiden Meßzeitpunkten nach dem Gespräch ist statistisch signifikant (Abb. 1).

Die Ergebnisse der Angstmessung fanden ihr physiologisches Korrelat im Verhalten von Blutdruck und Puls. Während vor dem Gespräch kein Unterschied in der Pulsfrequenz nachweisbar war, unterschieden sich die aufgeklärten Patienten von den beruhigten Patienten nach dem Gespräch signifikant, im Sinne einer höheren Pulsfrequenz. Auch der systolische und der diastolische Blutdruck stiegen bei aufgeklärten Patienten deutlich an, während es in der beruhigten Patientengruppe zu einem geringgradigen Abfall kam.

Sowohl intra-, als auch postoperativ im Aufwachraum wies die risikoaufgeklärte Gruppe einen deutlich höheren Anstieg des systolischen Blutdruckes auf, Zeichen eines erhöhten streßbedingten Sympathicustonus. Diese Tendenz setzte sich nach Rückkehr auf Station

ANGST

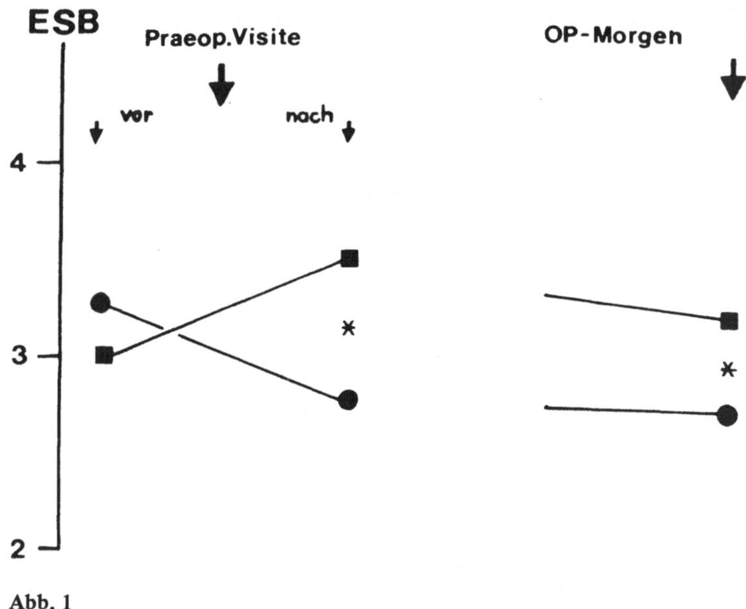

Abb. 1

fort. Der Unterschied war auf dem 4⁰/oo-Niveau signifikant (Abb. 2). Auch der Narkosemittel-
verbrauch war in der risikoaufgeklärten Gruppe signifikant höher als der in der beruhigten
Patientengruppe (Abb. 3).

Beide Faktoren, sowohl der erhöhte Sympathicustonus als auch der Mehrverbrauch an
Narkotika müssen als vermeidbare Erhöhung des Narkoserisikos angesehen werden.

Fassen wir die Ergebnisse dieser Studie zusammen, so müssen wir feststellen: Die Angst-
induktion durch Risikoaufklärung als emotionales Phänomen, sowie deren somatische Konsequenzen, kann vom anästhesiologischen Standpunkt nicht vorbehaltlos toleriert werden.
Es muß aus humanen und psychosomatischen Gründen als bedenklich angesehen werden,
durch die juristische Verpflichtung zur Risikoaufklärung dem Patienten das Anxiolyticum
Anaesthesist in dieser angstvoll erlebten Situation zu entziehen.

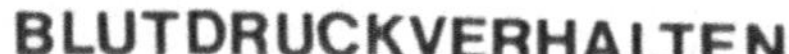

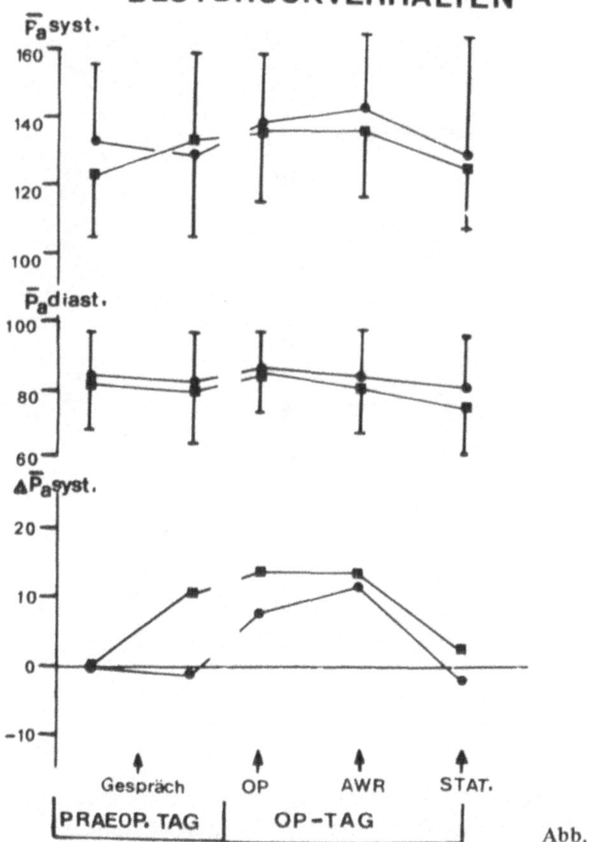

Abb. 2

MEDIKAMENTENVERBRAUCH

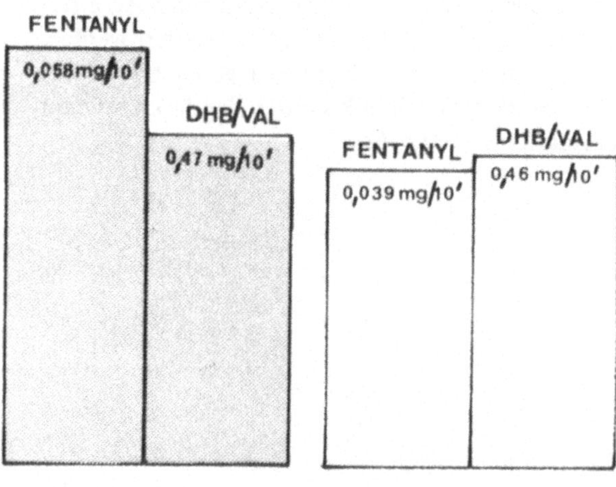

Abb. 3

Das hohe Lebensalter als Risikofaktor in der Neuroanaesthesie

R. Enzenbach und St. Lührmann

Die zunehmende Lebenserwartung unserer Bevölkerung und die Verbesserung der chirurgischen Therapie führen dazu, daß wir heute in steigendem Maße alte Patienten zu behandeln und zu anaesthesieren haben.

Die Überalterung macht sich besonders bemerkbar in den großen Städten, z.B. West-Berlin mit einem Einwohner-Anteil von 3% an über 80jährigen. V. Bramann und Herold berichteten von der Freien Universität schon 1969 einen Prozentsatz von 2,1% über 80jähriger in ihrer Operationsstatistik [3]. Mayrhofer gab für Wien im Jahre 1968 die gleiche Altersgruppe 1,7% an [8].

Auch in unserem Krankengut der Neurochirurgischen Klinik ist von 1968 bis 1978 eine ständige Zunahme der alten Patienten — wir haben bereits die über 70jährigen erfaßt — festzustellen (Abb. 1). Gegenüber dem Stand vor 10 Jahren beträgt die Steigerung jetzt das 3- bis 4fache. Im Vergleich dazu ist die Zunahme in der Operations-Gesamtstatistik, trotz Vermehrung der Bettenzahl von 60 auf 80, wesentlich geringer.

Im Gegensatz zu Mayrhofer, der für die Allgemeinchirurgie — allerdings bei den über 80-jährigen — ein dreifaches Überwiegen der Frauen gegenüber den Männern fand, ist das Geschlechterverhältnis in unserem Krankengut noch ausgewogen.

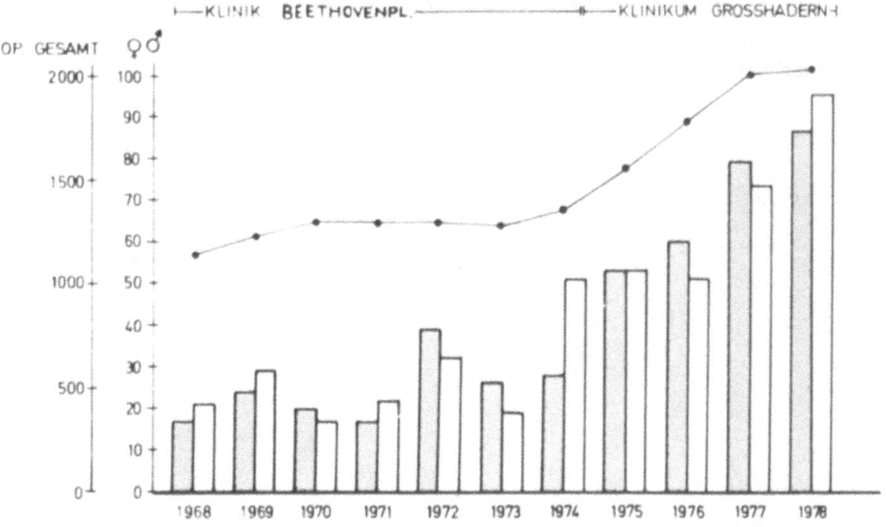

Abb. 1. Zunahme der über 70jährigen Patienten im Verlaufe der letzten 11 Jahre (Säulen) im Vergleich mit der Gesamt-Statistik (Punkte) neurochirurg. Eingriffe. n = 908

Auch bei den diagnostischen Eingriffen in Narkose, zu den Angiographien kommen ab 1975 noch die Computer-Tomographien hinzu, läßt sich die gleiche Zunahme alter Patienten feststellen (Abb. 2). Bei einem Großteil der alten, häufig verwirrten Patienten konnten exakte Tomographien meist mit Kontrastmittelinjektion nur unter völliger Ruhigstellung durch Narkose ermöglicht werden.

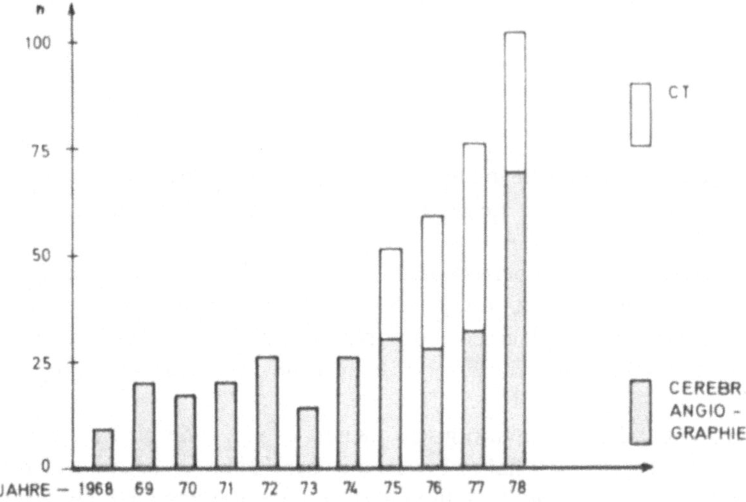

Abb. 2. Diagnostische Eingriffe in Narkose bei Patienten > 70 Jahre, ab 1975 zusätzlich Computer-Tomographie

Die Aufteilung nach der Art der neurochirurgischen Operationen bei 634 Patienten dieser Altersgruppe zeigt den hohen Prozentsatz von Schmerzeingriffen (Trigeminus-Eingriffe, Chordotomien etc.) (37,5%). Erst in großem Abstand folgen Operationen bei Hirntumoren (13,4%), Bandscheibenprolaps (9,3%) und Gefäßeingriffe und sonstiges (Extra-Intracranieller Bypass, Gefäßmißbildungen, Ventriculoatriale Ableitung durch Ventile, Tracheotomien etc.) (11,8%). Rückenmarktumoren und tumorbedingte Wurzelkompressionssyndrome, Eingriffe an peripheren Nerven, subdurale Haematome und Schädel-Hirn-Traumen liegen jeweils deutlich unter der 10%-Grenze (Abb. 3).

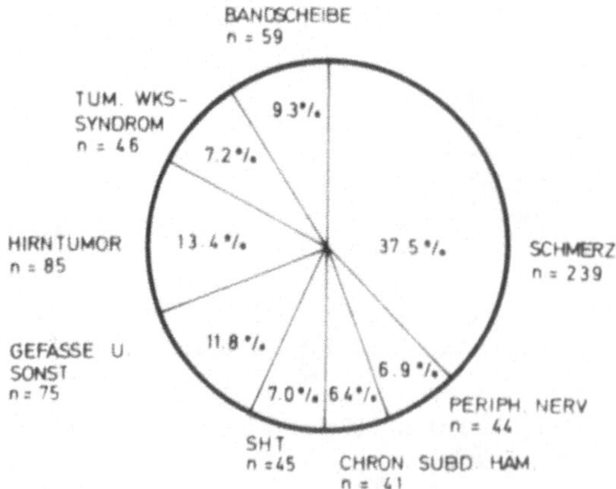

Abb. 3. Art der neurochirurgischen Eingriffe bei Patienten > 70 Jahre. n = 634

Alter und Allgemeinzustand der Kranken, sowie Art, Schwierigkeitsgrad und Dauer des Eingriffs bestimmen die Prognose. Die verminderte Belastbarkeit alter Patienten geht aus der Verschiebung des Blut-pH, Abweichung der Ionenkonzentration, Dehydratation mit Abfall des zentralen Venendrucks, Hypalbuminaemie, Fehlwerten beim Blutbild, Haematokrit und Defizit in den Gerinnungsfaktoren hervor [1, 2, 5].

Die praeoperativen Risikofaktoren, am Beispiel von 186 neurochirurgischen Patienten über 70 Jahren gezeigt, betreffen mit 63% überwiegend das Cardiovasculäre System, wobei Herzinsuffizienz, Coronarsclerose und abgelaufener Herzinfarkt in 43% pathologischen EKG's seinen Ausdruck findet. Ein Drittel aller Kranken war mit Hypertonie und 10% einer allgemeinen Gefäßsclerose belastet (Abb. 4).

		n	%	
HERZ:	Herzinsuffizienz	40	22	
	Coronarsklerose	21	11	
	Herzinfarkt	10	5	
	pathol. EKG	77	43	63%
KREISLAUF:	Hypertonie	60	32	
	allg. Arteriosklerose	18	10	
	Hypotonie	2	1	
	sonst.	7	4	
ATMUNG:	Ateminsuffizienz	15	8	
	Emphysem	13	7	13%
	sonst.	4	2	
STOFFWECHSEL:	Diabetes mell.	43	23	
	Fettstoffwechselst.	8	4	31%
	Adipositas	7	4	
ORGANE:	Leber	6	3	
	Niere	6	3	
	Struma	6	3	15%
	Hypophys. Insuff.	3	2	
	sonst.	3	2	

Abb. 4. Praeoperative Risikofaktoren bei 186 Kranken > 70 Jahre der Neurochirurg. Klinik

Demgegenüber erscheint die Häufung von respiratorischen Störungen und Insuffizienz in dieser retrospektiven Studie mit 13% nur gering dokumentiert. Sicher sind hier nur manifeste Krankheitsbilder — über das allgemeine Altersemphysem hinausgehend — erfaßt worden. In vergleichbaren Statistiken anderer Studien wird diese Belastung im Durchschnitt viel höher, etwa mit 21—37%, angegeben [9, 10].

Es fanden sich Stoffwechselstörungen in 31%, fast ein Viertel aller Kranken waren Diabetiker, 15% der Patienten wiesen manifeste Organinsuffizienzen, gleich oft verteilt auf Leber, Niere und Schilddrüse, auf. Hieraus resultieren Gerinnungsstörungen und verzögerter

Medikament-Abbau bzw. Ausscheidung, renale Insuffizienz, bei altersgemäß allgemein schon 50%iger Reduktion der Nierenfunktionsgrößen, neben hypophysärer Insuffizienz.

Der Vorbereitung auf den Eingriff — soweit diese der Krankheitsverlauf zuläßt, und möglichst im eigenen Hause — kommt daher bei den geriatrischen neurochirurgischen Operationen große Bedeutung zu.

Zur anschaulichen Gegenüberstellung wurden nach dem postoperativen Verlauf zwei Gruppen unterschieden: In die Bewertungsgruppe „gut" wurden alle Patienten eingereiht, die in gutem Zustand nach Hause entlassen oder zur Nachbehandlung in ein auswärtiges Krankenhaus verlegt werden konnten. Die Gruppe „schlecht" dagegen umfaßte alle in der Klinik verstorbenen Patienten und diejenigen, die in einem gegenüber dem Aufnahmebefund verschlechterten Zustand zurückverlegt wurden. Der Problematik dieser vereinfachenden Einteilung, in die auch andere Faktoren (individuelle Nachsorgemöglichkeit, Bettenmangel, Kapazität der Intensivpflegestation u.a.) eingehen, sind sich die Autoren bewußt.

Am Beispiel von 75 Hirntumor-Patienten kann gezeigt werden (Abb. 5): Bei den „guten" Verläufen (46 Kranken) ist der Anteil der längeren Vorbereitungszeit über 5 Tage mit 61% zu 39% kürzerer Vorbereitungszeit fast umgekehrt, wie bei den „schlechten" Verläufen mit 34% längerer und 66% kürzerer Vorbereitungszeit. Dabei ist jedoch zu berücksichtigen, daß in die „schlechte" Verlaufsgruppe teilweise Schwerkranke miteingehen, bei denen eine Notfallindikation zur sofortigen Operation (z.B. bei zunehmender Bewußtseinsstörung) gegeben ist.

Von entscheidender Bedeutung für den Verlauf sind die ersten Tage auf der Intensivstation, da bei den heutigen Möglichkeiten der intraoperativen Überwachung und Therapie, künstlicher Beatmung, Ausgleich von Flüssigkeits- und Ionenbilanz, großer Blutverluste, Beeinflussung des intracraniellen Drucks und der renalen Ausscheidung auch Schwerstkranke über den Eingriff selbst fast immer hinwegzubringen sind und der Tod im Operationssaal heute zu den ausgesprochen „seltenen Ereignissen" gehört. Von unseren insgesamt 908 Patienten haben alle den diagnostischen oder operativen Eingriff selbst überlebt.

Der Einfluß der praeoperativen Risikofaktoren auf die Prognose läßt sich am besten bei elektiven Eingriffen erkennen (Abb. 6). Während sich in der Gruppe mit gutem Ergebnis der Risikofaktor 0 oder 1 bei zwei Drittel aller Patienten findet, ist bei der Gruppe mit schlechtem Ausgang mehr als die Hälfte der Kranken mit 2, 3 oder noch mehr Risiken belastet.

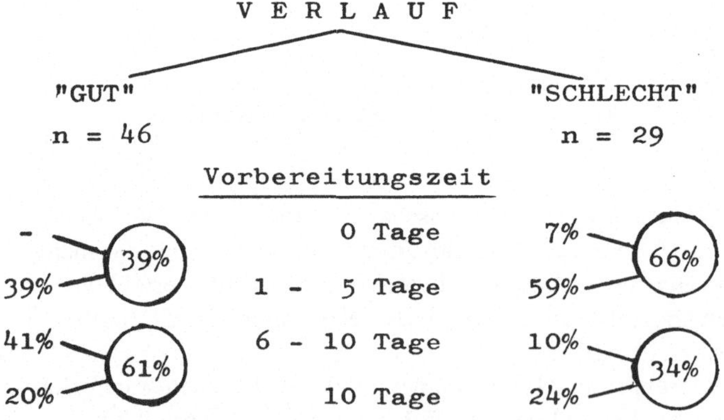

Abb. 5. Vorbereitungszeit bei Hirntumor-Patienten > 70 Jahre. n = 75

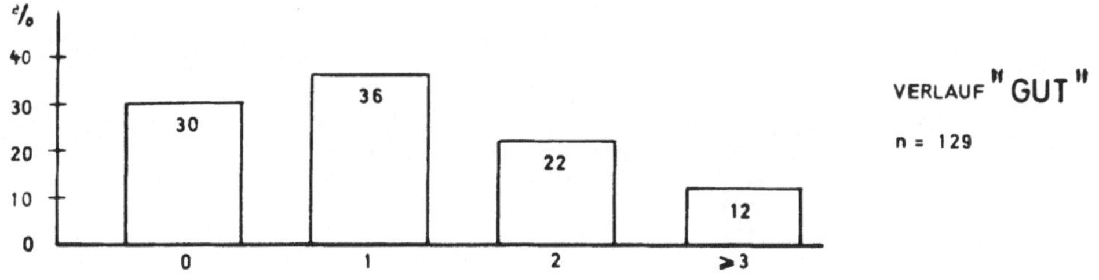

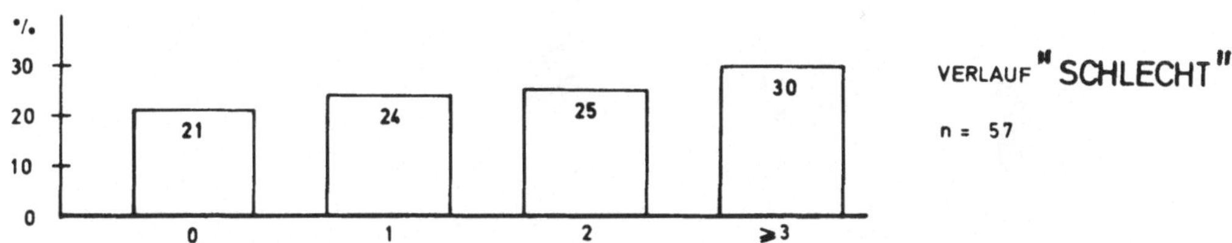

Abb. 6. Polymorbidität bei elektiven Eingriffen und ihre Zuordnung nach dem Verlauf. n = 186. Die Häufigkeit der Risikofaktoren (0 bis 3 und darüber – Abszisse) zeigt in der Gruppe „gute" Verläufe (oben) abnehmende, in der Gruppe „schlechte" Verläufe (unten) zunehmende Tendenz

In der Statistik läßt sich bei den günstigen Verläufen für die Häufigkeit und Kombination von Risikofaktoren (z.B. cardiale, respiratorische, Stoffwechsel- und Organstörung) eine deutlich abnehmende, bei den schlechten Verläufen dagegen eine ansteigende Tendenz feststellen. Als der für den postoperativen Verlauf auf der Intensivpflegestation der Neurochirurgie bei Eingriffen am Zentralnervensystem entscheidendste Faktor ist, im Gegensatz zu anderen operativen Fächern, die Bewußtseinsstörung anzusehen. Gerade beim alten Menschen, der bereits funktionell und organisch am Rande der Kompensationsmöglichkeit steht, führt eine Verschlechterung der Bewußtseinslage rasch zur Manifestation, vor allem pulmonaler Komplikationen. Die akute respiratorische Insuffizienz leitet dann den circulus vitiosus vegetativer und Organstörungen ein.

Bereits das Vorliegen einer praeoperativen Bewußtseinsstörung läßt nach unseren Erfahrungen beim alten Hirntumor-Kranken schon eine Beurteilung der Prognose zu (Abb. 7 links). Bei allen 46 Hirntumor-Patienten mit „gutem" Verlauf war keine Störung des Bewußtseins registriert, während sich unter den 29 „schlechten" Ausgängen mehr als ein Drittel bereits somnolenter oder bewußtloser Patienten befand. In dieser Gruppe stellte sich postoperativ noch in der Hälfte der Fälle eine weitere Verschlechterung der Bewußtseinslage ein. Facit: Keiner der bereits praeoperativ bewußtseinsgestörten Patienten mit Hirntumor über 70 Jahre konnte entlassen oder in gutem Zustand rückverlegt werden.

Im Gegensatz dazu beim chronisch subduralen Haematom (Abb. 7 Mitte): Das bessere Bewußtseinsniveau bestand bei den „guten" Verläufen; hier war mehr als die Hälfte der 23 Kranken wach. Durch den relativ kleinen Eingriff, meist nur eine Ableitung von einem kleinen Bohrloch aus, ließ sich unmittelbar postoperativ eine Verbesserung der Bewußtseinslage erreichen (38%). Unter den 10 „schlechten" Verläufen der hier vorwiegend somnolenten Patienten trat in 2 Fällen (10%) postoperativ eine weitere Verschlechterung ein.

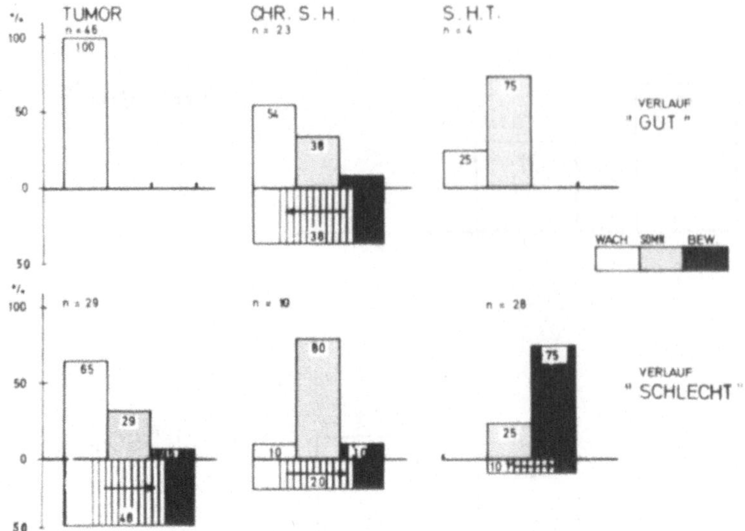

Abb. 7. Praeoperative Bewußtseinslage (obere Säulen: wach = weiß, somnolent = grau, bewußtlos = schwarz) und postoperative Änderung (unten mit Richtungspfeil) beim Hirntumor, chron. subduralem Haematom und Schädel-Hirntrauma. „Gute" Verläufe (1. Reihe), „schlechte" Verläufe (2. Reihe)

Beim Schädel-Hirn-Trauma (Abb. 7 rechts) dagegen standen nur 4 günstige Ergebnisse bei einem wachen und 3 somnolenten Kranken 28 „schlechten" Verläufen in dieser Altersgruppe gegenüber. Letztere waren zu 75% praeoperativ bereits tief bewußtlos, in 10% verschlechterte sich nach der Operation noch das Bewußtseinsniveau.

	HIRNTUMOR	lumb. BANDSCHEIBE
	n=75	n=44
	%	%
Cardiovasc. Stoerung	19	14
Respirat. Stoerung	27	14
Organ. Stoerung	19	11
Nachblutung	25	4
Sonstige	3	–

POSTOPERATIVE MANIFESTATION VON

PRAEOPERATIVEN RISIKOFAKTOREN

	HIRNTUMOR	lumb. Bandscheibe
	44 %	17 %

Abb. 8. Postoperative Komplikationen und Manifestation praeoperativer Risikofaktoren bei 119 Patienten > 70 Jahre. Gegenüberstellung Hirntumor und lumb. Bandscheibe

Das Bild der postoperativen Komplikationen ist nach der Art der neurochirurgischen Operation unterschiedlich. Der Vergleich zwischen extracraniellem und intracraniellem Eingriff ist an einer Gegenüberstellung von Patienten mit Hirntumor und lumbalem Bandscheibenvorfall zu erkennen (Abb. 8): Es zeigt sich, daß die hohe cardiovasculäre Vorbelastung (63%) in relativ geringerem Maße, und mehr beim zentralen Eingriff zum Ausdruck kommt, als die respiratorische. Letztere stellt vor allem beim Hirntumor im Zusammenhang mit der Bewußtseinsstörung beim zentralen Eingriff eine fast doppelt so hohe Komplikationsrate (27%) als nach Bandscheibenoperationen (14%) dar und erfordert stets eine Respirator-Therapie auf der Intensivstation. Daneben ist der hohe Prozentsatz von 25% erforderlichen Recraniotomien bemerkenswert, wobei sich die Tendenz zur Nachblutung aus dem Zusammentreffen von Gerinnungsstörungen, allgemeiner Gefäßsclerose, Hochdruck, möglicherweise auch Einfluß der Hirnatrophie erklären läßt. Daß dieser Komplikation für die postoperative

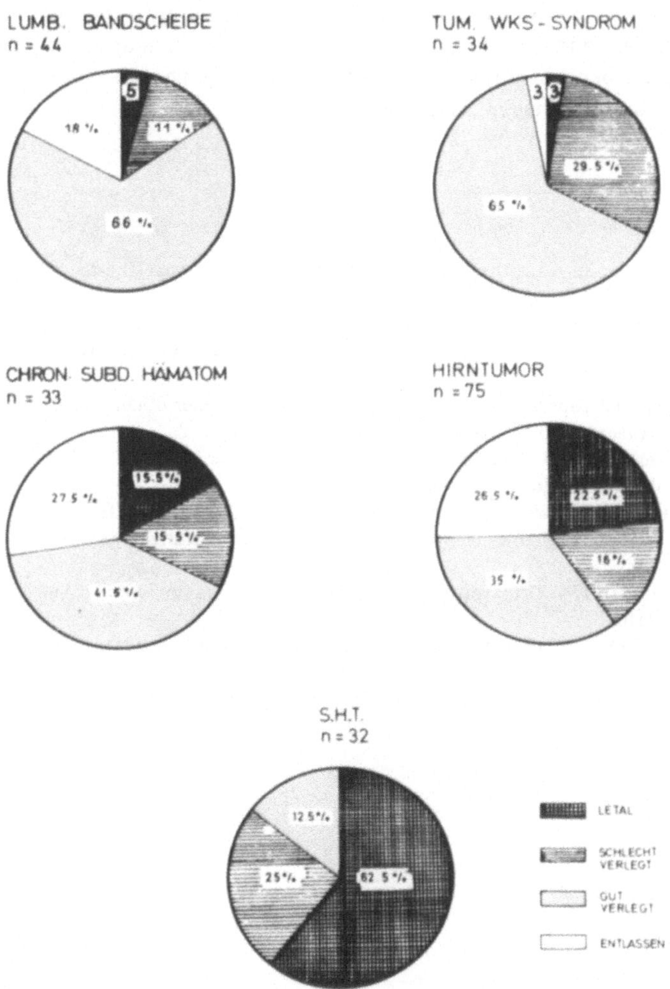

Abb. 9. Verläufe nach neurochirurgischen Eingriffen 1968–1978 bei 218 Patienten > 70 Jahre

Prognose eine wesentliche Bedeutung zukommt, geht aus der Tatsache hervor, daß in mehr als der Hälfte aller „schlechten" Verläufe eine Recraniotomie erforderlich war. Eine postoperative Manifestation der schon praeoperativ bekannten Risikofaktoren fand sich nach den Hirntumor-Eingriffen in 44%, nach der lumbalen Prolapsentfernung nur in 14%.

Einen Überblick über Verlauf und Ergebnisse nach verschiedenen neurochirurgischen Eingriffen bei 218 Patienten über 70 Jahre gibt Abb. 9. Nur insgesamt 16% „schlechte" Ergebnisse nach Bandscheibenoperation, 1 Kranker verstarb an Herzinfarkt bei schwerer Coronarstenose, eine Patientin an Uraemie im Gefolge allgemeiner Nephrosclerose. Ähnlich gute Ergebnisse, zumindest für die Kurzzeitprognose, wurden bei Rückenmarks- und Wurzelkompressionssyndromen durch Tumor, auch unter Einschluß der Wirbelmetastasen erzielt. Mehr als 2/3 günstige Verläufe ergaben sich noch beim chronisch subduralen Haematom, 3/5 auch bei Hirntumoren. Im Gegensatz dazu stehen die ausgesprochen schlechten Ergebnisse nach Schädel-Hirntraumen mit operativer Indikation beim alten Menschen, wobei in unserem Krankengut nur 12,5% aller Patienten eine gute Chance für das weitere Leben erreichten. Trotz aller operativen und therapeutischen Bemühungen auf der Intensivstation ist hier die Prognose meist schon bei der Aufnahme in die Klinik durch die Schwere des Traumas (meist Polytraumen), mangelnde Vorbereitungszeit durch sofort indizierte Operation und Umfang und Lokalisation der cerebralen Schäden festgelegt.

Literatur

1. Benke A (1970) Geriatrische Anaesthesie. Anaesthesie in extremen Altersklassen. Anaesthesie und Wiederbelebung 47:108
2. Bergmann H (1976) Die Auswahl der Anaesthesiemittel und -methoden bei kardiozirkulatorischen Risikofaktoren. Der Risikopatient in der Anaesthesie. Klinische Anaesthesiologie und Intensivtherapie 11:135
3. v. Bramann H, Herold G (1969) Die postoperative Früh- und Spätmortilität bei über 80jährigen (Auswertung von 910 Allgemein-Anaesthesien). Anaesthesist 18:321
4. Hamer Ph (1976) Das Alter als Narkoserisiko. Anaesthesiologische Informationen 17:334
5. Lawin P (1965) Alter Patient und Anaesthesie. Anaesthesist 14:103
6. Lorhan PH (1967) Anaesthesia Experiences with the Octagenarian. Curr Res Anesth 46:601
7. Lutz H, Klose R, Peter K (1976) Die Problematik der praeoperativen Risikoeinstufung. Anaesthesiologische Informationen 17:342
8. Mayrhofer O, Kreuzer M, Niessner G (1970) Grundprinzipien der Narkoseführung im Senium. Anaesthesie und Wiederbelebung 47:101
9. Munteanu S, Reinhardt T (1970) Erfahrungen bei der Anaesthesie alter Patienten in der Neurochirurgie. Anaesthesie und Wiederbelebung 14:131
10. Pulver KG, Otten M (1970) Die Allgemein-Narkose im Greisenalter. Anaesthesie und Wiederbelebung 14:114

Comparative Study of Long-acting Tranquilizers for Oral Administration as a Hypnotics on the Day Before Operation

S. Ishii, M. Shibata, K. Nishikawa, M. Doi, K. Terauchi and Y. Kubo

Derivatives of benzodiazepine have been introduced in the clinical field as an agent of tranquilizers and hypnotics in recent years, because the relative cardiovascular and pulmonary safety of these derivatives as compared to other types of sedatives and hypnotics is well documented.

Alprazolam, a new derivative of benzodiazepine, has been recently synthesized and developed as a hypnotic.

This present study was undertaken using a single blind study in order to appraise the efficacy of this drug as an agent of hypnotics and of minor tranquilizers for pre-operative medication, as compared to the other derivatives of benzodiazepine such as lorazepam and bromazepam.

The chemical structures of these three drugs are shown in Fig. 1. In this study, 0.4 mg and 0.8 mg of alprazolam, 0.5 mg of lorazepam and 4 mg of bromazepam were administered orally in adult patients on the pre-operative night.

The investigation was carried out by a subjective assessment of an anaesthetist and the results were analyzed by the anaesthetist-in-chief to compare the results of the assessments between each drug. The details of the number of subjects in each drug group are shown in Fig. 2. The total number of subjects was 103 cases and an even distribution of background factors such as age, sex, body weight, anaesthetic technique and risk was observed.

In order to perform this clinical experiment a questionaire was handed to each patient. The important items from these questionnaires are shown in Fig. 3. All subjects were questioned on their previous history, such as their experiences of operations and hypnotics, their sleeping condition on the previous night and any pre-operative anxiety noted by the anaesthetist at the pre-anaesthetic visit. On the day of the operation patients were questioned again about the administration of the drugs, sleeping condition, pre-operative anxiety and some other items.

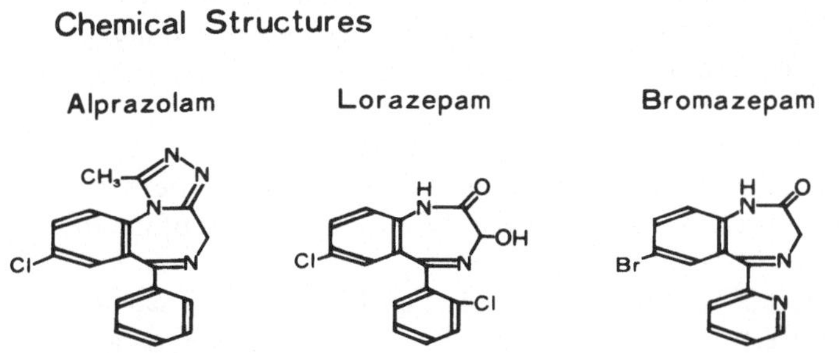

Chemical Structures

Alprazolam   Lorazepam   Bromazepam

Fig. 1

Backgrounds of Patients

Drugs		Alprazolam		Lorazepam	Bromazepam
Doses (mg)		0.4	0.8	0.5	4.0
No. of Patients		28	24	19	32
Sex	Male	13(46.4%)	9 (37.5%)	7 (36.8%)	16(50.0%)
	Female	15(53.6%)	15(62.5%)	12(63.2%)	16(50.5%)
Age ± S.D. (years)		46.0±12.5	45.1±10.5	46.5±14.8	43.2±11.1
Range		(17~66)	(23~65)	(13~65)	(24~67)
Body Weight ± S.D. (kg)		54.2± 8.2	50.5± 6.8	55.0+ 9.2	54.1± 9.8
Range		(30~68)	(35~66)	(40~74)	(39~74)
RISK	Good	17(60.7%)	9 (37.5%)	7 (36.8%)	15(46.9%)
	Fair	11(39.3%)	13(54.2%)	11(57.9%)	17(53.1%)
	Poor		2 (8.3%)	1 (5.3%)	
Method of Anesthesia	General Anesthesia	17(60.7%)	19(79.2%)	10(52.6%)	26(81.3%)
	Others	11(39.3%)	5 (20.8%)	9 (47.4%)	6 (18.7%)
Operations	Gyne.	10(35.7%)	8 (33.3%)	8 (42.1%)	11(34.4%)
	Surgery	12(25.0%)	12(50.0%)	9 (47.4%)	12(37.5%)
	Others	11(39.3%)	4 (16.7%)	2 (10.5%)	9 (28.1%)

Fig. 2

A general assessments was produced in five grades: excellent, good, fair, poor and very poor, according to the results of the questionnaires on the operation morning. The assessment of sleep and of interruption of sleep were assessed in four grade according to the duration of sleep.

Results

Fig. 4. This shows the results of global assessments of alprazolam, lorazepam and bromazepam as oral premedication. As shown in this figure, effectiveness of each drug on mental state on operation morning is as follows: 0.8 mg of alprazolam was the most effective, followed by 0.4 mg of alprazolam, 4 mg bromazepam and 0.5 mg of lorazepam. There were no poor or very poor grades with 0.8 mg of alprazolam.

Fig. 5. This shows global assessment of state of sleep on preoperative night. As shown in this figure, 0.8 mg of alprazolam was the most effective, followed by 4 mg of bromazepam, 0.4 mg of alprazolam and 0.5 mg of lorazepam. There were also no poor or very poor grades with 0.8 mg of alprazolam.

Fig. 6. Fig. a of this figure shows onset of sleep. As shown in this Fig., 0.8 mg of alprazolam was clearly superior to the other drugs in producing sleep. Fig. b shows interruption of sleep. As in Fig. a, 0.8 mg of alprazolam was seen to be the most efficacious of the four drugs in producing stable sleep.

Fig. 6 c and d. This shows sleeping patterns. Fig. c shows quality of sleep. There was little difference to be found in the efficacy of each of the drugs, each performing satisfac-

Questionaire for State of Sleep
and Preoperative Conditions

1) Did you fall asleep immediately last night ?
   1 : immediately
   2 : after a while
   3 : after a long time
2) Did you awake last night?
   How did you get back to sleep after you awoke?
   1 : did not awake
   2 : immediately
   3 : after a long time
   4 : impossible
3) Did you sleep well last night?
   1 : very well
   2 : well
   3 : a little
   4 : not at all
4) What time did you awake this morning?
5) How did you feel when you awoke?
   1 : better than usual
   2 : as usual
   3 : a little worse
   4 : much worse
6) Did you find anything unusual?
   1 : no
   2 : yes (drowsy. unsteady. dull. heavyheaded etc.)
7) How do you feel about the operation?
   1 : not anxious
   2 : somewhat anxious
   3 : very anxious
8) How many hours did you sleep last night?
   approximately________________hours.

Fig. 3

torily. Fig. d shows condition on awaking. The percentage of patients answering condition as usual was highest with 0.8 mg of alprazolam, followed by 0.5 mg of lorazepam, 0.4 mg of alprazolam and 4 mg of bromazepam. However, the percentage of patients answering better than usual was most with 4 mg of bromazepam, followed by 0.5 mg of lorazepam, 0.8 mg of alprazolam and 0.4 mg of alprazolam.

Fig. 7. This shows side effects. Fig. a shows incidence of side effects, 0.4 mg of alprazolam produced least side effect, followed by 0.5 mg of lorazepam, 4 mg of bromazepam and 0.8 mg of alprazolam. Fig. b shows the symptoms of side effect. Drowsiness was the most frequently observed symptom followed by unsteadiness, thickheadedness, enervation and heavyheadedness.

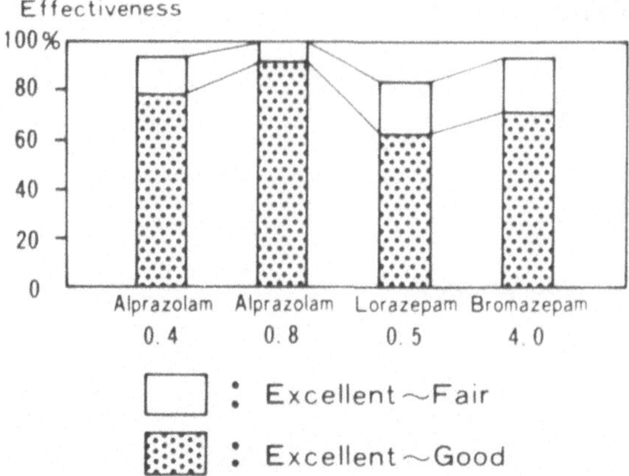

Fig. 4. Global Assessments of Alprazolam, Lorazepam and Bromazepam as Oral Premedication. Mental State on operating morning

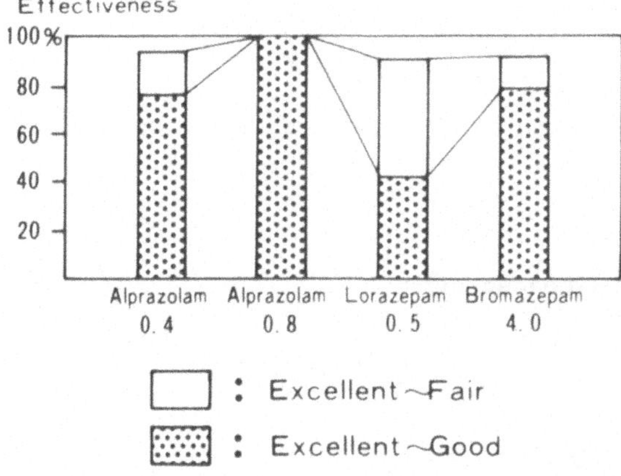

Fig. 5. Global Assessments of Alprazolam, Lorazepam and Bromazepam as Oral Premedication. State of sleep on preoperative night

Conclusion

1. It was proved that alprazolam was effective in global assessments of the state of sleep on the preoperative night and the mental state on the operating morning and that there was an apparent correlation in efficacy between 0.4 mg and 0.8 mg in single dosages.
2. Adverse effects of low-dose alprazolam were observed much less and appear to be nearly halve of those of the high-dose. Drowsiness was the most frequently observed adverse reaction followed by unsteadiness.
3. In efficacy, alprazolam at a single dose of 0.4 mg was superior to lorazepam at a single dose of 0.5 mg and almost equal to bromazepam at a single dose of 4.0 mg.
4. In safety, 0.4 mg alprazolam was found to have relatively lower incidence of adverse effects than lorazepam and bromazepam at the above-mentioned dosages.

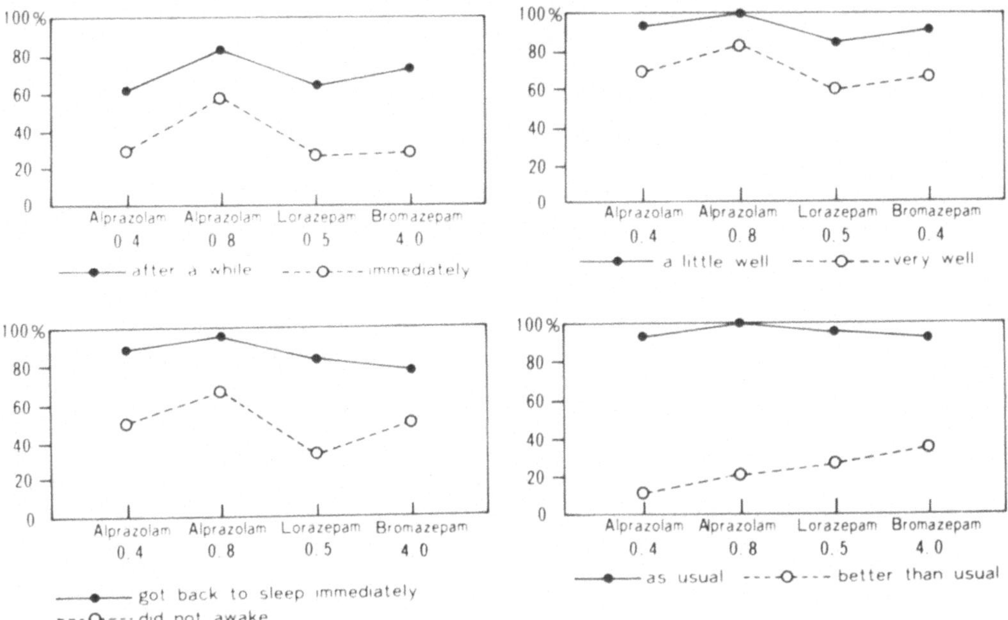

Fig. 6a–d. a Onset of sleep. b Interruption of sleep. c Quality of sleep. d Condition on awaking

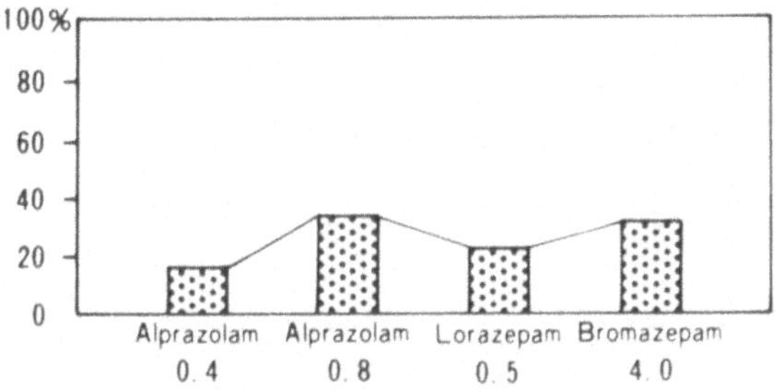

Drugs	Alprazolam		Lorazepam	Bromazepam
Doses (mg)	0.4	0.8	0.5	4.0
Drowsiness	3	6	1	4
Unsteadiness		3	1	3
Thickheadedness			1	3
Enervation			1	2
Heavyheadedness			1	1
Incidence (%)	3 / 19 (15.8)	8 / 24 (33.3)	4 / 18 (22.2)	10 / 32 (31.3)

Fig. 7a, b. Side Effects. a Incidence of side effects. b Symptome of side effects

Freie Themen
Allgemeinanaesthesie (Teil 1)

Vorsitz: K.-H. Weis und A. Benke

Ist eine Allgemeinanaesthesie bei Schrittmacherimplantation gerechtfertigt?

St. Necek, B. Szalay, B. Blauhut und H. Bergmann

Das anaesthesiologische Vorgehen bei Herzschrittmacherimplantationen ist 16 Jahre nach den ersten klinischen Erfahrungen noch immer nicht einheitlich [2, 5]. Anfangs wurden fast alle bekannten Anaesthetika dazu verwendet (Finck et al. [4], Howat [6]), derzeit befürworten einige die Regionalanaesthesie, andere die NLA. Warum wir der letzteren Gruppe angehören, wird an Hand unserer 10jährigen klinischen Erfahrung im folgenden gezeigt.

Krankengut

In den Jahren 1969 bis 1978 wurden an unserem Krankenhaus insgesamt 503 Schrittmachereingriffe durchgeführt, deren Art — in Neuimplantation und Revisionen unterteilt — in Tabelle 1 dargestellt ist.

Eine *Altersübersicht* zeigt Tabelle 2; 53% aller Patienten waren über 70 Jahre alt.

Unsere *Indikations*gruppen für eine Neuimplantation sind in Tabelle 3 angegeben. Naturgemäß steht dabei der totale AV-Block mit 64,3% zahlenmäßig an der Spitze. Aus der hohen Altersbelastung heraus sind zahlreiche Schrittmacherpatienten auch durch eine hohe Frequenz von Begleitkrankheiten besonders gefährdet. In Tabelle 4 sind diese zusätzlichen Risikofaktoren, die zum Teil auch additiv zu werten sind, zusammengestellt, wobei 57% manifeste Linksinsuffizienzen und 50% koronare Herzkrankheiten besonders auffallen.

Tabelle 1. Art der Schrittmachereingriffe

Neuimplantationen			258 (51,3%)
Revisionen			245 (48,7%)
Generatorwechsel		144	
Ermüdung	138		
Perforationsgefahr	6		
Sondenwechsel		52	
Dislokation	38		
Kabelbruch	12		
Hautperforation	2		
Generator/Sondenwechsel		31	
(Verlagerung)			
Epikardiale Elektroden		18	
	Summe	503	

Tabelle 2. Altersverteilung der Patienten

(277 Männer/54%; 233 Frauen/46%)	n	%
21–30 a	4	0,80
31–40 a	7	1,39
41–50 a	17	3,38
51–60 a	38	7,55
61–70 a	170	33,80
71–80 a	212	42,15
81–90 a	55	10,93
	503	100,00

Tabelle 3. Indikationen zur Neuimplantation (n = 258)

	n	%
Totaler AV-Block	166	64,34
Absolute Bradyarrhythmie	57	22,09
Sick Sinus Syndrom	17	6,59
Intermittierender AV-Block	10	3,88
Brady-Tachyarrhythmie	8	3,10
	258	100,00

Tabelle 4. Begleitkrankheiten bei 503 Schrittmacherpatienten

	n	%
Herzinsuffizienz	285	56,7
Koronare Herzkrankheit	250	49,7
Hypertonie		
(> 170 mmHg syst.)	193	38,4
Diabetes mellitus	82	16,3
Nierenfunktion ↓		
(Kreatinin ↑, BUN ↑)	65	12,9
Vitien	13	2,6

Anaesthesieverfahren

Und nun zum Anaesthesieverfahren (Tabelle 5): Die *Prämedikation* bestand aus Pethidin-Atropin, bei 479 Fällen (d.s. 95,3%) wurde eine Valium-NLA mit Intubation und Beatmung bei N_2O/O_2 angewandt, bei nur 24 Patienten (4,7%) vorwiegend Batteriewechsel, wurde in Lokalanästhesie operiert. Der Chirurg infiltrierte dazu bis zu 30 ml 1 bis 2 % Xylocain, insgesamt also bis zu 500 mg.

Tabelle 5. Anaesthesieverfahren

(503 Schrittmachereingriffe)

1. **Praemedikation**   Pethidin 100 mg > 60 a   50 mg > 60 a
   (i.m.)   Atropin   0,5 mg   0,25 mg

2. **Allgemeinanaesthesie**   479 (= 95,3%)

   Einleitung: 2,5–10 mg Diazepam, 0,1–0,3 mg Fentanyl
                       (2,5 mg DHB)
                       40 mg Succinylcholin   orotracheale
                             oder   Intubation
                       10–15 mg Alloferin   (nach LA 1% Novesin)

   Aufrechterhaltung: N_2O/O_2 4:2, Alloferin,
                       manuelle Beatmung

3. **Regionalanaesthesie**   24 (= 4,7%)
   (durch Chirurgen)

                       Xylocain ~30 ml (2/3 2%, 1/3 1%)
                                  500 mg
                       O_2 Insufflation (Brille)

4. **Überwachung**
   RR (unblutig), EKG (f-periphere Pulswelle)
   Bereitgestellt: Xylocain, Alupent, Atropin, Defibrillator
   98% aller Patienten kommen mit temporärem Schrittmacher zur Operation !!!

Alle Patienten wurden mittels EKG und unblutiger Druckmessung *überwacht*, Xylocain, Alupent, Atropin und ein Defibrillator sind bereitgestellt. 98% der Fälle kamen bereits mit einem vom Internisten gelegten temporären Schrittmacher zur Operation.

Komplikationen (Tabelle 6)

Wert und Berechtigung eines gewählten Verfahrens zur operativen Schmerzausschaltung werden nun nicht zuletzt von der Komplikationsrate bestimmt.

Bei unseren in Valium-NLA narkotisierten Patienten kam es zweimal bei liegendem temporären Schrittmacher zu einer Asystolie von etwa 30 Sekunden; 63 Patienten, also 12,5%, zeigten einen systolischen Druckabfall um mehr als 25% des Ausgangswertes, der mit Plasma-

Tabelle 6. Intraoperative Komplikationen (n = 503)

	Allgemeinanaesthesie	Regionalanaesthesie
Asystolie (~30 sec.)	2	1
RR ↓ (> 25% des Ausg. Wertes) (Plasmaersatzmittel)	63 (12,5%)	(?)
Ventrikuläre Extrasystolie	2	–
Letalität erste 24 Stunden	0	0

ersatzmitteln gut zu korrigieren war. Vorübergehende ventrikuläre Extrasystolen waren bei zwei Patienten zu beobachten. In *Regionalanaesthesie* kam es ebenso durch Dislokation der temporären Schrittmacherelektrode einmal zu einer Asystolie. Drei Patienten waren intraoperativ unruhig und klagten über Schmerzen.

Kein Patient kam während der ersten 24 postoperativen Stunden ad exitum. Am zweiten postoperativen Tag verstarb ein in Allgemeinanaesthesie operierter Patient an einer schon präoperativ bestandenen schweren Herzinsuffizienz.

Diskussion und Schlußfolgerung

Diskutieren wir nun unsere Ergebnisse, so ist zunächst darauf hinzuweisen, daß sich unsere niedrige Komplikationsrate vor allem durch den großzügigen Einsatz des temporären Schrittmachers erklären läßt. Das Anaesthesierisiko wird damit wesentlich verringert, die ASA-Gruppe 4 des kompletten AV-Blockes wird zu einer Gruppe 2 oder 3.

Drei Probleme sind es nun, die bei Anaesthesien zur Schrittmacherimplantation anfallen:
1. Die Vermeidung jeder zusätzlichen Störung von Reizbildung und -leitung durch die Anaesthesie, wenn ein AV-Block mit Kammerautomatie und ohne temporären Schrittmacher vorliegt.
2. Eine unzureichende Anpassung des HZV bei anaesthesiebedingter Änderung des peripheren Widerstandes und
3. ein technisch bedingter intraoperativer Ausfall eines schon liegenden temporären Schrittmachers.

Ad 1. Die Vermeidung zusätzlicher Reizbildungs- und Leitungsstörungen bestimmt nun die Wahl der Anaesthesietechnik. Die bei der NLA verwendeten Substanzen sind dabei am ehesten inert und werden auch von Befürwortern der Regionalanaesthesie als einzige Anaesthetika bei Schrittmacheroperationen akzeptiert. Halothan und Thiopental verlängern hingegen die Refraktionsperiode der AV-Überleitung, erhöhen die ventrikuläre diastolische Reizschwelle [7, 8, 9] und sind daher zu vermeiden.

Aber auch der Regionalanaesthesie werden spezifische Effekte nachgesagt: 400–500 mg Xylocain s.c. führen zu einem Blutspiegel von 2 μg/ml, 2–5 μg/ml Xylocain verlängern aber bereits die effektive Refraktionsperiode. EKG-Effekte und toxische hämodynamische Folgen sind allerdings erst bei über 5 μg/ml zu sehen [3], was bei unkontrollierter Infiltration auch nicht mit Sicherheit ausgeschlossen werden kann.

Atropin zur Prämedikation von 0,5 mg einschließlich Oberflächenanaesthesie des Larynx schützen vor Arrhythmien bei der Einleitung.

Ad 2. Die nächste potentielle Anaesthesiekomplikation bei Patienten mit temporärem Schrittmacher und konstanter Herzfrequenz kann daraus resultieren, daß eine plötzliche anaesthesiebedingte Erweiterung des peripheren Strombettes nicht rasch genug durch eine Erhöhung des HZV kompensiert werden kann. 12,5% unserer in Allgemeinanaesthesie betreuten Schrittmacherimplantationen hatten denn auch bei der Einleitung Druckabfälle um mehr als 25% des Ausgangswertes. Volumenersatzmittel und protrahierte Induktion genügen zur Kompensation. Im Gegensatz zu Hollinger und Richter [5], die von 9% tiefen Druckabfällen nach hochdosierter Prämedikation berichten, halten wir eine Vasokonstriktorengabe jedoch für nicht erforderlich.

Ad 3. Eine technisch bedingte intraoperative Asystolie bei liegendem temporären Schrittmacher ist schließlich, wie in unseren drei Fällen, durch eine Dislokation der Elektrode, aber auch bei unkontrolliertem Gebrauch des Kauters ([1], Simon) möglich. Unsere Fälle waren mit Thoraxkompressionen und Relokation der Elektrode ohne Schwierigkeit zu beherrschen. Die Wiederherstellung der Herzaktion unter Regionalanaesthesie hat allerdings am nicht bewußtlosen Patienten stattgefunden. Ein Kauter wird intraoperativ bei uns nicht verwendet. Wir sind also *zusammenfassend* der Meinung, daß auf Grund unserer klinischen Erfahrungen und der dabei beobachteten Zahl und Art von Komplikationen die Durchführung von Allgemeinanaesthesien zur Schrittmacherimplantation nicht nur gerechtfertigt ist, sondern auch befürwortet werden kann, wenn grundsätzlich temporäre Schrittmacher vor der Operation gelegt werden. Begründen läßt sich dieser Standpunkt 1. damit, daß bei entsprechender Auswahl des Anaesthesieverfahrens praktisch keine negativen Auswirkungen auf Reizbildung und -leitung zustande kommen und hämodynamisch nachteilige Veränderungen während der Induktion durch sorgfältige Überwachung der Patienten und Verlängerung der Einleitungsphase abgeschwächt sowie ohne Schwierigkeiten volumsmäßig kompensiert werden können, und 2. sich die negativen psychischen Auswirkungen einer Operation in Regionalanaesthesie gerade bei der in Frage stehenden Patientengruppe besonders nachteilig bemerkbar machen können, was durch eine Narkose zu vermeiden ist. Sedierungsmaßnahmen allein, insbesondere bei höherer Dosierung, sehen wir eher als problematisch an. Die Allgemeinanaesthesie schaltet schließlich nicht zuletzt auch ein teilweises Miterleben etwaiger Reanimierungsmaßnahmen aus.

Literatur

1. Ackermann R, Frohmüller H (1976) Transurethrale Resektion bei Herzschrittmacherpatienten. Urologe A 15:185–187
2. Blaum U, Schmidt H, Pflüger H (1977) Anästhesie bei Herzschrittmacherimplantation. Fortschr Med 95:1219
3. Covino BC, Vasallo HG (1976) Local Anesthetics, Mechanism of Action and Clinical Use. Grune-Stratton, New York San Francisco London
4. Finck AJ, Frank HA, Zoll PM (1969) Anesthesia in Relation to Permanently Implanted Cardiac Pacemakers. Anesth Analg 48:1043
5. Hollinger I, Richter JA (1978) Anästhesie bei der Schrittmacherimplantation. Herz 3:166–171
6. Howat DDC (1963) Anesthesia for the Insertion of Indwelling Artificial Pacemakers. Lancet I:855
7. Laver MB, Turndorf H (1963) Atrial Activity and Systemic Blood Pressure during Anesthesia in Man. Circulation 28:63
8. Pratila MG, Pratila V (1976) Sick-Sinus Syndrome Manifested during Anesthesia. Anesthesiology 44:5
9. Smith NT, Smith P (1972) Circulatory Effects of Modern Inhalation Anesthetic Agents. In: Chenoweth MB (ed) Modern Inhalation Anesthetics. Springer

Althesin-Effekt auf dem Ketamin-induzierten erhöhten Liquordruck

P. Vadon und F. Eckhart

1. Untersuchungen physiologischer Veränderungen am Gesunden durch Pharmaka, die bei Routineanaesthesien verwendet werden, sollen ihre Anwendbarkeit zur Narkoseeinleitung und zur Narkoseaufrechterhaltung auch bei bestimmten Erkrankungen ermöglichen. Die durch die Prüfung der Wirkung eines Anaesthesiemittels auf den CSFP gewonnenen Aussagen haben für Patienten mit erhöhtem intracraniellem Druck besondere Bedeutung. Eine Steigerung des Hirndruckes während der Operation kann zu Mangeldurchblutung, Hypoxie und Oedem des Hirngewebes führen. Dies gilt vor allem für die große Zahl von Patienten, deren Hirndurchblutung auch ohne primäre intracranielle Raumforderung gefährdet ist. Alphaxalon + Alphadolon-Azetat ist nach Ketamine, Flunitrazepam, Methohexital-Natrium und Etomidate das letzte in der Serie der i.v. Anaesthetik, das in einem standardisiertem Untersuchungsverfahren in seiner Wirkung auf den Hirndruck untersucht wurde. Unsere Untersuchungen betreffen die für die Hirnblutung bestimmenden Größen: mittlerer arterieller Blutdruck (MAP), Liquordruck (CSFP), Pulsfrequenz (BMP) und Kohlendioxydpartialdruck im kapillären Blut (pCO_2).

Bei unseren Untersuchungen der Wirkung von Anaesthesiemitteln auf den CSFP haben wir Ketamine zur Erzeugung reproduzierbarer CSFP-Steigerungen verabreicht. Der beim liegenden Patienten im Lumbalbereich gemessene CSFP zeigt bei freier Liquorpassage Veränderungen des intracraniellen Druckes direkt proportional an. — Die Hauptursache für die Wirkung von Anaesthesiemitteln auf den intracraniellen Druck ist die Veränderung des intracraniellen Blutvolumens. Die Anaesthesiemittel beeinflussen das intracranielle Blutvolumen durch ihre allgemeine Herz-Kreislaufwirkung und durch Änderung des Hirngefäßwiderstandes. Der Hirngefäßwiderstand, also der Durchmesser der Hirngefäße, kann durch direkte Wirkung auf die Hirngefäße oder durch Einfluß auf den Stoffwechsel des Gehirnes ebenfalls verändert werden. Eine Stoffwechseländerung ist die Folge einer geänderten cerebralen Funktion und als Summe des Stoffwechsels von aktivierenden und hemmenden neuronalen Formationen aufzufassen. Die Durchblutung des Gehirnes paßt sich dem der Stoffwechselaktivität der Ganglienzellen entsprechenden Sauerstoffbedarf an. Eine Stoffwechselsteigerung oder eine Verminderung des Sauerstoffangebotes z.B. durch Blutdruckabfäll, Erythrocytenverlust oder Ventilationsstörung bewirkt eine Zunahme der Hirndurchblutung durch Gefäßerweiterung. Eine Stoffwechselsenkung oder eine Erhöhung des Sauerstoffangebotes führen zur Abnahme der Hirndurchblutung.

2. Anaesthesiemittel, die das intracranielle Blutvolumen vergrößern, wie z.B. Ketamine und solche, die zusätzlich den Blutdruck durch Gefäßerweiterung und durch Verminderung der Herzleistung senken, wie die volatilen halogenierten Kohlenwasserstoffe, sollten bei Verdacht auf erhöhten intracraniellen Druck nicht verwendet werden. Es liegt nahe, bei Anaesthesien und bei der Intensivbehandlung von Patienten mit gefährdeter Hirndurchblutung nur solche

Mittel zu verwenden, die insgesamt den Stoffwechsel des Gehirnes senken. Die Ergebnisse von eigenen Untersuchungen verschiedener Narkosemittel haben gezeigt, daß neben der erwünschten Wirkung der Senkung des intracraniellen Druckes die Beeinflussung der Herz-Kreislauffunktion ebenso wichtig ist. Der CCP, die entscheidende Größe der Hirndurchblutung im Ganzen, ergibt sich aus der Differenz: MAP minus intracranieller Druck (ICP). Die Hirndurchblutung bei hohem ICP kann trotz vermindertem Sauerstoffbedarf nicht ausreichen, wenn bei cardial vorgeschädigten Patienten der Mitteldruck stärker gesenkt wird als der ICP. In dieser Situation sind Narkosemittel zu empfehlen, die die Herz-Kreislauffunktion wenig beeinflussen und den intracraniellen Druck senken. Diese Anforderungen erfüllen am besten die zur Neuroleptanalgesie verwendeten Mittel.

3. a) Aus insgesamt 18 Patienten mit normalem Liquordruck im Alter von 31–76 Jahren, die zur Operation eines Diskusprolapses im Lumbalbereich vorgesehen waren, wurden 3 Gruppen zu je 6 Patienten gebildet. Es wurden nur Patienten, bei denen keine Herz-Kreislauf- oder Lungenerkrankung feststellbar war, ausgewählt. Alle Patienten erhielten 30 Minuten vor Untersuchungsbeginn als Praemedikation 0,1 mg Atropin je 10 kg KG i.m.

Gruppe I: Bei diesen 6 Patienten im Alter von 40–60 Jahren (im Mittel 49,5) sollte die Wirkung von Alphaxalon + Alphadolon-Azetat auf den Liquordruck geprüft werden.

Gruppe II: Bei diesen 6 Patienten im Alter von 31–50 Jahren (im Mittel 41,5) sollte die Wirkung von Alphaxalon + Alphadolon-Azetat auf den ketaminbedingt erhöhten Liquordruck geprüft werden. Alphaxalon + Alphadolon-Azetat wurde zum Zeitpunkt des höchsten Liquoranstieges nach Ketamin injiziert.

3. b) Gruppe III: Bei diesen 6 Patienten im Alter von 40–67 Jahren (im Mittel 49,5) sollte geprüft werden, ob eine vorherige Alphaxalon + Alphadolon-Azetat-Gabe die ketaminbedingte Liquordrucksteigerung abschwächen kann und ob eine allenfalls resultierende Liquordrucksteigerung durch nochmalige Gabe von Alphaxalon + Alphadolon-Azetat vermindert werden kann. Ketamin wurde 2 Minuten nach der 1. Alphadolon-Azetat-Gabe verabreicht. Die 2. Alphaxalon + Alphadolon-Azetat-Gabe erfolgte wieder zum Zeitpunkt des höchsten Liquordruckanstieges nach Ketamine. Die i.v. Dosierung betrug bei Alphaxalon + Alphadolon-Azetat immer 0,05 ml/kg und bei Ketamin immer 2 mg/kg KG.

Untersuchungsablauf

3. c) Der Liquordruck wurde nach Lumbalpunktion über ein Druckaufnehmersystem kontinuierlich aufgezeichnet. Die Lumbalpunktion erfolgte in Seitenlage in der Etage über dem Diskusprolaps. Zur Vermeidung eines Liquorverlustes war die Spinalnadel bei der Punktion des Subarachnoidalraumes mit dem gefüllten Druckaufnehmersystem verbunden. Atem- und hustensynchrone Liquorschwankungen ergaben den Nachweis der freien Liquorpassage. Die Herzaktion und die Pulsfrequenz wurden mit Hilfe eines EKG-Sichtgerätes kontinuierlich überwacht. Die unblutige Messung des systolischen und des diasystolischen Blutdruckes erfolgte vor Untersuchungsbeginn und weiter in Minutenabständen. Die Blutgase der spontan atmenden Patienten wurden vor Untersuchungsbeginn und zu den Zeitpunkten der größten Liquorveränderungen aus kapillär abgenommenem Blut bestimmt. Die Errechnung der Differenz aus mittlerem arteriellen Blutdruck und Liquordruck ergab den Hirnperfusionsdruck (CPP).

4. a) Abb. 1 zeigt uns den typischen Ablauf des Liquormomentandruckes in der Gruppe I, bei der mit nur Althesin untersuchten Gruppe.

Abb. 2 faßt die Ergebnisse dieser, nur allein mit Althesin behandelten Gruppe zusammen. Auffallend ist die Eintönigkeit des Kurvenablaufes. Außer der Zunahme der Pulsfrequenz im Mittel mit 11 Schlägen führte die Alfathesingabe zu keiner nennenswerten Änderung.

Abb. 3 ist der Druckablauf bei einem Patienten der Gruppe II. Bei diesen Patienten haben wir Althesin erst auf dem Höhepunkt des mit Ketamingabe ausgelösten Liquordruckanstieges verabreicht. Die Mittelwertkurven zeigen einen signifikanten Anstieg des Liquordruckkes um 16,5 mmHg, des mittleren arteriellen Druckes um 18 mmHg, des Hirnperfusionsdruckkes um 1,5 mmHg gegenüber den Ausgangswerten. Alfathesin senkte die Werte nach durchschnittlich 2 Minuten ausgeprägt, ausgenommen Pulsfrequenz, welche um 27 pro Minute gleich hoch blieb.

Abb. 5 repräsentiert die Druckverhältnisse typischerweise bei der Gruppe III. Hier haben wir Ketamin nach vorheriger Gabe von Alfathesin gespritzt, um zu sehen, ob der Ketamin induzierte Druckanstieg zustande kommen kann. Ja, so war es, wie es zu sehen ist, zeitlich verzögert. Eine wiederholte Alfathesingabe vermochte allerdings auch diesen Anstieg des Liquordruckes zu blockieren, gleich wie in der Gruppe 2.

Abb. 6 zeigt uns die errechneten Werte. Bemerkenswert ist, daß der Ketamineffekt erst später zur Geltung kam, sowie die ebenso prompte Normalisierung der Lage nach der zweiten Althesingabe, wie bei der Gruppe II. Es bestand außerdem eine etwas deutlichere Steigerung des pCO_2 im Schnitt von 5 mmHg, als bei den vorhergehenden Gruppen.

4. b) Alphaxalon + Alphadolon-Azetat, ein Steroidnarkotikum mit kurzer Wirkungsdauer, bewirkt einen ausgeprägten Abfall des CSFP, dem wahrscheinlich eine Zunahme des cerebralen Gefäßwiderstandes bei Senkung des Hirnstoffwechsels zugrunde liegt. Die CSFP-Senkung erfolgt auch bei geringgradigem Anstieg des pCO_2-Wertes, der die Weite der Hirngefäße ebenfalls beeinflußt und die Hirndurchblutung dem Gasaustausch anpaßt. Der CSFP-Abfall kann einen Abfall des arteriellen MAP in der gleichen Größenordnung kompensieren und so den CPP konstant halten. Eine ausreichende Sauerstoffversorgung der Ganglienzellen wird sicher auch bei geringem Abfall des Hirnperfusionsdruckes garantiert, da die vasokonstriktorisch bedingte Abnahme des cerebralen Blutflusses eine Anpassung an den verminderten Sauerstoffbedarf des Gehirns darstellt. Alphaxalon + Alphadolon-Azetat ist in seiner Wirkung ähnlich den Barbituraten und es ist wie diese zur Verwendung bei Patienten mit gefährdeter Hirndurchblutung mit oder ohne gesteigerten intracraniellen Druck geeignet.

Rohypnol/Ketanest Kombinationsanaesthesie bei kleinen und mittleren gynäkologischen Eingriffen

K.F. Rothe und R. Schorer

Der in den letzten Jahren zu beobachtende Trend, die Anwendung von Narkosegasen einzuschränken um Gesundheitsschäden von Patienten, Anaesthesie- und OP-Personal zu verhindern, führte zu verstärkten Bemühungen in der Weiterentwicklung intravenöser Anaesthesietechniken.

Unseres Wissens wurde die Anaesthesiekombination Rohypnol/Ketanest 1973 erstmals von de Castro erwähnt und als „Ataranalgesia" vorgestellt. Sie wurde von Vontin in Tübingen aufgegriffen, der dann die Methodik verfeinerte und systematisierte. Als „Ataranalgesie" wird sie heute bei uns in allen operativen Bereichen angewendet.

Nach Vontin ist der Begriff Ataranalgesie als Kombination von Flunitrazepam + Analgetika definiert (Abb. 1). Grundsätzlich ist die Ataranalgesie bei Spontanatmung oder auch bei Beatmung möglich. Unter Spontanatmung ist sie zunächst als Typ I (Analgosedierung) bei Operationen mit zusätzlicher Lokalanaesthesie z.B. im HNO- oder ZMK-Bereich indiziert, wobei der Patient ansprechbar und kooperativ bleibt.

Typ II der Ataranalgesie, auf den nachher noch eingegangen wird, kommt bei uns inzwischen in allen operativen Bereichen und bei Patienten aller Altersklassen zur Anwendung, wo eine Intubation nicht erforderlich ist. Auch als Ergänzung bei partieller oder nachlassender Leitungsanaesthesie ist sie gut geeignet. Eingriffe, bei denen auf eine Intubation und künstliche Beatmung nicht verzichtet werden kann, erfolgen in Ataranalgesie Typ III.

Induktion der Ataranalgesie Typ II
Nach Vontin werden 0,2—2,0 mg Rohypnol *langsam* i.v. nach Wirkung verabreicht (0,2 mg/ 20 sec). Der Patient soll schlafen, aber noch auf Anruf reagieren. Anschließend wird Ketanest 0,3—2,0 mg/kg injiziert. Beim Nachlassen der Analgesie erfolgt die Nachinjektion von kleinen Dosen Ketanest (0,3—0,8 mg/kg).

Nun zu einigen Ergebnissen aus einer retrospektiven Auswertung von 978 Narkosen in Rohypnol/Ketanest Kombinationsanaesthesie, die bei kleinen und mittleren gynäkologischen Eingriffen durchgeführt wurden. Das Alter der Patientinnen lag zwischen 13 und 78 bei 37,3 Jahren. An Zeitintervallen wurden ausgewertet: Injektions- und OP-Beginn mit 6,2 Minuten und Injektionsbeginn und OP-Ende mit 23,9 Minuten. Die Praemedikation bestand aus Atropin oder Atropin/Pentazocin. Wesentliche Bedeutung hatte für uns das Verhalten von systolischem Blutdruck und Herzfrequenz nach Ataranalgesie vom Typ II.

Eine zusammenfassende Darstellung des Kreislaufverhaltens unter der angewandten Anaesthesieform gibt Abb. 2. Auf der Abszisse ist die Zeit aufgetragen, auf der Ordinate die Abweichung des Blutdrucks oder der Herzfrequenz gegenüber dem Ausgangswert in Δ RR% bzw. Δ HT%. Auf die Darstellung der Streuungen wurde der Übersichtlichkeit halber verzichtet. Hypotone Ausgangslage < 100 mm Hg, normotone Ausgangslage 101—149 mm Hg, hypertone Ausgangslage > 150 mm Hg.

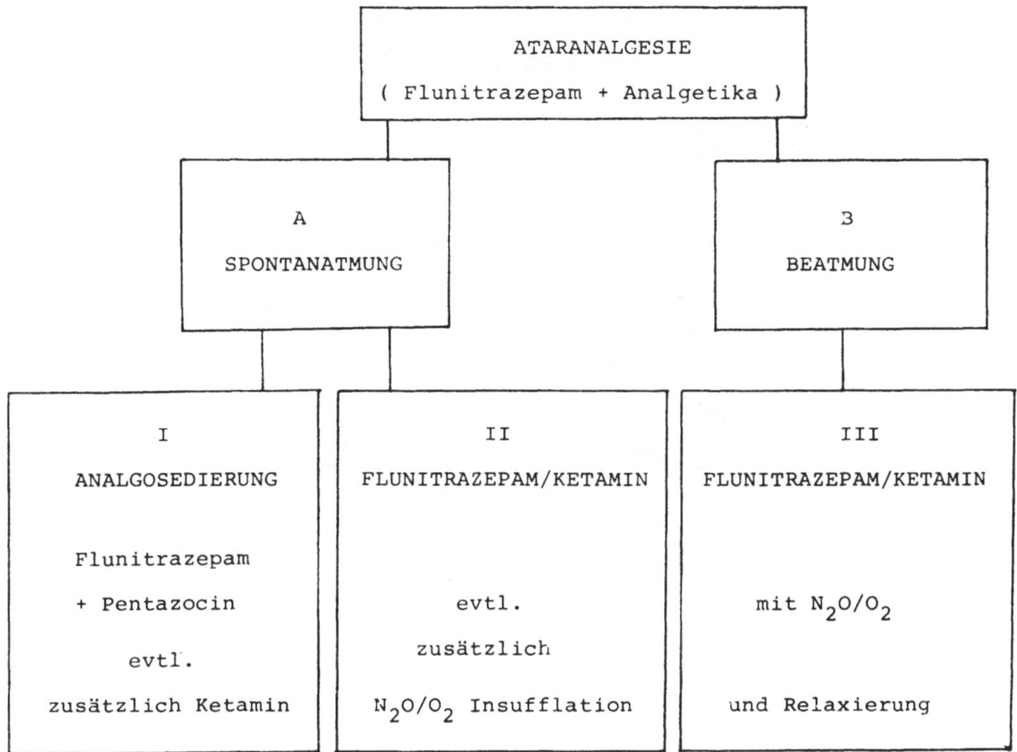

Abb. 1

Nach Vontin werden bei richtiger Dosierung und Injektionstechnik die Kontraindikationen von Ketamin und Flunitrazepam aufgehoben. Soweit das die durch Ketamin bedingte Steigerung von Blutdruck und Herzfrequenz betrifft, deckt sich diese Aussage nicht mit unseren klinischen Erfahrungen, denn es trat stets, von Einzelfällen abgesehen, nach der Injektion von Flunitrazepam/Ketanest ein Anstieg beider Kreislaufparameter auf, der bereits nach 5 Minuten und somit noch vor OP-Beginn dem Ausgangswert gegenüber signifikant erhöht war und noch weiterhin anstieg. Er erreichte für den Blutdruck nach 15 Minuten und für die Herzfrequenz bereits nach 10 Minuten den Höhepunkt, um dann zum Ende der Operation hin wieder abzufallen. Verlauf und Ausmaß beider Kreislaufparameter waren über den untersuchten Zeitraum von 20 Minuten hinweg von der praeoperativen Ausgangslage des systolischen Blutdrucks abhängig. Der prozentual und auch absolut stärkste Anstieg fand sich bei hypotoner Ausgangslage.

Um den Einfluß der von uns angewendeten Praemedikation auf die Kreislaufverhältnisse zu überprüfen, wurden die Ergebnisse von mit Atropin und Atropin/Pentazocin praemedizierten Patienten miteinander verglichen. Der Verlauf des Anstiegs der Kreislaufparameter war in beiden Gruppen sehr ähnlich, jedoch lagen die Werte der nur mit Atropin praemedizierten Patientinnen bei nahezu gleichen Ausgangswerten stets über denen der Kontrollgruppe. Der Unterschied war aber nicht statistisch signifikant. Diese Befunde stehen im Einklang mit den Ergebnissen von Szappanyos et al. (1970). Sie fanden das Ausmaß des Blutdruckanstieges nach Ketanestinjektion ebenfalls vom praeoperativen Ausgangswert abhängig.

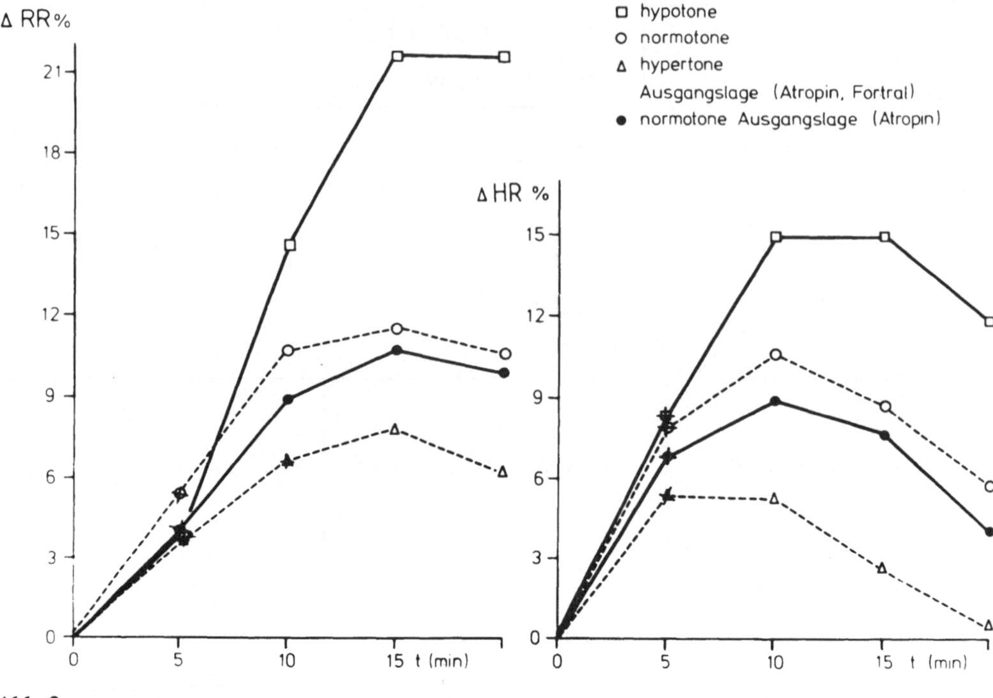

Abb. 2

Je höher der initiale Blutdruckwert war, desto geringer war der nachfolgende Blutdruckanstieg. Diese Ergebnisse zeigen, daß der Blutdruckabfall aufgrund der peripheren Vasodilatation nach Flunitrazepam zumindest bei der von uns angewendeten Dosierung den Blutdruckanstieg der nachfolgenden Ketanestinjektion nicht aufzuheben vermag. Auch bei der Ataranalgesie Typ II handelt es sich um eine modifizierte Ketanestanaesthesie und selbst Kombinationen von Droperidol oder Diazepam mit Ketamin vermögen die kreislaufspezifischen Merkmale der Ketanestanaesthesie nicht zu verschleiern.

Direkte Kontraindikationen der Ataranalgesie sind uns bisher noch nicht bekannt. Beim Vorliegen einer exzessiven Hypertonie, eines amnestisch erfaßbaren apoplektischen Insultes oder bei Myasthenia gravis ist Vorsicht geboten. Gerade die stabilen Kreislaufverhältnisse und die erhaltene Spontanatmung unter der Ataranalgesie Typ II lassen den Einsatz in der Katastrophenmedizin sinnvoll erscheinen.

Ataranalgesie I (Analgosedierung – Spontanatmung)
15–30 mg Pentazocin dreizeitig, 0,5–2,5 mg Flunitrazepam langsam (0,2 mg/20 sec)
Nachinjektion: 15–30 mg Pentazocin und 0,3–0,5 mg Flunitrazepam, bei Bedarf Übergang
auf Ataranalgesie II
Ataranalgesie II (Flunitrazepam/Ketamin – Spontanatmung)
0,4–2,0 mg Flunitrazepam, 0,3–2,0 mg/kg Ketamin, bei Nachinjektion 0,3–0,8 mg/kg
Ketamin, bei Bedarf Übergang auf Ataranalgesie III
Ataranalgesie III (Flunitrazepam/Ketamin – Beatmung)
0,3–2,0 mg Flunitrazepam, 0,3–1,5 mg/kg Ketamin + N_2O/O_2 + Relaxierung
bei Nachinjektion 0,3–0,8 mg/kg Ketamin

Ergebnisse

1359 Narkosen, davon 12,1% Halothan, Lachgas-Maske; 15,9% Ataranalgesie I; 72% Atar-
analgesie II
Alter zwischen 13 und 78 Jahren, Mittel 37,3 Jahre
Gewicht im Mittel 62,7 kg
Zeitintervalle Injektion bis OP-Beginn 6,2 Minuten, Injektion bis OP-Ende 23,9 Min
Praemedikation 51,6% Atropin, 48,4% Atropin/Pentazocin
Versagerquote 4,2% unabhängig von Praemedikation
Narkotikaverbrauch je nach Praemedikation
Atropin: Flunitrazepam 0,00045 mg/kg Min; Ketamin 0,072 mg/kg Min
Atropin/Pentazocin: Flunitrazepam 0,00039 mg/kg Min; Ketanest 0,066 mg/kg Min

Anaesthesie bei Skolioseoperationen

G. Kessler

Einleitung

Von den 73 aus den Jahren 1972 bis 1979 an der Orthopädischen Universitätsklinik Hamburg-Eppendorf operierten Skoliosen konnten 55 ausgewertet werden. Bei den Operationen handelt es sich um hintere Spondylodesen, die mittels des Harrington-Instrumentariums ausgeführt wurden. Hierbei wird durch einen ca. 5 mm starken Distraktionsstab die Konkavseite der Wirbelsäulenkrümmung extendiert (Abb. 1 und 2). Der Distraktionsstab wird über zwei Haken an der Wirbelsäule eingesetzt. Die Distraktion hemmende Bandverbindungen werden gelöst, Querfortsätze osteotomiert, Rippen teils gelöst, und Muskeln, Sehnen und Fascien eingekerbt. Bei doppelseitigen Krümmungen werden zwei oder drei Distraktionsstäbe verwandt. Ausgeprägte Rippenbuckel werden zusätzlich reseziert. In vorliegendem Patientengut wurden zudem 22 Gibben reseziert [1].

Der Sinn der Harrington-Operation liegt in der Begradigung der Wirbelsäule und gleichzeitig in der Verhinderung des Fortschreitens bereits vorhandener Lungenfunktionsstörungen.

Aspekte der Narkoseführung, des Blutersatzes, des intraoperativen Aufwachens, der postoperativen Respirator-Therapie und der Spätergebnisse der Lungenfunktionen werden erörtert.

Patientengut: Das Patientengut besteht aus 55 Skoliose-Patienten mit Fehlbildungs-, idiopathischen und Lähmungsskoliosen. Das Alter der operierten Patienten liegt zwischen 7 und 42 Jahren, dabei kommen 3 weibliche Patienten auf einen männlichen (Abb. 3). Bei 26 Patienten wurde im Thorakalbereich, bei 22 im Thorakal-Lumbal- und bei 7 im Lumbalbereich eine Spondylodese nach Harrington durchgeführt.

Methodik, Ergebnisse, Diskussion

Die präoperativen Vorbereitungen sind in Tabelle 1 aufgeführt.

Alle Patienten wurden in der sogenannten Hocklagerung operiert; es wurde darauf geachtet, daß die Vena cava caudalis nicht komprimiert wurde. Obligatorisch für die Narkosen sind zwei großkalibrige Venenzugänge, ein Venenkatheter, ein Ösophagus-Stethoskop, arterielle Druckmessung, EKG und Urinkatheter. Die Narkosen dauerten im Durchschnitt 7,1 Stunden (Tabelle 2), der intra- und postoperative Blutverbrauch lag im Mittel bei 8,5 Konserven Blut insgesamt (Abb. 4). Die postoperativ transfundierten Konserven wurden innerhalb der ersten 12 Stunden der Überwachungsperiode gegeben. Die Menge des transfundierten Blutes hat sich in den letzten Jahren parallel zu den längerdauernden Narkosen erhöht. Diese wurden notwendig durch kompliziertere Operationstechniken bei Rippenbuckelplastiken.

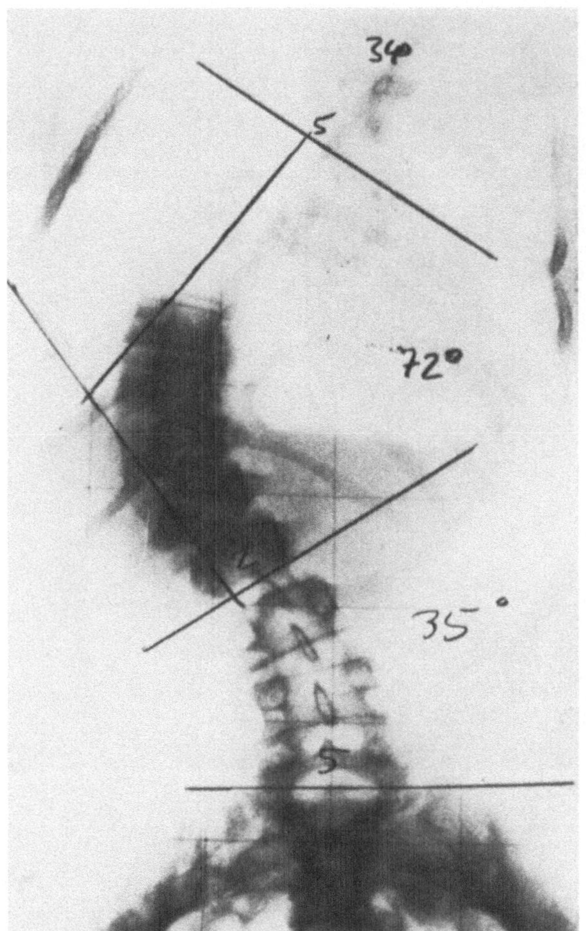

Abb. 1. Röntgenbild eines 15jährigen Patienten mit idiopathischer Thorakalskoliose

Massentransfusionen von 15 oder mehr Konserven wurden nachweislich durch Gerinnungsstörungen verursacht. In unserem Krankengut wurden 2 Fälle mit einer Verbrauchskoagulopathie und 7 weitere Fälle gefunden, die therapiert werden mußten. Um den Blutverbrauch
zu senken, wurden die Narkosen so geführt, daß der systolische Blutdruck den Wert von 100
mmHg nicht überschritt. In 7 Fällen wurde die Methode der Hämodilution angewandt. Das
Ergebnis war eine Bluteinsparung von 2 Konserven pro Patient. Die Untersuchungen von
Sunder-Plaßmann et al. [10] bestätigen dies, während Weidriger et al. [11] die tatsächliche
Einsparung sehr kritisch beurteilen (Tabelle 3).
    Die Methode der Autotransfusion mit dem Bentley-Retransfusionsgerät wurde nur in 3
Fällen angewandt. Die Einsparung betrug hier 2 Konserven pro Patient. Jedesmal wurde eine
Hämoglobinurie und Hämoglobinämie — wie von Kieninger et al. [7] beschrieben — beobach-
tet. Die dritte Autotransfusion komplizierte sich durch eine unmittelbar nach der Gabe von
1500 ml Blut aufgetretene Verbrauchskoagulopathie.

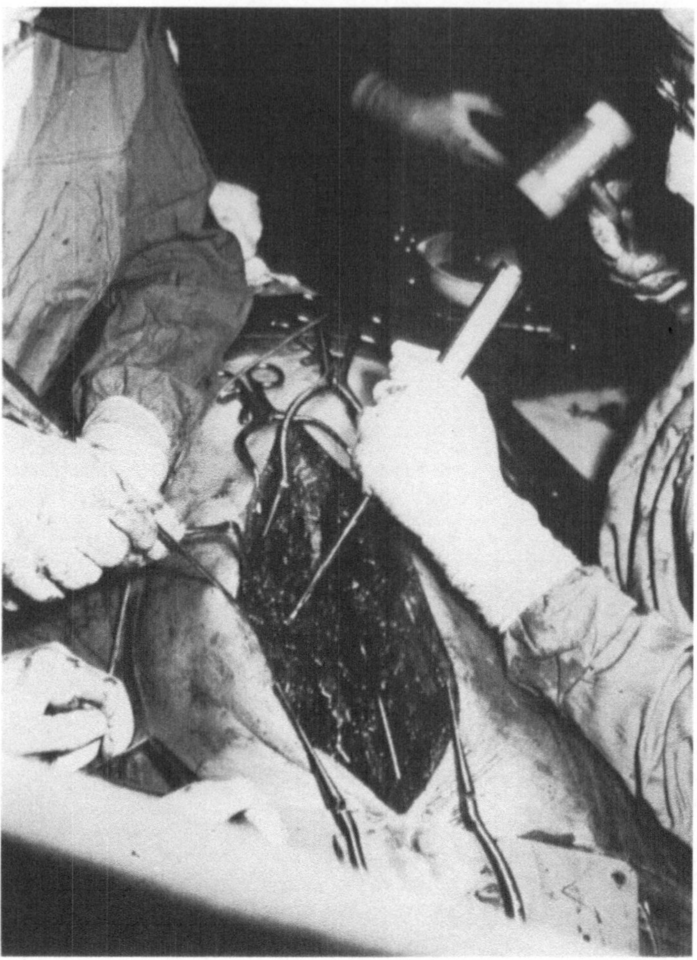

Abb. 2. Intraoperativer Situs einer Spondylodese nach Harrington nach Einsetzen des Distraktionsstabes

Tabelle 1. Routinemäßige Voruntersuchung bei Spondylodesen (nach Harrington)

1) Blutbild, BSG, Elektrolyte, Transaminasen, Gerinnungsstatus, Blutgruppe
2) Elektrokardiogramm
3) Lungenfunktionsprüfungen
4) Röntgen-Thorax

Routinemäßige präoperative Übungen

1) Bewegen von Fingern, Händen, Armen und Beinen auf Aufforderung zum intraoperativen Ausschluß
   eines Querschnitts (besonders wichtig bei fremdsprachigen Patienten)
2) Blähen mit Beatmungsgerät (Bennett-Respirator PR 2)

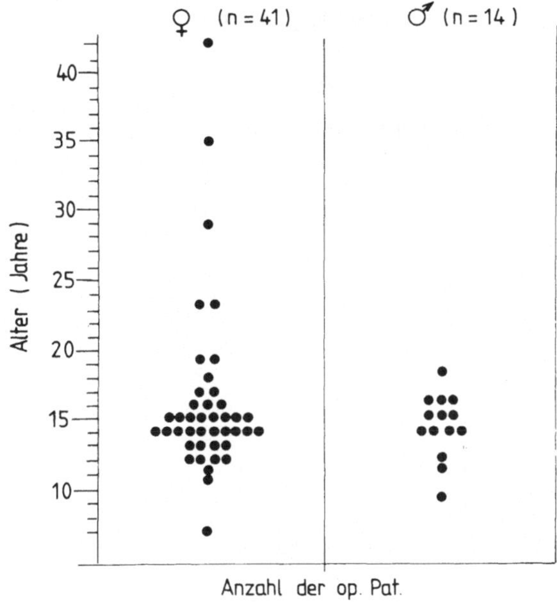

Abb. 3. Anzahl und Altersverteilung der nach Harrington operierten Patienten

Tabelle 2. Dauer der bei den Spondylodesen nach Harrington von 1972–1979 durchgeführten Narkosen

Dauer d. Narkosen in Std.	3	4	5	6	7	8	9	10	11	12
Anzahl d. Narkosen	1	8	9	18	9	4	4	2	–	–

Tabelle 3. Durch Hämodilution und Autotransfusion eingesparte Konserven

Methode	Zahl der Fälle	Eingesparte Konserven
a) Hämodilution	7	14
b) Autotransfusion (n. Bentley)	3	6

Trotz aller Schwierigkeiten müssen wegen des noch vorhandenen Hepatitis-Risikos weitere Möglichkeiten gefunden werden, Blut einzusparen. 2 unserer Patienten erkrankten leider postoperativ an einer Hb_SAg-positiven Hepatitis.

Nun zur eigentlichen Besonderheit dieser Anaesthesie, dem intraoperativen Aufwachen. Der Patient wird intraoperativ erweckt, um grobneurologisch einen iatrogenen Querschnitt auszuschließen. Fünf Forderungen sind an das Aufwachen zu stellen, sie sind in Tabelle 4 zusammengefaßt. Bereits präoperativ wird wegen des narkosebedingten verminderten Wachheitsgrades in der Aufwachphase das Bewegen der Hände, Arme, Beine und Füße auf Auffor-

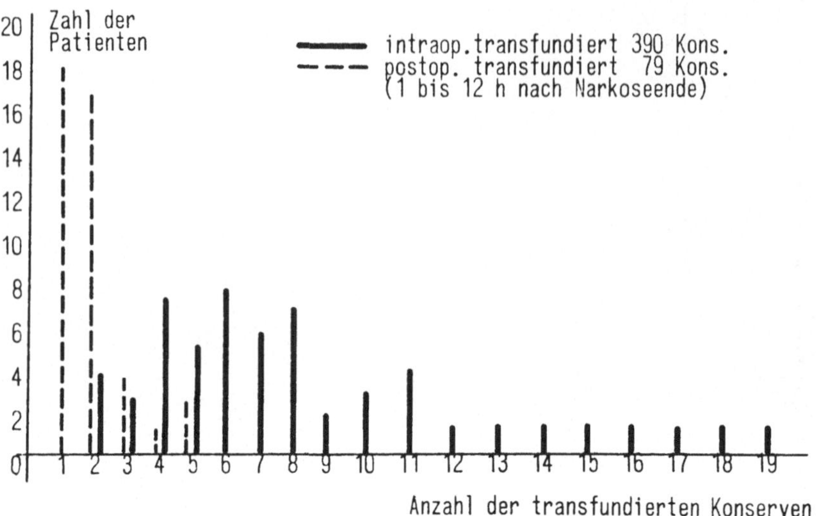

Abb. 4. Intra- und postoperativer Blutverbrauch bei 55 Spondylodesen nach Harrington

derung geübt. Die Sprachbarriere bei ausländischen Patienten kann so überwunden werden. Damit der Patient gezielt aufwacht, wird das gut steuerbare Halothan mit Fentanyl in der Narkoseführung kombiniert. Nach Messungen an Kurznarkosen mit Halothan wurde festgestellt, daß die Aufwachzeiten vom chirurgischen Stadium bis zur Ansprechbarkeit ca. 6 Minuten dauern. Blutspiegel-Bestimmungen nach Drosselung der Halothan-Zufuhr ergaben 10 Minuten später noch Werte von 2,5 mg% Halothan im venösen Blut [6]. Ein bestimmter Fentanylspiegel ist zur Ausschaltung des intraoperativen Wundschmerzes nötig. In diesem fortgeschrittenen Operationsstadium ist der Distraktionsstab bereits eingesetzt, Querfortsätze reseziert, Rippen, Muskeln und Fascien eingekerbt. Die Relaxation muß zur grobneurologischen Überprüfung fast aufgehoben sein. Der Patient beginnt unter kontrollierter manueller Beatmung spontan zu atmen, bewegt jetzt auf Aufforderung Hände, Arme, Beine und Füße, öffnet die Augen (Abb. 5). Blutdruck und Pulsfrequenz steigen (Abb. 6). Ein durch einen starken Wundschmerz bedingtes Aufbäumen könnte in diesem Stadium das Ausbrechen des Distraktionsstabes und im ungünstigsten Fall die Ausbildung eines traumatischen Querschnitts zur Folge haben. Werden die Anzeichen einer beginnenden Lähmung diagnostiziert, so wird durch Verkürzung des Distraktionsstabes die Extension vermindert. Das Risiko eines iatroge-

Tabelle 4. An das intraoperative Aufwachen müssen 5 Forderungen gestellt werden

---

1) Der Patient muß gezielt erweckt werden können.
2) Der Patient darf nur so weit relaxiert sein, daß er auf Aufforderung noch Hände, Arme und Beine bewegen kann.
3) Der Patient muß den Tubus tolerieren (Gefahr der Extubation).
4) Der Patient darf sich nicht aufbäumen (Gefahr des Querschnitts).
5) Der Patient darf keine Schmerzen haben.

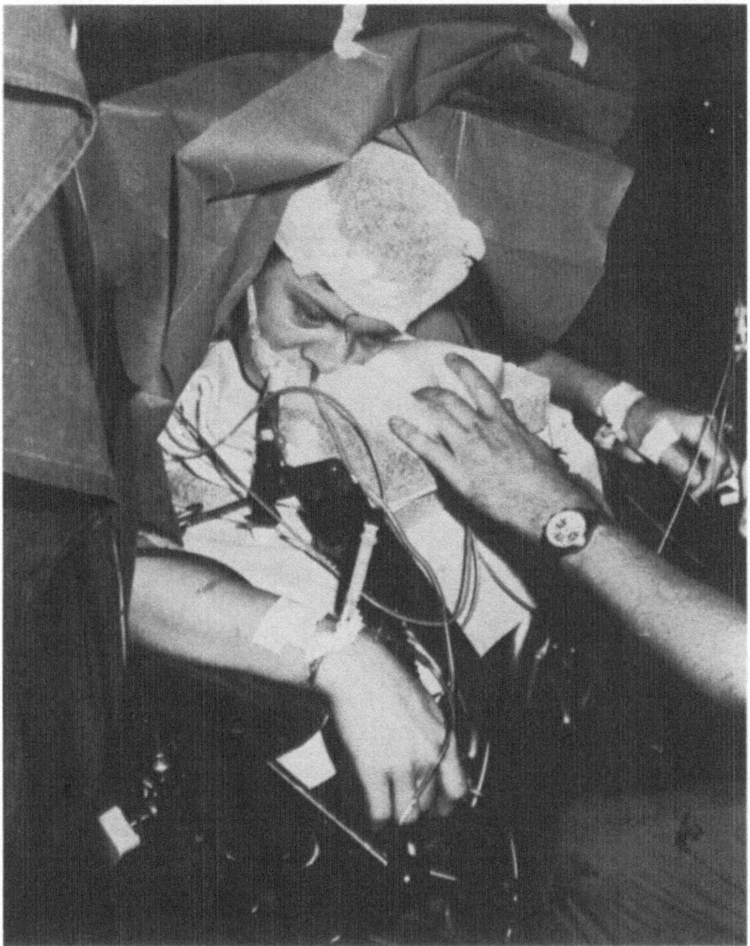

Abb. 5. Intraoperativ aufgewachter Patient

nen Querschnitts wird so erheblich verringert, aber nicht ausgeschlossen. Im Zweifelsfall
kann das Aufwachen mehrmals wiederholt werden.

Ein weiterer wichtiger Punkt ist die postoperative Respirator-Therapie. Nach 6- bis 10-
stündigen Narkosen ist eine postoperative Ateminsuffizienz zu erwarten. Sie wird durch drei
Umstände begünstigt:

1. Wundschmerzen, hauptsächlich im Gebiet der resezierten Gibben, dadurch schnelle und
flache Atmung.

2. Mechanische Behinderung der Atmung durch das Gipsbett.

3. Narkotika-Überhang.

Postoperativ wurden in 50% der Fälle respiratorische Azidosen und in einigen Fällen
Atelektasen nachgewiesen. Seit 1977 werden alle Patienten nach einem Bläh-Schema behandelt. Der Patient wird postoperativ viertelstündlich 5mal gebläht, nach 6 Stunden halbstündlich 5mal, nach 12 Stunden stündlich 5mal gebläht usw. Seit Anwendung dieses Schemas
wurden keine pulmonalen Komplikationen mehr beobachtet. Nach den Ausführungen von

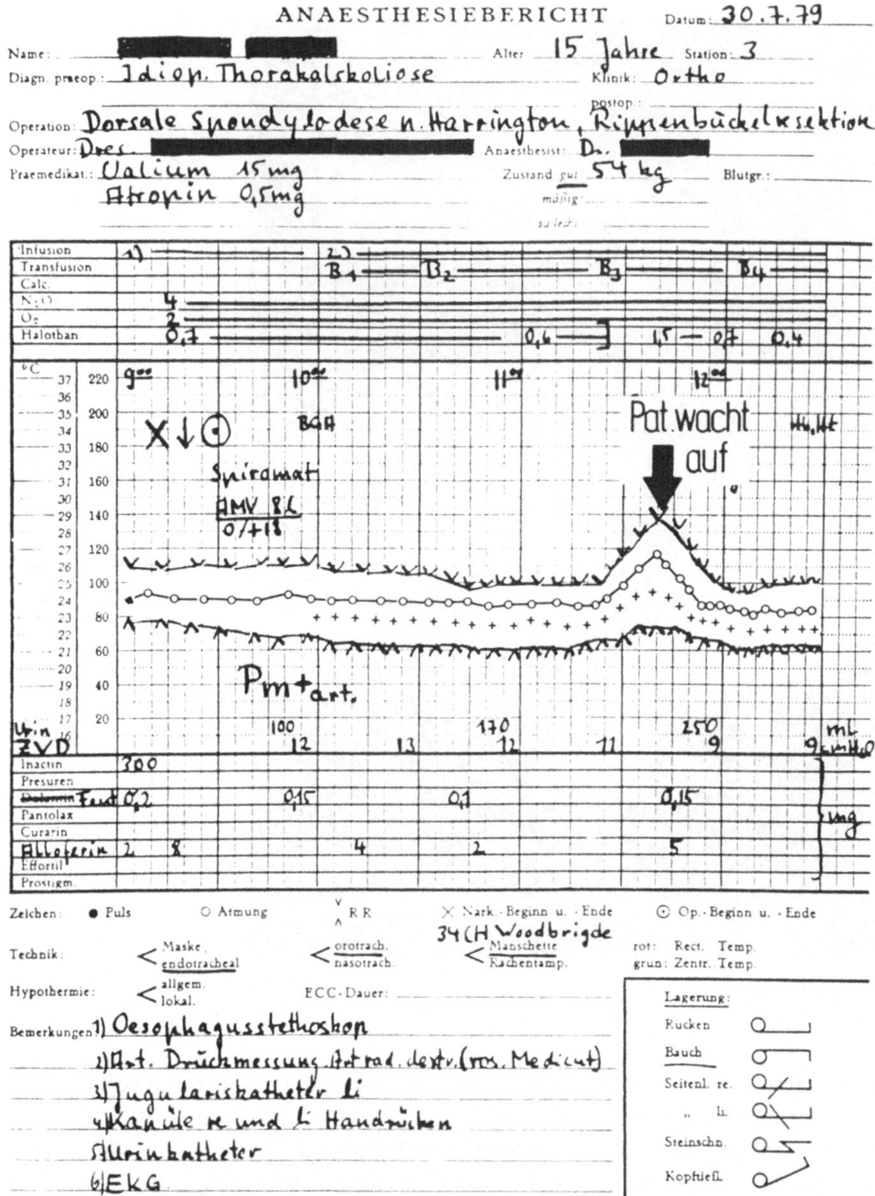

Abb. 6. Puls- und Blutdruckkurve während des Aufwachens

Rodewald [8] ist eine Langzeitbeatmung nur beim instabilen Thorax angezeigt. Die postoperative Behandlung des auch noch nach Rippenbuckelresektion stabilen Thorax ist eine Domäne der krankengymnastischen Behandlung mit Respiratoren und Totraumvergrößerern. Fasol et al. [2] gehen sogar soweit, selbst den instabilen Thorax mit Ateminsuffizienz konservativ zu behandeln.

Zu den Spätergebnissen der Lungenfunktionen — ausgehend von den präoperativen Werten (restr. Ventilationsstörungen in 80% der Fälle, Totalkapazität im Mittel 79% des Sollwertes, Lungenemphysem in 25%, gestörter Gasaustausch für O_2 und CO_2 in Ausnahmefällen) — wird festgestellt, daß sich keine gerichteten Veränderungen ergeben haben. Die postoperativen Kontrolluntersuchungen fanden nach im Mittel drei Jahren statt (Minimum 12 Monaten, Maximum 7 Jahren). Wie auch von Henche et al. [5] berichten, führen die Spondylodesen nach Harrington bezüglich der Lungenfunktion weder zu einer Verbesserung noch zu einer Verschlechterung der Situation.

Zusammenfassung

Es wird über 55 Anaesthesien bei Harrington-Operationen berichtet. Es handelt sich hierbei um Versteifungsoperationen der Wirbelsäule mit teils ausgedehnten Rippenbuckel-Plastiken. Interessante Aspekte ergeben sich aus der Länge und dem Blutverbrauch der Narkose sowie dem intraoperativen Aufwachen, der postoperativen Atemtherapie und dem Ergebnis der Nachuntersuchungen der Lungenfunktionen.

Im Schnitt dauerten die Narkosen 7,1 Stunden. Pro Patient wurden 8,5 Konserven Blut gebraucht. In wenigen Fällen wurden zur Blutersparnis die Methoden der Hämodilution und Autotransfusion angewandt. Das Aufwachen ließ sich mit der Kombinationsnarkose (Halothan/Fentanyl) erreichen. Alle Patienten sind zeitgerecht erwacht. Postoperativ wird seit 1977 ein hier entworfenes Bläh-Schema benutzt. Die pulmonale Komplikationsrate ist deutlich gesunken. Zuletzt sei gesagt, daß sich durch die Spondylodesen nach Harrington die Lungenfunktionen der Patienten weder verschlechtert noch verbessert hatten.

Literatur

1. Dahmen G (1976) Skoliose-seitliche Wirbelsäulenverkrümmung. In: Bernbeck, Dahmen G (Hrsg) Kinderorthopädie. Thieme Stuttgart
2. Fasol P, Benzer H, Haider W, Lackner F, Politzer P, Stöger A (1975) Die Therapie der Atemstörung beim schweren Thoraxtrauma. Anästhesist 24:367
3. Hall JE, Levine CK, Sudhir KG (1978) Intraoperative awakening to monitor spinal cord function during Harrington instrumentation and spine fusion. J Bone Jt Surg 60:533
4. Harrington Pr (1972) Instrumentation techniques in spine surgery. Orthop Clin North Amer 3:49
5. Henche HR, Morschner E, Rutishauer M (1977) Die Entwicklung der Lungenfunktion nach Skoliosebehandlung durch Harrington-Instrumentarium. Z Orthop 115:816
6. Kessler G, Haferkorn D (1977) Vergleichende Untersuchungen über die postnarkotische Phase nach Kurznarkosen mit Halothan und Ethrane. Prakt Anästh 12:269
7. Kieninger G, Junger H, Neugebauer W, Schmidt K (1976) Die intraoperative Autotransfusion. Prakt Anästh 11:203
8. Rodewald G (1969) Rippenbrüche, Sternumbrüche, der instabile Brustkorb. In: Baumgartl F, Kremer K, Schreiber HW (Hrsg) Spezielle Chirurgie für die Praxis. Bd 1, Teil 12, Thieme Stuttgart
9. Sudhir KG, Smith RM, Hallund JE, Hansen DD (1976) Intraoperative awekening for early recognition of possible neurologic sequelae during Harrington-rod spinal fusion. Anesth Analg Curr Res 55: 526
10. Sunder-Plassmann L, Klövekorn WP, Messner K (1976) Präoperative Hämodilution: Grundlagen, Adaptionsmechanismen und Grenzen klinischer Anwendung. Anästhesist 25:124
11. Weidriger G, Hasselbring H, Steinlein H (1976) Wie groß ist der Nutzeffekt der präoperativen Hämodilution wirklich? Anästhesist 25:189

Anaesthesie für computerisierte Tomographie des Schädels: 5 Jahre Erfahrung mit EMI Scanner

J. Bläss und K. Skarvan

Seit 1971 der erste EMI Scanner der Welt vorgestellt wurde, hat sich die cerebrale Computertomographie schnell als ein führendes und vor allem nicht invasives Verfahren in der neuroradiologischen Diagnostik von intrakraniellen Krankheitsprozessen durchgesetzt. Beim Schädel-Hirn-Trauma ist die cerebrale Angiographie heute weitgehend durch die computerisierte Tomographie ersetzt worden, die als empfindlichste Methode zum Nachweis posttraumatischer intrakranieller Blutungen oder anderer Komplikationen (z.B. Hirnödem) gilt. Um Bilder der gewünschten Qualität und hoher diagnostischer Aussagekraft zu erhalten, ist es eine unabdingbare Voraussetzung, daß der untersuchte Patient während jedes Scanvorganges den Kopf vollständig ruhig hält. Diese Bedingung wird von den meisten Patienten erfüllt. Bei motorisch unruhigen oder bewußtlosen Patienten, bei wenig kooperativen Patienten sowie bei Kindern unter 6 Jahren ist in der Regel zur absoluten Ruhigstellung ein Anaesthesieverfahren notwendig.

Methodik und Fragestellung

Seit 1973 wurden auf der neuroradiologischen Abteilung des Kantonsspitals Basel nahezu 14 000 cerebrale Computertomographien durchgeführt. Wir haben retrospektiv die Narkoseprotokolle von 339 EMI Scan Patienten unter mehreren Gesichtspunkten ausgewertet. In einem ersten Untersuchungszeitraum von 14 Monaten in den Jahren 1976—1977 wurden 209 Anaesthesieprotokolle berücksichtigt, die als repräsentativ für den EMI Scanner der ersten Generation anzusehen sind. Seit August 1978 ist bereits ein EMI Scanner der 2. Generation in Betrieb, so daß wir für eine Zeitspanne von 10 Monaten (September 1978 — Juni 1979) die Narkoseprotokolle (n = 120) unter dem neuen EMI auswerten konnten. Wir haben die Ergebnisse dieser beiden Untersuchungsreihen miteinander verglichen und unsere Resultate den Angaben der Literatur gegenübergestellt. Gleichzeitig suchten wir zu klären:
1. welche Auswirkungen der EMI Scanner der 2. Generation auf die Anaesthesiedauer und das Anaesthesieverfahren hat,
2. ob sich ein generell empfehlenswertes Anaesthesieverfahren herauskristallisiert hat.

Ergebnisse

Die Untersuchung der Auswirkungen des neuen EMI auf die Untersuchungsdauer und Anaesthesiedauer im Vergleich zum EMI der 1. Generation (Abb. 1) ergab einen hochsignifikanten Unterschied (p 0,001). Basierend auf wesentlich kürzeren Scanzeiten (Standardscan-

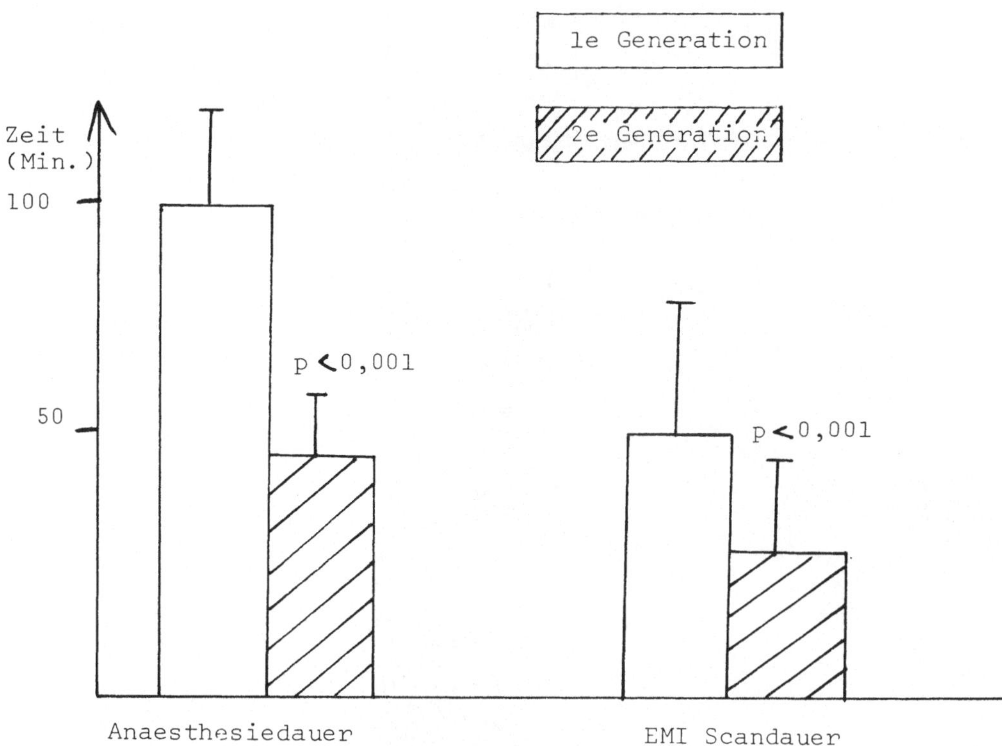

Abb. 1. Anaesthesie- und Untersuchungsdauer für den EMI-Scanner der ersten und zweiten Generation

dauer beim EMI 1. Generation 6 min., beim EMI 2. Generation 80 sec.) hat sich die Anaesthesiedauer von durchschnittlich 98 Min. (range 30–225 Min.) früher auf jetzt 42 Min. (range 18–85 Min.) verringert. Auch die Kopflagerung hat sich mit dem EMI Scanner der 2. Generation entscheidend geändert. Während beim alten EMI Scanner ein Wasserbehälter aus Gummi als Absorptionsausgleich und zur Fixierung des Kopfes diente (Abb. 2a), erfolgt die Kopflagerung beim neuen Scanner auf einer Stütze (Abb. 2b).

Was Art und Häufigkeit der angewandten Anaesthesieverfahren anbelangt, so steht beim Erwachsenen die Intubationsnarkose mit 78,5% an erster Stelle, wobei es sich in 55% der Fälle um Patienten mit akutem Schädel-Hirn-Trauma handelte (Abb. 3).

Bei Erwachsenen wurde im Vergleich zu früheren Jahren vermehrt ein intravenöses Anaesthesieverfahren ohne Intubation in Spontanatmung durchgeführt (Abb. 3: unter Sedation).

Zur Anwendung kamen Althesin sowie Diazepam in Kombination mit Methohexital oder Dehydrobenzperidol. In größerem Umfang als beim EMI der 1. Generation wurde unter dem EMI Scan der 2. Generation bei Kindern ohne Hirndruckzeichen mit Erfolg eine intramuskuläre Ketaminnarkose (46%) angewandt. Bei den übrigen Kindern kam eine Intubationsnarkose mit Beatmung zur Anwendung. Komplikationen (Tabelle 1) während und kurz nach der Untersuchung traten in 16 Fällen auf, dabei überwogen bedrohliche, meist tachykarde Herzrhythmusstörungen (ein Fall mit Asystolie) und respiratorische Probleme (3 Laryngospasmen, 1 CO_2-Retention). In einem Falle kam es bei einem Säugling zur Abkühlung mit einer Rektaltemperatur unter 34 °C. Den beiden Todesfällen lag in einem Falle ein ma-

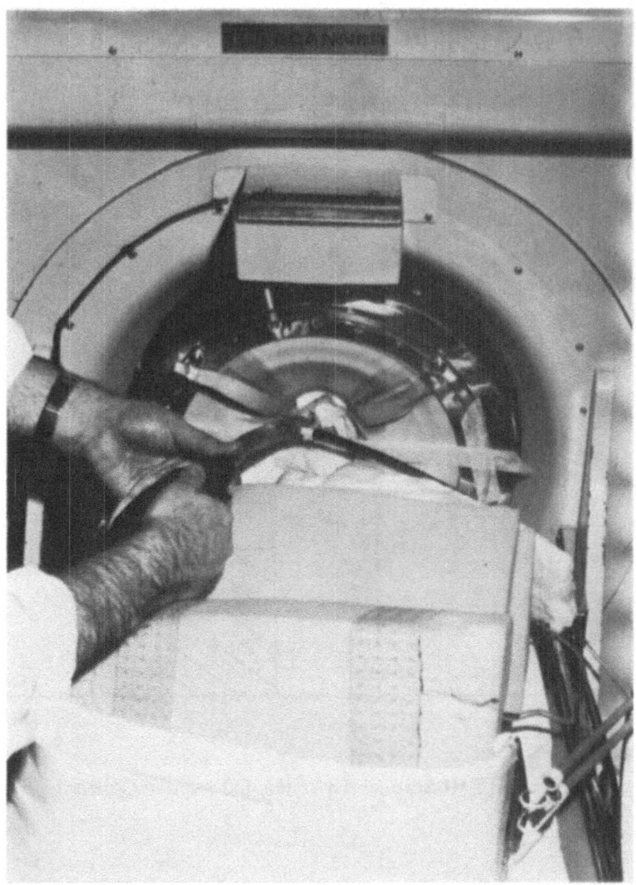

Abb. 2a. Kopflagerung beim EMI Scanner der ersten Generation. Beim alten Scanner ist der Kopf des Patienten weitgehend von einem mit Wasser gefüllten Gummibehälter eingeschlossen. Wie auf der Abbildung ersichtlich ist, ist vor allem bei Kleinkindern der Zugang zum Kopf des Patienten sehr erschwert

lignes Hirnödem, im anderen Falle eine nicht beherrschbare Blutung bei schwerem Polytrauma zugrunde.

Was das Patientengut anbelangt, das einer Betreuung durch den Anaesthesisten bedarf, so stellten Patienten mit akutem Schädel-Hirn-Trauma den größten Prozentsatz dar (Tabelle 2). Einen hohen Prozentsatz stellen Kinder unter 10 Jahren dar, die 1976/1977 noch 27%, in den Jahren 1978/1979 aber schon fast 40% des Patientengutes ausmachten.

Sowohl bei Schädel-Hirn-Verletzten als auch nicht traumatisierten Patienten fanden sich Krankheitszustände mit schwerwiegender Beeinträchtigung der Lungenfunktion wie Aspiration und akute respiratorische Insuffizienz. (Tabelle 3). Dazu kommen beim Schädel-Hirn-Trauma noch massive Gerinnungsstörungen und einseitige Intubationen, wobei letztere bei auswärtig intubierten und dann per Luft- oder Bodentransport eingelieferten Patienten festgestellt wurden. In beiden Patientengruppen sind außerdem Herzrhythmusstörungen ein bekanntes Nebensymptom bei Hirnblutungen [10], und chronische Lungenfunktionsstörungen zu erwähnen.

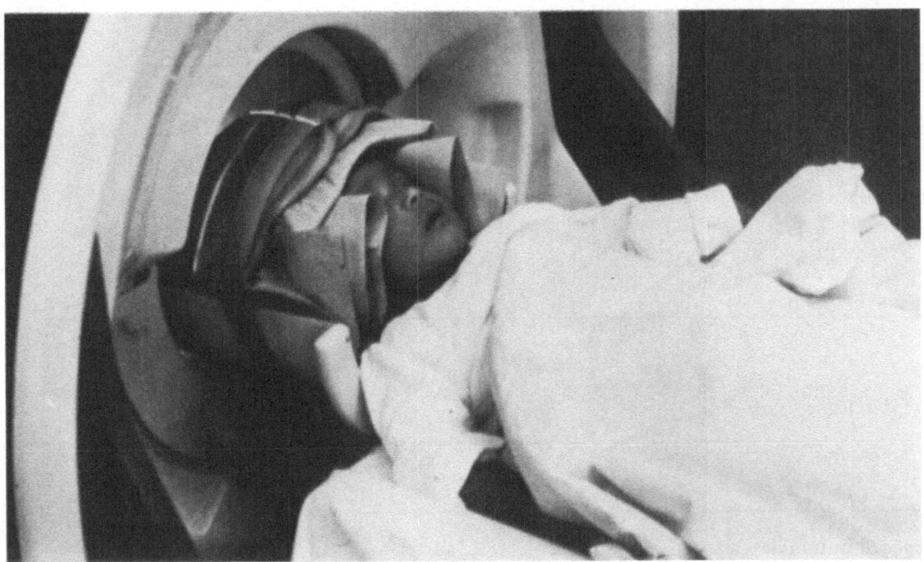

Abb. 2b. Kopflagerung beim EMI Scanner der zweiten Generation. Beim neuen Scanner wird der Kopf auf einer Stütze gelagert. Zur besseren Fixierung ist bei Kindern zusätzlich eine Haltevorrichtung angebracht. Zwischen Patient und Apparat besteht ein deutlicher Freiraum, der einen leichten Zugang zum Kopf des Patienten erlaubt

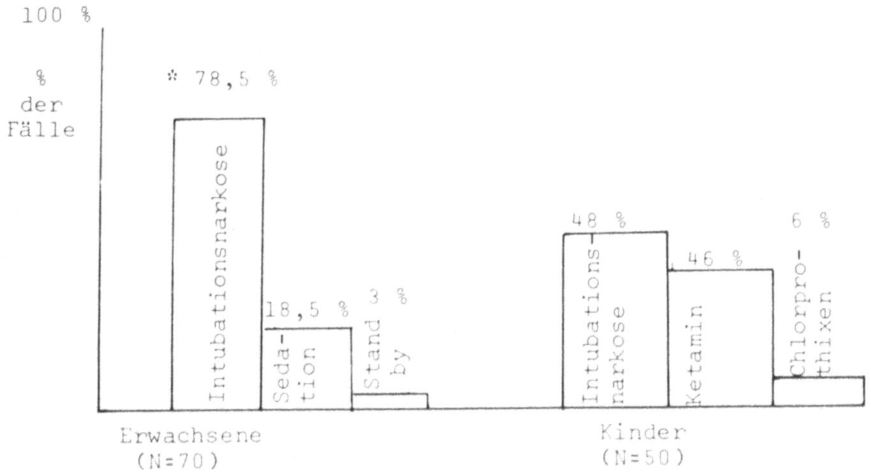

Abb. 3. Art und Häufigkeit der Anaesthesieverfahren unter dem EMI Scanner der zweiten Generation (1978/1979)

Eine Allgemeinanaesthesie unter dem neuen EMI war in 4,2%, und unter dem EMI der 1. Generation in 6,4% der total untersuchten Patienten notwendig (Tabelle 4). Über die herkunftsmäßige Zusammensetzung beziehungsweise den Aufenthaltsort der Patienten unseres Krankengutes nach der EMI Scan-Untersuchung gibt Abb. 4 Auskunft.

Tabelle 1. Komplikationen während und kurz nach der Anaesthesie

	Zahl der Fälle (n = 339)
Herzrhythmusstörungen	8
Rspiratorische Probleme	5
Abkühlung (< 34 °C)	1
Exitus	2
	16

Tabelle 2. Einweisungsdiagnosen

	Zahl der Fälle (n = 339)	%
Akutes Schädelhirntrauma	136	40%
Nicht traumatische subarachnoidale und intracerebrale Blutung	42	12%
Intrakranielle Tumore	47	11%
Hydrocephalus internus	29	9%
Andere	95	28%

Tabelle 3. Zustand der Patienten vor der Anaesthesie

	Nicht traumatisierte Patienten (n = 205)	Schädel-Hirn Trauma (n = 134)
Schwerwiegende Lungenfunktionsstörung	32	35
Einseitige Intubation	–	5
Arrhythmien	11	8
Herzinsuffizienz	10	–
Säure-Base-Elektrolyt Störung	9	23
Massive Gerinnungsstörung	–	9

Tabelle 4. Allgemeinanaesthesie für EMI Scan

	Total Patienten untersucht	Zeitspanne in Monaten	In Allgemein- anaesthesie
Basel (1976/77)	3281	14	6,4%
Basel (1978/79)	2565	10	4,2%
San Diego (Aidinis 1976)	2502	23	6,7%
UCLA (Ferrer 1977)	4000	19	2,0%

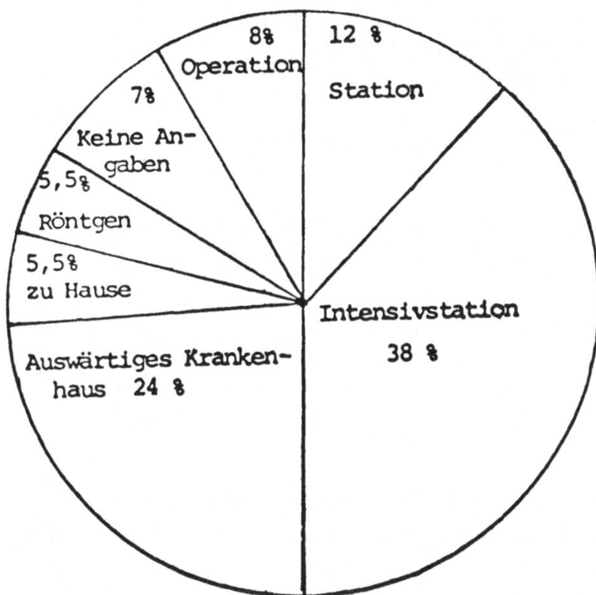

Abb. 4. Aufenthaltsort der Patienten nach EMI Scan Untersuchung

Diskussion

Eine fünfjährige Erfahrung mit dem EMI Scanner der 1. Generation und 2. Generation ergab deutlich verkürzte Scan- und Anaesthesiezeiten sowie eine wesentlich verbesserte Patientenlagerung bei dem Scanner der 2. Generation. Im Vergleich mit dem Scanner der 1. Generation ist die Kopflagerung beim neuen EMI bequemer und sicherer geworden. Beim Scanner der 1. Generation hatte der Anaesthesist kaum einen Zugang zum Gesicht beziehungsweise zu den Atemwegen des Patienten. Dieser Umstand war bei den jüngsten Patienten mit einer ausgeprägten Anteflexionshaltung des Kopfes verbunden. Mit der dadurch bedingten Gefahr der Verlegung der Atemwege ohne sofortige Zugangsmöglichkeit zum Kopf des Patienten waren wir bei Kindern unter vier Jahren in der Regel zur Intubationsnarkose gezwungen. Eine weitere Indikation dafür stellte die mögliche Ruptur des Wasserbehälters dar mit der Gefahr der ausgeprägten Aspiration beim nicht intubierten, narkotisierten Patienten [4].

Mit den weit besseren Lagerungsbedingungen beim EMI Scanner der 2. Generation ist auch bei Säuglingen und Kleinkindern ohne Schwierigkeiten ein Anaesthesieverfahren in Spontanatmung ohne Intubation möglich. Wenn auch ein Sedationsverfahren (Abb. 5) der nicht invasiven cerebralen Computertomographie am ehesten entsprechen würde, hat diese Methode zur Ruhigstellung von motorisch unruhigen Patienten sowohl bei Erwachsenen als auch bei Kindern kein befriedigendes Ergebnis erbracht [3, 11]. Während mit Diazepam alleine keine ausreichende Immobilisation erzielt werden kann, ist dies mit einer Kombination von Diazepam und Pentazozin schon eher möglich. Doch auch damit kommt es häufig zu unvorhergesehenen Patientenbewegungen beziehungsweise sind zu hohe Dosen mit der Gefahr der Atemdepression und des zu starken sowie zu lange dauernden Überhanges nötig. Eine generelle Empfehlung dieser Methode ist daher auf keinen Fall möglich. Aufgrund unse-

Erwachsene   Kinder

Diazepam u. Pentazozin	SEDATION	?
Althesin (fraktioniert oder Infusion)	SPONTANATMUNG OHNE INTUBATION	Ketamin oder Althesin
Althesin/Thiopental Muskelrelaxans N_2O-O_2	INTUBATION UND BEATMUNG	Althesin/Thiopental Muskelrelaxans oder HALOTHAN/N_2O-O_2

Abb. 5. Anaesthesieverfahren für EMI Scan

rer bisherigen Erfahrungen wird bei Kindern Ketamin den oben angeführten Ansprüchen am ehesten gerecht [12]. Zu beachten ist eine ausreichende Dosierung von Ketamin intramuskulär (10 mg/kg KG). Bei Kontrastmittelgabe, was eine Verdoppelung der Untersuchungszeit bedeutet, sind in der Regel intravenöse Repetitionsdosen von Ketamin (1—2 mg/kg KG) nötig. Bei auswärtigen und ambulanten Patienten, die immerhin in unserem Krankengut einen Prozentsatz von über 25% ausmachen, wirkt sich die allerdings nicht selten verlängerte Aufwachphase nachteilig aus. Eine alternative Methode vor allem bei Kontraindikationen für Ketamin (klinische Hirndruckzeichen) stellt die intravenöse Althesingabe beim spontanatmenden, nicht intubierten Kind dar. Stuart hat die Althesininfusion mit Erfolg auch bei Säuglingen und Kleinkindern angewandt [9]. Nicht vergessen werden darf jedoch die Intubationsnarkose die jedoch den invasivsten Charakter von den bisher angeführten Methoden hat und von uns daher meist nur noch bei Kindern mit klinischen oder anamnestischen Hirndruckzeichen angewendet wurde.

Beim nicht traumatisierten erwachsenen Patienten hat sich uns die fraktionierte Althesingabe gut bewährt, wobei in Anbetracht des kurzdauernden Abtastvorganges beim Scanner der 2. Generation (80 sec.) in der Regel 1—2 ml Althesin pro Schicht genügen. Entsprechend positive Erfahrungen liegen von Stuart mit der Althesin Infusionsmethode vor [9]. Zur Ruhigstellung von motorisch unruhigen Schädel-Hirn-Verletzten empfiehlt sich die Intubation und die Gabe von Hirndruck senkenden Anaesthetika wie Thiopental oder Althesin [8] sowie die Gabe eines Muskelrelaxans, zusätzlich eventuell ein intravenöses Analgetikum, das natürlich immer dann indiziert ist, wenn Schmerzen offensichtliche Ursache der Unruhe des Patienten sind. Mit Rücksicht auf eine mögliche intracranielle Drucksteigerung empfiehlt sich bei akuten Schädel-Hirn-Traumen auf Halothan, Enflurane und Lachgas zu verzichten.

Neben dem Narkoseverfahren, in Anbetracht des nicht seltenen kritischen Zustandes des Patientengutes, gilt es ein adäquates Monitoring zu beachten: EKG, Blutdruck ev. direkt gemessen, neurologischer Status und nasale Temperaturkontrolle. Dazu kommen beim Traumapatienten die Überwachung der Diurese, der arteriellen Blutgasanalyse und des Gerinnungsstatus.

Komplikationen während oder unmittelbar nach der Anaesthesie für EMI Scan scheinen von der Narkose selbst, der Anaesthesiedauer, dem Zustand des Patienten und von der apparatbedingten Kopflagerung des Patienten abhängig zu sein. Drei Komponenten davon werden vom Scanner der 2. Generation positiv beeinflußt:

1. Auf der Grundlage wesentlich verkürzter Scan Zeiten hat sich die Anaesthesiedauer deutlich vermindert.
2. Die Kopflagerung ist sicherer geworden.
3. Letzteres und die kürzere Anaesthesiedauer erlauben weniger invasive Anaesthesieverfahren und eine geringere Narkotikamenge.

Diese Einflüsse des EMI Scanner der 2. Generation scheinen wesentlich zu einer Senkung der Komplikationsrate im Rahmen der Anesthesie beizutragen. Erwähnenswert ist in diesem Zusammenhang die Kontrastmittelgabe (Telebrix), die in unserem Krankengut immerhin bei etwa 40% der total untersuchten Patienten zur Anwendung kommt. Trotz fehlender Zwischenfälle unter dem vom Anaesthesisten betreuten eigenen Patientengut ist dabei doch immer an die Möglichkeit von allergischen oder gar anaphylaktischen Reaktionen zu denken [5].

Im Hinblick auf die zunehmende Inbetriebnahme neuer EMI Scanner dürfen für den Anaesthesisten relevante organisatorische Probleme nicht übersehen werden. Dazu gehört eine großzügige Planung des Untersuchungsraumes sowie das Vorhandensein eines mit zentralen Leitungsanschlüssen ausgestatteten Einleitungsraumes.

In Anbetracht der je nach Örtlichkeiten mehr oder weniger großen Zahl von akuten Traumapatienten mit Schädel-Hirn-Verletzung stellt der Transport, sei es von der Notfallstation zum Scan Labor oder vom Scanner in den Operationssaal, eine Phase mit Risiken dar. Die Berücksichtigung von möglichst kurzen Transportwegen bei der Planung ist daher von Vorteil.

Zusammenfassung

Zur optimalen Ausnützung der cerebralen Computertomographie mit dem EMI Scanner ist eine absolut ruhige Lage des Kopfes während des Abtastvorganges erforderlich. Bei motorisch unruhigen bewußtlosen Patienten, bei unkooperativen Patienten sowie bei Kindern unter sechs Jahren ist in der Regel ein Anaesthesieverfahren zur Ruhigstellung notwendig. Mit der Einführung eines EMI Scanners der 2. Generation konnten wir dessen Auswirkungen auf den Untersuchungsverlauf und Anaesthesie im Vergleich zum EMI der 1. Generation abklären.

Unter dem neuen EMI Scanner ergaben sich deutlich kürzere Scan- und Anaesthesiezeiten; seine weit besseren Lagerungsbedingungen erlauben es bei nicht traumatisierten Patienten einschließlich Kindern weitgehend auf eine Intubationsnarkose zu verzichten. Als geeignetes Anaesthesieverfahren hat sich uns die fraktionierte Althesingabe beim Erwachsenen sowie die Ketaminnarkose bei Kindern ohne Hirndruckzeichen erwiesen. Bei traumatisierten Patienten hat sich uns eine Intubationsnarkose mit Thiopental, einem nicht depolarisierenden Muskelrelaxans und Sauerstoff bewährt.

Literatur

1. Aidinis SJ, Zimmerman RA, Shapiro HM, Bilanvick LT, Broennle AM (1976) Anesthesia for brain computer tomography. Anesthesiology 44:420–425
2. Ambrose J (1973) Computerized transverse axial scanning (tomography) Part Z Clinical application. Brit J Radiol 46:1023–1047
3. Anderson RE, Soborn AG (1977) Efficacy of simple sedation for pediatric computer tomography. Radiol 124:739–740

 4. Cordes RA, Eagle T (1978) Near drowing: a complication of computerized axial tomography of the head. Anesth Analg 57:358–360
 5. Elke M, Ferstl A (1974) Notfallsituationen in der Röntgendiagnostik. Georg Thieme Stuttgart
 6. Ferrer-Brechner Th, Winter J (1977) Anesthetic considerations for cerebral computer tomography. Anesth Analg 56:344–347
 7. Michenfelder JD, Theye RA (1973) Cerebral protection by thiopental during hypoxia. Anesthesiology 39:510–517
 8. Shapiro HM (1975) Elevated Intracranial Pressure. Anesthesiology 43:455
 9. Stuart HO (1979) Total intravenous anesthesia for computerized axial tomography. Anesthesia 34: 509–512
10. Weidler DJ (1974) Myocardial damage and cardiac arrhythmias after intracranial hemorrhage. Stroke 5:759–764
11. Weisberg LA (1979) CT and acute head trauma Computerized tomography. 3:15–28
12. Welborn SG (1976) Anesthesia for emi scanning in infants and small children. South Med J 69: 1294–1295

Wann hat Fentanyl einen atemdepressiven Effekt?

H. Stoeckel, J. Schüttler und J.H. Hengstmann

Bei 10 Probanden wurde die atemdepressive Wirkung nach Bolusinjektion von 0,5 mg Fentanyl untersucht und über einen Zeitraum von 4 Stunden gemessen: spirometrische Größen, in- und exspiratorische Strömungsgeschwindigkeit, endexspiratorischer CO_2, Blutgasanalysen sowie die CO_2-Antwort mittels Rückatmungsversuch. Zusätzlich wurden die Fentanylkonzentrationen im Serum radioimmunologisch bestimmt.

Es zeigte sich folgendes Verhalten der Atmungsgrößen:

1. Eine starke primäre Atemdepression, die nach ca. 4 Minuten z.T. in einer Apnoe resultierte;

2. Eine geringer ausgeprägte Atemdepression, die zu unterschiedlichen Zeitintervallen nach Injektion sekundär auftritt und mit einem Fentanyl-Rebound gut korrelierte.

3. Eine Verminderung der „Erregbarkeit" des Atemzentrums zeigte sich im Rückatmungsversuch durch eine Parallelverschiebung und Steigungsänderung der CO_2-Antwortkurve.

Continuous Infusion of Ketamine for Thoracic Surgery Using One-lung Ventilation

G. Silvay, A. Weinreich, P. Lumb and H. Shiang

The study was undertaken to determine whether ketamine could be used during one lung anesthesia as an alternative to the commonly used halothane, for the following reasons: 1. In abolishing ventilation to the upper lung, the hypoxic vasoconstrictor reflex is initiated and blood is shunted to the well ventilated, dependent lung. However, the volatile anesthetic agents abolish this reflex and permit the return of pulmonary blood flow to this nonventilated region producing a true intrapulmonary shunt with unacceptably low PaO_2 in 20% of cases. The intravenous anesthetic agents appear not to have this effect. 2. Depressive effect of halothane on cardiac output and venous desaturation. 3. The potential hepato-toxic effect of halothane enhanced by: a) previous radiotherapy, or chemotherapy; b) repeated halothane anesthesia; c) elevated liver function tests. 4. The immunosuppressive action of halothane in cancer surgery. 5. Operating room pollution with halothane. 6. The effect of 100% oxygen on shunt fraction. Anesthetic technique: Seventy-five unselected patients for thoracotomy, using an endobronchial technique were anesthetized with ketamine 2 mg/kg, preceded by diazepam and droperidol i.v. and maintained on continuous ketamine, 2 mg/kg per hour, by means of an IVAC infusion pump supplement by 50% N_2O/O_2 and incremental doses of d-tubocurarine. Arterial cannulation was routinely employed for continuous monitoring of systemic pressure and blood gas analysis. In 25 of these patients, mixed venous samples were obtained and the shunt fractions calculated.

All patients made uneventful post-operative recoveries. Significant elevation of arterial blood pressures (above 20 torr) did not occur, and there were no instances of emergence delirium, hallucinations or dreams recalled by patients. In all cases the arterial saturation remained above 90%, and the mean shunt fraction was 23.2% at FiO_2 0.5.

It is suggested that ketamine provides a satisfactory alternative to halothane in patients where the preoperative PaO_2 values are low or where relative hypoxemia intraoperatively might be unacceptable, as in patients with cerebrovascular or myocardial insufficiency, or anemia.

Freie Themen
Allgemeinanaesthesie (Teil 2)

Vorsitz: H. Lutz und H.W. Opderbecke

Gegenüberstellung der Plasmakatecholaminwerte bei Halothan-N$_2$O-Anaesthesie und NLA

D. Balogh, H. Hortnagel, A. Hammerle, Th. Brücke und R. Stadler-Wolffersgrün

Einleitung

Die Halothan-N$_2$O-Anaesthesie und die NLA zählen heute zu den gebräuchlichsten Anaesthesieverfahren, deshalb erscheint eine genaue Kenntnis ihrer Wirkung auf das vegetative Nervensystem von großer Bedeutung.

Das Ziel unserer Untersuchung war es, einen weiteren Einblick in den Funktionszustand des sympathischen Nervensystems und dessen Auswirkung auf Blutdruck und Herzfrequenz bei diesen beiden Anaesthesieverfahren zu gewinnen.

Patienten und Methodik

Die Untersuchung wurde an 2 Gruppen von je 10 Patienten mit ausgedehnten abdominellen Eingriffen durchgeführt. Die durchschnittliche Operations-Dauer lag zwischen 2 1/2 und 3 h.

Halothan-N$_2$O-Anaesthesie

Bei Halothan-N$_2$O-Anaesthesie erfolgte die Prämedikation mit 1 mg Pethidin/kg KG und 0,5 mg Atropin i.m. 1 h vor Operations-Beginn. Zur Einleitung wurden etwa 3,5 mg Thiopental/kg KG injiziert. Zur Intubation wurden 1 mg Suxamethonium/kg KG verabreicht, zur weiteren Muskelrelaxierung wurde Alcuronium mit einer Initialdosis von 0,2 mg/kg KG verwendet, bei Bedarf wurde nachinjiziert. Die Anaesthesie wurde mit N$_2$O-O$_2$ im Verhältnis 2:1 und Halothan, bei einem mittleren Halothanindex von 0,67%, weitergeführt.

Neuroleptanalgesie

Die Prämedikation für die NLA erfolgte mit etwa 0,2 mg Piritramid/kg KG sowie 0,5 Atropin i.m. 1^h vor Operations-Beginn. Eingeleitet wurde mit 0,15 mg DHP/kg KG sowie etwa 7,5 μg Fentanyl/kg KG, anschließend wurde mit 0,25 mg Alcuronium/kg KG relaxiert und nach 3 Minuten N$_2$O-O$_2$-Beatmung intubiert. Die Anaesthesie wurde mit N$_2$O-O$_2$ im Verhältnis 2:1, sowie einer halbstündlichen i.v. Gabe von 0,1 mg Fentanyl fortgeführt, Alcuronium wurde bei Bedarf nachinjiziert.

Die Patienten beider Gruppen erhielten bei Operations-Ende 2 mg Neostigmin mit 0,5 mg Atropin i.v. Während der Operation wurde pro Stunde etwa 500 ml Ringerlactat oder 5% Glukose zugeführt. Blutverluste bis 500 ml wurden mit 3,5% Humanalbuminlösung ersetzt, jeder weitere Blutverlust durch Bluttransfusionen.

Die Feststellung der Anaesthesietiefe ist bei vollrelaxierten Patienten nur schwer objektivierbar. Wir versuchten bei dieser Studie Herzfrequenz und Blutdruck möglichst konstant zu halten. Die Herzfrequenz wurde kontinuierlich am Oszillogramm verfolgt, der Blutdruck alle 5 Minuten manuell gemessen.

Die Blutabnahmen zur Bestimmung von A und NA erfolgten jeweils vor Einleitung der Anaesthesie, bei Operations-Beginn, 10 Minuten nach dem Schnitt, in der Folge halbstündlich sowie postoperativ 1 Stunde und 4 Stunden nach Operations-Ende.

Ergebnisse

Herzkreislaufparameter

In Abb. 1 (Halothan-N$_2$O) und Abb. 2 (NLA) sind Herzfrequenz sowie die Differenz des systolischen und diastolischen Blutdruckes vom jeweiligen Ausgangswert dargestellt.

In beiden Gruppen kam es initial zu einem Blutdruckabfall, im weiteren Verlauf der Anaesthesie wurde der Ausgangswert nahezu wieder erreicht. Bei der NLA allerdings rascher als bei Halothan-N$_2$O. Postoperativ lag der Blutdruck bei der NLA über dem Ausgangswert, während er bei Halothan-N$_2$O kaum davon abwich. Die Herzfrequenz blieb in beiden Gruppen relativ konstant, ein Frequenzabfall in der frühen postoperativen Phase könnte durch Neostigmin bedingt sein.

Plasmakatecholamine

Abb. 3 (Halothan-N$_2$O) und Abb. 4 (NLA) zeigen die intra- und postoperativen Adrenalin-(A) und Noradrenalinwerte (NLA).

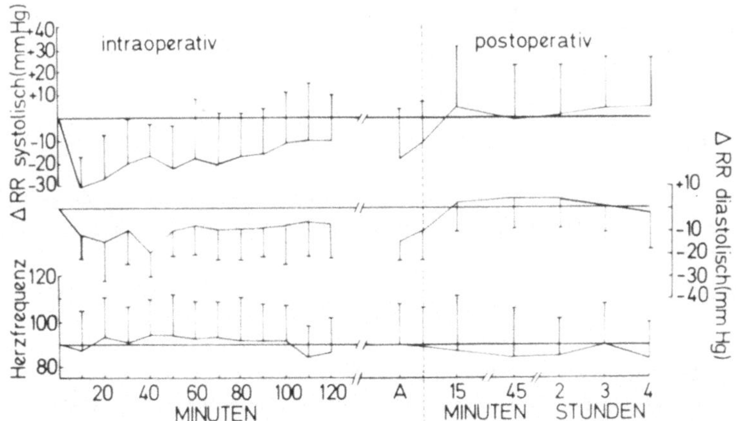

Abb. 1. Bei Halothan-N$_2$O-Anaesthesie. Herzfrequenz sowie Differenz des systolischen und diastolischen Blutdruckes vom jeweiligen Ausgangswert. Die Basislinien entsprechen dem errechneten mittleren Ausgangswert des systolischen (120 ± 40 mmHg) und des diastolischen (80 ± 11 mmHg) Blutdruckes und der Herzfrequenz (90 ± 13/min). Die strichlierte Linie deutet das Operationsende an. A = 10 min. vor Operationsende

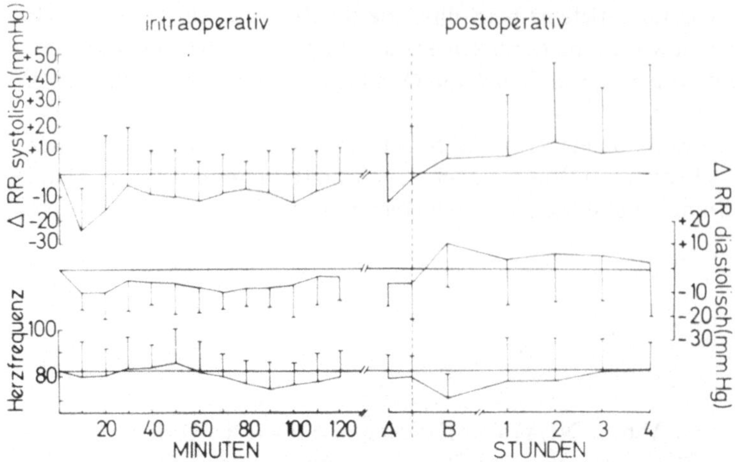

Abb. 2. Neuroleptanalgesie. Herzfrequenz sowie Differenz des systolischen und diastolischen Blutdruckes vom jeweiligen Ausgangswert. Die Basislinien entsprechen dem errechneten mittleren Ausgangswert des systolischen (130 ± 31 mmHg) und diastolischen (70 ± 27 mmHg) Blutdruckes und der Herzfrequenz (83 ± 12/min.). Die strichlierte Linie deutet das Operationsende an. A = 10 min. vor Operationsende, B = 15 min. nach Operationsende

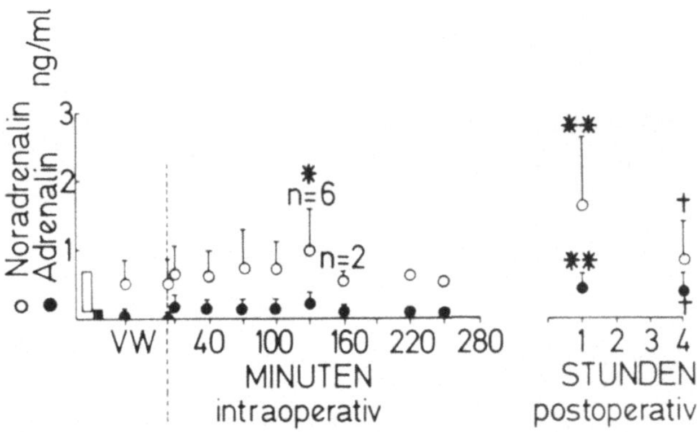

Abb. 3. Bei Halothan-N_2O-Anaesthesie. Mittelwerte des NA und A im Plasma. Die offene Säule zeigt den Normbereich für NA, die gefüllte Säule für A. Die strichlierte Linie markiert den Operationsbeginn VW = Vorwert, *p<0,02, **p<0,02, +p<0,05

Bei der Halothan-N_2O-Anaesthesie verändern sich die A-Werte kaum; bei NA kommt es intraoperativ zu einem geringfügigen kontinuierlichen, jedoch nicht signifikanten Anstieg. Postoperativ war sowohl A wie NA signifikant gegenüber dem Ausgangswert erhöht.

Bei der NLA fällt sofort der von der Operationsdauer abhängige kontinuierliche NA-Anstieg auf; auch bei der A kommt es schon intraoperativ zu einem signifikanten Anstieg, der jedoch unabhängig von der Operationsdauer ist. Postoperativ besteht kein wesentlicher Unterschied gegenüber der Halothan-N_2O-Gruppe [1, 4].

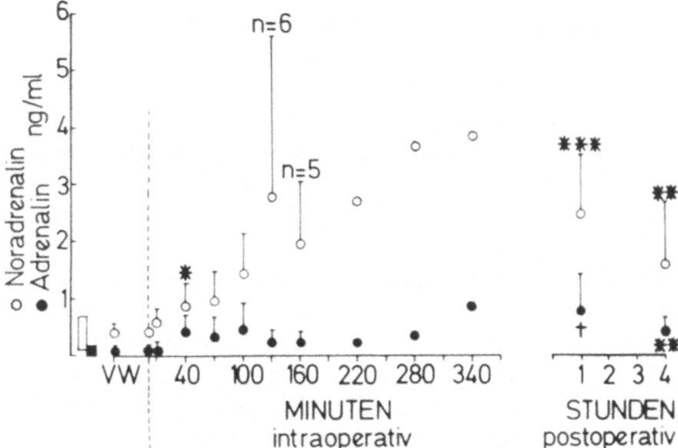

Abb. 4. Bei Neuroleptanalgesie. Mittelwerte des NA und A im Plasma. Die offene Säule zeigt den Normbereich für NA, die gefüllte für A. Die strichlierte Linie markiert den Operationsbeginn. VW = Vorwert, *p<0,01, **p<0,01, ***p<0,001, ⁺p<0,02

Diskussion

Die Ergebnisse dieser Untersuchung zeigen, daß zwei vergleichbare kombinierte Allgemeinanaesthesien ein unterschiedliches Verhalten des sympathischen Nervensystems auslösen [2, 5].

Durch wiederholte intraoperative Messung konnten wir erstmals zeigen, daß insbesondere die NA-Konzentration bei der NLA mit der Dauer der Operation zunimmt. Dies könnte einerseits dadurch bedingt sein, daß die Dosis von Fentanyl, die im Verlauf der Operation nachinjiziert wurde für die Aufrechterhaltung der anfänglich bestehenden Analgesie nicht ausgereicht hat, andererseits aber auch, daß bei der NLA eine Anpassung an den momentanen Operationsreiz viel schwerer möglich ist als bei Inhalationsnarkotika [6, 7].

Wie wiederholt beschrieben [10, 13, 14] blieb auch in unserer Untersuchung Herzfrequenz und Blutdruck im Wesentlichen konstant und geben so nur eine geringe Aussage über die tatsächliche Aktivität des sympathischen Nervensystems. Es läßt sich an Hand dieser Parameter nur schwer feststellen, ob die Narkosetiefe ausreicht, den Organismus vor dem Operations-Streß zu schützen [3, 8].

Da die Höhe der NA-Konzentration bei NLA von der Dauer der Operation abhängt, erhebt sich die Frage, ob gerade bei Risikopatienten langdauernde Eingriffe in NLA durchgeführt werden sollen [12, 14]. Ich möchte hier auf die Untersuchungen von Knitza und Ma [9] hinweisen, wo die Auswirkungen der NLA auf den Stoffwechsel aufgezeigt werden. Die Tatsache, daß die Aktivierung des sympathischen Nervensystems nicht mit einer entsprechenden Erhöhung von Herzfrequenz und Blutdruck einhergeht, sollte nicht darüber hinwegtäuschen, daß möglicherweise andere Systeme wie z.B. der Stoffwechsel davon betroffen werden.

Literatur

1. Ahnefeld FW, Frey R (1965) Untersuchungen über den Plasmakatecholaminspiegel nach Operationen und Traumen. Anaesthesist 14:36
2. Betléri I (1970) Katecholaminbestimmungen während verschiedener Narkoseverfahren. Anaesth 19:257

3. Edmonds-Seal J, Prys-Roberts C (1970) Pharmacology of drugs used in neuroleptanalgesia. Br J Anaesth 42:207
4. Eisele R, Lohmann W, Kötter D, Nasseri M (1974) Das Verhalten der Plasmakatecholamine nach Bauchoperationen beim Menschen. Langenbecks Arch Chir 336:103
5. Gött U, Klensch H (1970) Plasmakatecholaminänderungen bei verschiedenen Anaesthesietechniken. In: Neue klinische Aspekte der Neuroleptanalgesie. Schattauer, Stuttgart New York
6. Hamelberg W, Sprouse JH, Mahaffey JE, Richardson JA (1960) Catecholamine levels during light and deep anesthesia. Anaesthesiology 21:297
7. Halter JB, Pflug AE, Porte D (1977) Mechanism of plasma catecholamine increases during surgical stress in man. J Clin Endocrinol Metab 45:936
8. Havers L, Kreppel E (1966) Über die Wirkung der Neuroleptanalgesie auf die sympathische Aktivität. Acta Anaesthesiol Scand 23:12
9. Knitza R, Obermann M, Fischer F, Bässler KH (1978) Kreislaufverhalten, Blutgasanalysen, Säure-Basen- und Stoffwechselveränderungen unter Neuroleptanalgesie mit und ohne Betarezeptorenblocker bei der Elektrokoagulation des Ganglion Gasseri. Anaesth 27:213
10. Nikki P, Takki S, Tammisto T, Jäättelä A (1972) Effects of operative stress on plasma catecholamine levels. Ann Clin Res 4:146
11. Prys-Roberts C, Gersh BJ, Baker AB, Reuben SR (1972) The effects of halothane on the interactions between myocardial contractility, aortic impedence and left ventricular performance. I. Theoretical considerations and results. Br J Anaesth 44:634
12. Stoelting RK, Gibbs PS, Creasser CW, Peterson C (1975) Hemodynamic and ventilatory responses to fentanyl, fentanyldroperidol, and nitrous oxide in patients with aquired valvular heart disease. Anaesthesiology 42:319
13. Taggart P, Hedworth-Whitty R, Carruthers M, Gordon PD (1976) Observations on electrocardiogram and plasma catecholamines during dental procedures: The forgotten vagus. Br Med J 2:787
14. Tammisto T, Takki S, Nikki P, Jäättelä A (1973) Effect of operative stress on plasma catecholamine levels during neuroleptanalgesia. Anaesthesist 22:158

Zur Frage des Einflusses einer Enflurananaesthesie auf das intra- und postoperative Verhalten der Plasma-Renin-Aktivität sowie von Plasma-Aldosteron und Plasma-Cortisol bei orthopädischen Eingriffen

G. Hack, V. Pless und H. Vetter

Bisher veröffentlichte Studien über die Plasma-Renin-Aktivität (PRA) unter verschiedenen Anaesthesie- und Operationsbedingungen haben zu teilweise divergenten Ergebnissen geführt [1, 7, 11, 13, 14]. Besondere Aktualität gewinnt diese Fragestellung im Hinblick auf die Beobachtung, daß Angiotensin-Antagonisten wie das Saralasin im Tierexperiment unter Halothan- und Enflurananaesthesie einen Blutdruckabfall zu induzieren vermögen, dagegen nicht unter Fluroxen- oder Ketamin-Narkose [7].

In früheren Studien [13] fanden wir unter normotensiver Halothannarkose über den Normbereich hinaus erhöhte Werte für die Plasma-Renin-Aktivität, das Plasma-Aldosteron (PA) und Plasma-Cortisol (PC). In Weiterführung dieser Untersuchungen sollte in der vorliegenden Arbeit Aufschluß über das Verhalten des Renin-Angiotensin-Aldosteron-Systems (RAAS) unter Enfluran/N_2O-Anaesthesie gewonnen werden. Die zusätzliche Bestimmung von Plasma-Cortisol sollte darüber Auskunft geben, inwieweit die ACTH-Sekretion an der Regulation des PA-Spiegels beteiligt ist.

Zur Untersuchung kamen 10 weibliche und 5 männliche, endokrin gesunde Patienten im Alter von 19—39 Jahren, welche sich orthopädischen Eingriffen von im Durchschnitt 85 Minuten Dauer im Bereich der unteren Wirbelsäule oder der Extremitäten unterziehen mußten.

Zur Prämedikation erhielten die Kranken ausnahmslos 10—20 mg Diazepam am Vorabend sowie 0,5 mg Atropin und 2 ml Thalamonal 1 Stunde vor Narkosebeginn. Die Anaesthesie wurde mit 1 mg Brevimytal/kg KG intravenös eingeleitet und nach Intubation (3—6 mg d-Tubocurarin + 75—100 mg Succinyldicholin) mit einem Enfluran/N_2O/O_2-Gemisch bei im Durchschnitt 1,5 MAC unter Normoventilation aufrechterhalten.

Zur perioperativen Infusionstherapie verwendeten wir 5%ige Glucose, Ringerlösung und Kolloide, letztere in der Regel bereits präoperativ zur Aufrechterhaltung einer Normovolämie. Die Gesamt-Na^+-Zufuhr belief sich bei diesem Infusionsschema auf durchschnittlich 1,1 mval Na^+/kg Körpergewicht/h Op-Zeit. Schwankungen des Blutdrucks überstiegen nicht 15% des Ausgangswertes.

Am präoperativen Tag wurde gegen 8.00 Uhr morgens nach Bettruhe die basale PRA, das PA, PC sowie der Serum-Na^+ und -K^+-Wert ermittelt (Abb. 1). Eine 2. Bestimmung erfolgte nach 2stündiger Orthostase und zusätzlicher Stimulation der PRA durch 40 mg Furosemid. Am Op-Tag erfolgten Hormonanalysen vor und nach der Prämedikation, 30 Minuten nach Narkosebeginn vor dem Hautschnitt, intraoperativ in 15—30 Minuten Abstand sowie postoperativ 1, 2 und 3 Stunden nach Op-Ende. Weitere Bestimmungen führten wir jeweils nach einer nächtlichen Ruheperiode am 1., 3., 6. und 9. postoperativen Tag durch.

Die PRA wurde radioimmunologisch nach Haber et al. [5] ermittelt (Normbereich: 0,3—3 ng/ml · 3 h), PA bestimmten wir ebenfalls mittels Radioimmunoassay nach Vetter et al.

<u>Modus der Blutentnahmen:</u>

<u>1. Am Tage vor der OP:</u>

R   RUHEWERT gg. 8^{00} h
        (Plasma-Renin, -Aldosteron und -Cortisol,
        sowie Serum-Na^+ und -K^+)
        Anschließend Injektion von 40 mg Lasix ^{R} i. v.
S   nach STIMULATION

<u>2. Am OP-Tag:</u>
VP   Vor Prämedikation
NP   Nach Prämedikation (kurz vor Narkoseeinleitung)
NA   Nach Narkoseeinleitung (vor OP-Beginn)
OP   Ab OP-Beginn in Abständen von 15-30 Min. (Je nach Dauer)

1.   Std.
2.   Std.
3.   Std.   nach OP-Ende

<u>3. Postoperative Tage:</u>
1.   Tag   Serum-Na^+ und K^+-Kontrolle
3.   Tag
6.   Tag
9.   Tag   nach OP

Abb. 1. Übersicht über die Zeitpunkte der Blutentnahmen zur Bestimmung von Plasma-Renin-Aktivität, Plasma-Aldosteron, Plasma-Cortisol sowie Serum-Natrium und -Kalium

[12] (Normbereich: 20–120 pg/ml) und die PC-Analysen erfolgten nach der Methode von Murphy et al. [9] (Normbereich: 2–25 µg/100 ml).

Auf Abb. 2 ist das Verhalten der PRA während der verschiedenen Abnahmezeitpunkte dargestellt. Die Gerade markiert hier wie auf den beiden folgenden Abbildungen die obere Grenze des Normbereiches. Der Stimulationstest am präoperativen Tag führte zu einer deutlichen Zunahme der PRA, während sich unter dem Einfluß der Prämedikation eine leichte, wenn auch nicht signifikante Abnahme des Hormonspiegels nachweisen ließ. 30 Minuten nach Einleitung der Anaesthesie findet sich unter 1,5 MAC Enfluran + Na_2O/O_2 eine gegenüber dem Wert nach Prämedikation (NP) 2fach höhere PRA, welche bei zusätzlichem Op-Trauma nicht weiter zunimmt. Postoperativ bleibt die PRA am 1. und 3. Tag mittelgradig, am 6. und 9. Tag nurmehr leicht erhöht.

Die PA-Werte korrespondierten, wie aus Abb. 3 zu entnehmen ist, weitgehend mit der jeweils ermittelten PRA: Zunahme nach Stimulation, dämpfender Effekt der Prämedikation auf die Aldosteron-Sekretion, deutliche Anstiege 30 Minuten nach Einleitung der Enfluran-Anaesthesie sowie unter zusätzlichem Op-Streß. Postoperativ zeigten sich mäßig erhöhte Werte bis zum 6. postoperativen Tag.

Grundlegend anders verhielt sich das PC (Abb. 4): Die Werte blieben nicht nur, wie dies auch von anderen Autoren beschrieben wurde, unter alleiniger Enflurananaesthesie unverändert, sondern lagen auch bei zusätzlichem Op-Trauma bei deutlichem Aufwärtstrend um im Durchschnitt 50% gegen Ende des Eingriffs sowie während der ersten 3 postoperativen Stunden unterhalb der oberen Normbereichsgrenze.

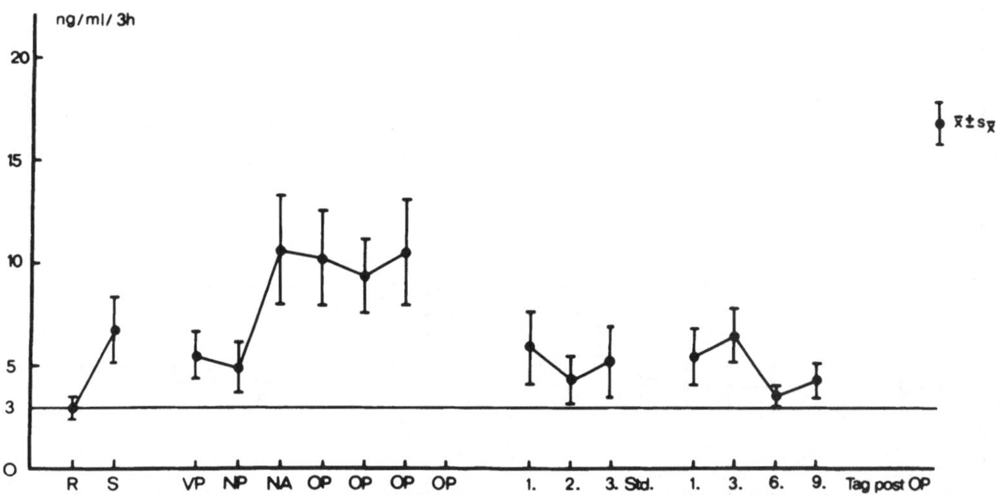

Abb. 2. Mittelwerte und Standardabweichungen der Mittelwerte für die Plasma-Renin-Aktivität (PRA) während der verschiedenen Abnahmezeitpunkte. Obere Normbereichsgrenze: 3 ng/ml · 3 h

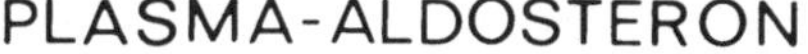

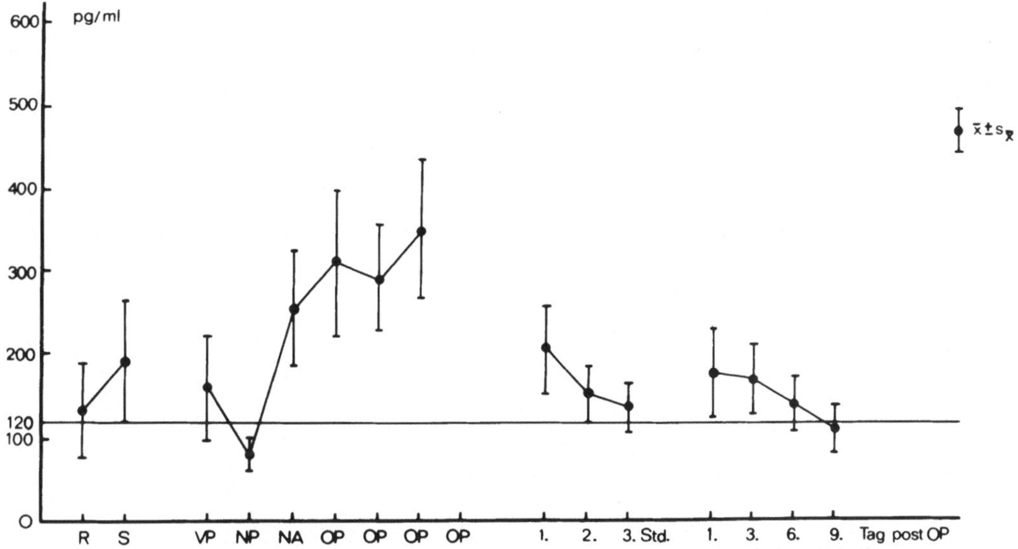

Abb. 3. Mittelwerte und Standardabweichungen der Mittelwerte für das Plasma-Aldosteron (PA) während der verschiedenen Abnahmezeitpunkte. Obere Normbereichsgrenze: 120 pg/ml

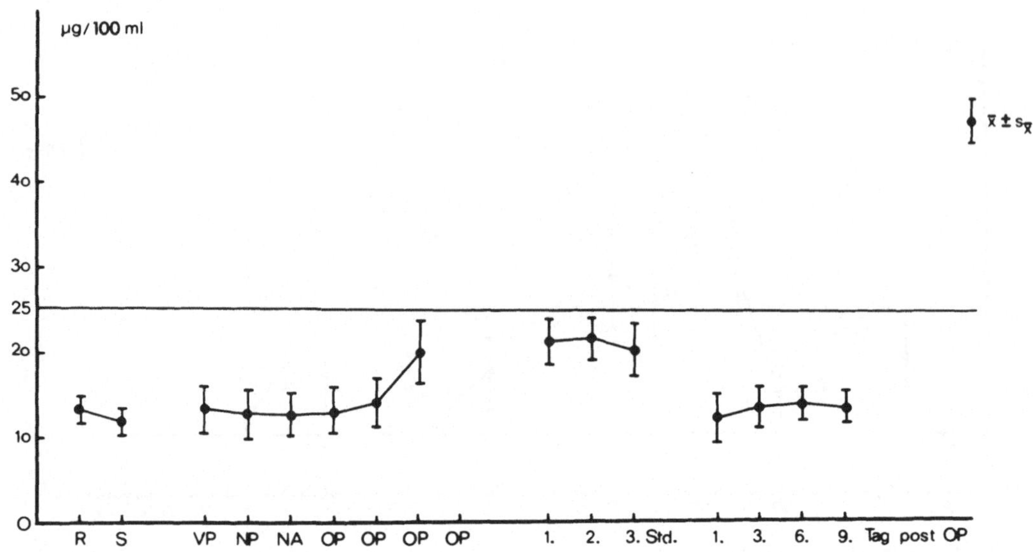

Abb. 4. Mittelwerte und Standardabweichungen der Mittelwerte für Plasma-Cortisol (PC) während der verschiedenen Abnahmezeitpunkte. Obere Normbereichsgrenze: 25 µg/100 ml

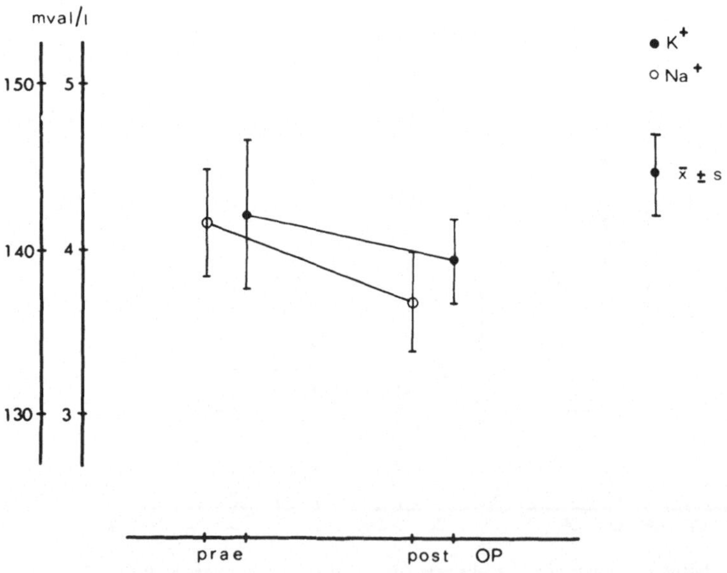

Abb. 5. Mittelwerte für Serum-Natrium und -Kalium am präoperativen sowie 1. postoperativen Tag

Ein Vergleich der Serum-Elektrolyte Na^+ und K^+ (Abb. 5) am präoperativen und 1. postoperativen Tag zeigt eine geringe Abnahme um 4,8 mval/l für Na^+ sowie 0,3 mval/l für K^+.

Auf die abschließende Diskussion unserer Befunde kann im Rahmen dieses Vortrages nur kurz eingegangen werden:

1. Die von uns nachgewiesene Erhöhung der PRA unter Enfluran erklärt sich aus der Änderung der Nierenhämodynamik: So fanden Cousins et al. [2] bei 1,0 MAC Enfluran eine Reduktion der Nierendurchblutung sowie der GFR auf 77 bzw. 79% des Kontrollwertes. Die nur geringen Abnahmen der Serumspiegel von Natrium und Kalium vom präoperativen zum 1. postoperativen Tag machen eine Stimulation der Reninfreisetzung über die Chemoreceptoren der Macula densa in diesem Zeitraum wenig wahrscheinlich. Nach Studien von Ganong [3] am Hund muß die Serum-Natrium-Konzentration wenigstens um 20 mval/l fallen, um einen Reiz auf die Reninsekretion zu bewirken. Postoperativ, möglicherweise auch intraoperativ muß dagegen zusätzlich eine katecholamininduzierte Erhöhung der PRA angenommen werden, wenngleich hohe Enflurankonzentrationen die Katecholamin-Freisetzung aus dem Nebennierenmark zu hemmen vermögen [4].

2. Aus der fehlenden Korrespondenz von PA- und PC-Werten geht hervor, daß die unter Enfluran erhöhten PA-Spiegel nicht ACTH-bedingt sind, die Aldosteronsekretion somit ausschließlich über das Renin-Angiotensin-System getriggert wird. Neben einer vermehrten Sekretion aus der Nebennierenrinde muß grundsätzlich als weitere Ursache für die von uns nachgewiesenen erhöhten PA-Werte eine verminderte metabolische Clearancerate für Aldosteron in der Leber diskutiert werden. Inwieweit mögliche Änderungen der Leberdurchblutung unter Enfluran, wie sie für Halothan nachgewiesen wurden, zu einer klinisch relevanten Abnahme der Aldosteron-Metabolisierungsrate führen können, ist unseres Wissens nicht bekannt.

3. Überrascht haben uns die auch bei zusätzlichem Op-Trauma im Normbereich liegenden PC-Werte, wenngleich von der 30. Op-Minute an ein deutlicher Trend zur Erhöhung nachweisbar war. Im Gegensatz zu kürzlich veröffentlichten Befunden der Mainzer Arbeitsgruppe [6] sowie von Oyama et al. [10], welche die PC-Spiegel unter Enfluran und großen abdominalchirurgischen Operationen untersuchten, waren die von uns herangezogenen orthopädischen Eingriffe mit erheblich kürzerer Op-Zeit im Bereich der unteren Wirbelsäule oder der Extremitäten vom Streß-Ausmaß her offensichtlich zu gering, um eine vermehrte ACTH- und damit Cortisol-Sekretion zu induzieren.

Literatur

1. Bailey DR, Miller ED Jr, Kaplan JA, Rogers PW (1975) The renin-angiotensin-aldosterone system during cardiac surgery with morphine-nitrous oxide anesthesia. Anesthesiology 42:538
2. Cousins MJ, Greenstein LR, Hitt BA, Mazze RI (1976) Metabolism and renal effects of enflurane in man. Anesthesiology 44:44
3. Ganong WF (1969) Review of medical physiology. 4th edition, Lange Medical Publications, Los Altos, California
4. Göthert M, Wendt J (1977) Inhibition of adrenal medullary catecholamine secretion by enflurane: I. Investigations in vivo. Anesthesiology 46:400
5. Haber E, Koerner T, Page LB, Kliman B, Purnode A (1969) Application of a radioimmunoassay for angiotensin I to the physiologic measurements of plasma renin activity in normal human subjects. J clin Endocrin 29:1349
6. Lanz E, Sinterhauf K, Müller T, Bregenzer M (1979) Enflurane-Narkose und Plasma-Cortisol. Anästhesist 28:111

7. Miller ED Jr, Bailey DR, Kaplan JA, Rogers PW (1975) The effect of ketamine on the renin-angiotensin system. Anesthesiology 42:503
8. Miller MD Jr, Longnecker DE, Peach MJ (1978) The regulatory function of the renin-angiotensin system during generel anesthesia. Anesthesiology 48:399
9. Murphy BEP, Pattee OJ (1964) Determination of plasma corticoids by competitive protein-binding analysis using gel filtration. J clin Endocr 24:919
10. Oyama T, Matsuki A, Kudo T (1972) Effects of ethrane anesthesia and surgery on adrenocortical function. Can Anaesth Soc J 19:394
11. Robertson D, Michelakis AM (1972) Effects of anesthesia and surgery on plasma renin activity in a man. J clin Endocr Metab 34:831
12. Vetter W, Vetter H, Siegenthaler W (1973) Radioimmunoassay for aldosterone without chromatography. Acta Endocr 74:548
13. Vetter H, Hack G, Marx M, Witassek F (im Druck) Effects of anaesthesia and surgery on the renin-angiotensin-aldosterone-system. In: Stoeckel H, Oyama T: Endocrinology in anaesthesia and surgery. Anästhesiologie und Intensivmedizin. Springer, Berlin Heidelberg New York
14. Wernze HM, Hilenhaus I, Rietbrock, Schüttke R, Kühn K (1975) Plasma-Renin-Aktivität und Plasma-Aldosteron unter Narkose sowie Operationsstreß und Beta-Receptoren-Blockade. Anästhesist 24:471

Evaluation of Blutorphanol (Stadol) as a Supplement to Balanced Anesthesia in Cesarian Section

H. Henriksen, T.K. Abboud and M. Shnider

Butorphanol tartrate is a new potent, synthetic parenteral analgesic with low addictive properties. At high doses it produces less respiratory depression than equi-analgesic doses of morphine or meperidine. It has received extensive clinical trials for relief of post-operative and chronic pain. It has been reported to be safe effective supplement to nitrous oxide-relaxant anesthesia in non-obstetric operations. Studies have not previously been done to evaluate the efficacy, safety and side effects of butorphanol as a supplement to nitrous oxide for cesarian section anesthesia.

Approximately 100 patients undergoing cesarian section under nitrous oxide-relaxant anesthesia were studied. Ventilation was controlled through-out the operation. Immediately after delivery of the baby, nitrous oxide concentration was increased from 55 to 66%, and patients were given butorphanol 2 mg or alphaprodine 30 mg, with additional increments as needed. Blood pressure and heart rates were monitored. At completion of the operation, patients were evaluated for necessity of narcotic antagonists, time of awakening, emergence reactions, nausea and vomiting, other untoward side-effects, and amount of analgesic administered in the recovery room. At 24 to 48 hours, patients were interviewed to determine incidence of awareness of surgery, and their evaluation of the anesthetic.

In the 50 patients who received butorphanol (mean total dose 4.7 mg) there was no intraoperative hypotension and most patients awakened promptly (mean time 2.8 ± 5 min). Three patients required narcotic antagonist, none developed nausea or vomiting. One patient had dizziness, one had undesirable hallucinations, one had partial recall of the surgery. Butorphanol is an effective supplement to nitrous oxide-relaxant anesthesia and compares favorably to standard narcotics used in balanced anesthesia for cesarian section.

Das Verhalten der Streßhormone hGH und Cortisol unter verschiedener Fentanyl-Dosierung

J. Schüttler, H. Stoeckel und P.M. Lauven

Bei Patienten, die sich einer abdominellen Hysterektomie unterzogen, wurde eine Fentanyl-Infusion-Stickoxydul-Narkose durchgeführt. Bei der Fentanyl-Infusion verwendeten wir zwei unterschiedliche Dosierungsintervalle von 250 μg/min über 5 min zur Einleitung und von 9 μg/min zur Aufrechterhaltung der Narkose. Bei den Bolusinjektionen wurden Dosierungen von 7 μg/kg bis zu 30 μg/kg Körpergewicht gewählt. Gemessen wurden mittels Radioimmunoassay die Fentanylkonzentrationen sowie die hGH- und Cortisol-Spiegel im Serum.

Bei dem Nebennierenrindenhormon Cortisol ließ sich ausgehend von Werten, die im tageszeitlichen Normbereich lagen, ein kontinuierlicher Anstieg feststellen, der sich während und nach Operationen fortsetzte.

Bei den hGH-Konzentrationen fanden wir ein deutlich unterschiedliches Verhalten. Es kam 10 Minuten nach Narkosebeginn zu einem steilen Anstieg der Konzentrationen mit einem Maximum nach 60 Minuten. Der mittlere Anstieg belief sich auf das 100fache des Ausgangswertes. Anschließend zeigte sich während der Operation ein kontinuierlicher Abfall der hGH-Spiegel mit einer Halbwertszeit von 30 Minuten, der sich auch nach Ende der Narkose fortsetzte.

Die möglichen Ursachen für das unterschiedliche Verhalten der beiden Hormone im Serum bei verschiedener Dosierung werden diskutiert.

Anaesthesieprobleme bei Bifurkationsresektionen der Trachea

D. Balogh, E. Kornberger, E. Leitner und G.M. Salzer

Bifurkationsresektionen werden selten durchgeführt, und so bietet sich jedem Anaesthesisten nur selten die Gelegenheit, eigene Erfahrungen über Besonderheiten und Zwischenfälle bei diesen Operationen zu gewinnen. Wir möchten deshalb hier von 6 Eingriffen dieser Art berichten.

Sie sehen hier eine Tabelle (1) der operierten Patienten. Bei vier von ihnen wurde zusätzlich zur Bifurkation die rechte Lunge resiziert, bei einem wurde die Bifurkation mit dem rechten Oberlappen entfernt, beim letzten Fall handelt es sich um eine ausgedehnte Resektion der distalen Trachea. Es wurden verschiedene Anaesthesieverfahren gewählt; diesbezüglich hat es bei keinem nennenswerte Probleme gegeben.

Die Wahl des Narkotikums erscheint uns von untergeordneter Bedeutung, sie kann dem jeweiligen Allgemeinzustand, sowie etwaigen zusätzlichen Risikofaktoren angepaßt werden. Schwierigkeiten können eventuell entstehen, wenn zeitweise mit sehr hohem O_2-Anteil bzw.

Tabelle 1. Bifurkationsresektion. Charakterisierung der Patienten

	Alter Geschlecht	Art des Tumors	Durchgeführte Operation	Anästhesieverfahren	postoperative Komplikationen
1	60 a ♂	Zylindrom	Resektion Carina + re Lunge	Ketalar Fluothan O_2	Malacie li HB
2	64 a ♂	Carcinom	Resektion Carina + re Lunge	Fluothan $N_2O - O_2$	
3	59 a ♂	Carcinom	Resektion Carina + re Lunge	NLA	Sekretstau Anastomosen-Leck
4	34 a ♀	Zylindrom	Resektion Carina + re Lunge	Fluothan $N_2O - O_2$	
5	49 a ♂	Carcinom	Resektion Carina + re OL	NLA	
6	42 a ♀	Zylindrom	Resektion dist. Trachea Prothesen-interposition	NLA	

mit reinem O_2 beatmet wird, und man auf die analgetische Wirkung von Lachgas vorüberge-
hend verzichten muß.

Ein technisches Problem ist zweifellos die Beatmung während der Bifurkationsresektion,
die deshalb an Hand des detaillierten Operationsplans mit dem Chirurgen schon frühzeitig be-
sprochen werden sollte. Bei zwei unserer Patienten (Fall 1, 4) war mehrere Tage vor dem
Eingriff eine bronchoskopische Verkleinerung des Tumors notwendig, da sonst eine ausreichende endotracheale Beatmung während der Präparation, bis zur Durchtrennung der Trachea, nicht möglich gewesen wäre.

Intraoperativ haben wir die von Grillo [3] angegebene Methode angewandt. Bis zur Frei-
legung der Trachealbifurkation, wird in endotrachealer Intubationsnarkose operiert, dann
wird der linke Hauptbronchus im Bereich der pars membranacea durchtrennt und ein steriler
Spiral-Tubus durch das Operations-Feld eingeführt, um so die Beatmung während der Bifurkationsresektion sicherzustellen. Nach Legen eines Teiles der Anastomosennähte wird der
Tubus wieder aus dem Operations-Feld entfernt, der in der Trachea verbliebene, wird nun
über die Anastomose in den Bronchus vorgeschoben. Nach Verschluß der Anastomose muß
der Tubus in die Trachea zurückgezogen werden, denn nur so kann die Dichte der Anastomo-
sennaht geprüft werden.

Bei dieser Vorgangsweise ist folgendes zu beachten: 1. daß bei der orotrachealen Intubation ein langer, schlanker Tubus mit schmalem Ballon, also ein Endobronchial-Tubus verwendet wird. Nur so ist das spätere Vorschieben in den Bronchus ohne Gefährdung der Anastomose möglich. 2. Für die Beatmung durch das Operations-Feld müssen mehrere Spiral-Tubus-
se in verschiedenen Größen mit passenden Zwischen- und Ansatzstücken, sowie Beatmungs-
schläuche steril vorbereitet werden. All das darf erst nach Beendigung der Operation unsteril
gemacht werden, da eine nochmalige Beatmung durch das Operations-Feld notwendig werden kann. Bei einem der vorher erwähnten Eingriffe (Fall 4) wurde der Ballon des orotrachealen Tubus bei den letzten Anastomosennähten durchstochen. Es konnte dann trotz ex-
tremer Flowerhöhung keine ausreichende Beatmung erzielt werden, so daß das nochmalige
Einführen des Tubus in den Bronchusstumpf notwendig wurde, um die in Seitenlage nicht
ganz leichte Umintubation vornehmen zu können. 3. Vor Durchtrennung des Bronchus muß
das gesamte sterile Beatmungssystem vorbereitet werden. Mit besonderer Sorgfalt soll der
Tubus ausgewählt, der Cuff geprüft und eventuell die Spitze unterhalb des Cuffes gekürzt
werden, damit sie keinen Lobärbronchus verschließt [2, 3, 4, 8].

Die Anwendung der extrakorporalen Zirkulation, die in einigen Publikationen angeführt
wird, erschien uns nie notwendig [1].

Das wesentliche Problem aber erscheint uns die postoperative Betreuung, die abermals
eine enge Zusammenarbeit zwischen Chirurg und Anaesthesisten erfordert. Wir glauben,
entgegen dem Wunsch der Chirurgen, daß eine postoperative Nachbeatmung in den meisten
Fällen notwendig ist, doch versuchen wir sie auf ein Mindestmaß zu reduzieren; (Blutgaswerte, Thoraxröntgen und jeweilige Kooperationsbereitschaft des Patienten sind unsere Kriterien). Zur Beatmung verwenden wir ein volumengesteuertes Gerät, achten aber genau darauf,
daß der Druck, wenn möglich 30 cm H_2O-Säule nicht überschreitet. Eine Druckbegrenzung
wie sie beim Engström möglich ist, erscheint uns hier sehr gut geeignet. Das Absaugen soll
mit weichen Saugern gemacht werden, und, wenn auskultatorisch kein Sekret festgestellt
wird, nur 1 X stündlich erfolgen. Bei einem unserer Patienten (Fall 3) mußten wir wegen
eines postoperativen Apoplex' mit Hemiparese besonders häufig absaugen, und mußten leider bei der Obduktion eine Perforation im Anastomosenbereich feststellen.

An Spätkomplikationen sahen wir 1 X eine Malazie des linken Hauptbronchus (Fall 1), die nur durch einen Tubus offen gehalten werden konnte. Seit 8 Jahren trägt der Patient einen Tubus zur Schienung des Bronchus, den er durch ein Tracheostoma selber wechselt. Eine seitliche Öffnung ist zur Ventilation des Oberlappenbronchus ausgeschnitten und eine zweite proximale ermöglicht dem Patienten das Sprechen [6].

Bei einigen unserer Patienten (Fall 2, 6) traten nach Wochen Atembeschwerden auf, die durch Granulome bedingt waren, die dann bronchoskopisch entfernt wurden. Die Patientin mit der Trachealresektion (Fall 6) hatte mehrmals dramatische Blutungen, die jedesmal eine Notintubation, Absaugen und anschließend maschinelle Beatmung notwendig machten.

Aus diesem Bericht ersehen Sie, daß die Bifurkationsresektion für den Anaesthesisten zahlreiche Probleme bieten kann. Sie sehen aber auch, daß diese Patienten zu den wenigen gehören, mit denen der Anaesthesist über längere Zeiträume in Kontakt bleibt. Wir achten darauf, daß ein Patient immer durch denselben Kollegen betreut wird, da nur so sich ein Vertrauensverhältnis zwischen Patient und Anaesthesist aufbauen läßt; was für den Patienten gerade bei Auftreten bedrohlicher Komplikationen sehr wichtig ist.

Literatur

1. Adkins PC, Izawa EM (1964) Resection of Tracheal Cylindroma using Cardiopulmonary Bypass. Arch Surg 88:405
2. Gefin B, Blaud J, Grillo HC (1969) Anaesthetic Management of Tracheal Resection and Reconstruction. Anaesth Analg Curr Res 48:884
3. Grillo HC, Bendixen HH, Gephart T (1963) Resection of the Carina and Lower Trachea. Ann Surg 158:889
4. Lee P, English JCW (1974) Management of Anaesthesia during Tracheal Resection. Anaesthesia 29: 305
5. Neville WE, Bolanowski P, Soltanzadeh H (1976) Prothetic Reconstruction of the Trachea and Carina. J thor cardiovasc surg 72:525
6. Salzer GM, Scharfetter H, Leitner E (1972) Resektion der Trachealbifurkation. Thoraxchirurgie 20: 107
7. Salzer GM (1974) Weitere Erfahrungen mit der Resektion der Trachealbifurkation. Thoraxchirurgie 22:147
8. Theman TE, Kerr JH, Nelems JM, Pearson FG (1976) Carinal resection. A report of two cases and a description of the anaesthetic technique. J of thoracic and cardiovasc Surg 71:314

Anaesthesierisiko bei urologischen Eingriffen an der Restniere

E. Salehi

Bei Ausfall einer Niere in Folge von Aplasie, Erkrankung oder Nephrektomie, übernimmt eine gesunde Restniere die Funktion zweier Nieren. Die Narkosebelastbarkeit dieser Patienten ist in der Regel nicht wesentlich eingeschränkt und bedeutet bei einem evtl. operativen Eingriff kein großes Risiko; vor allem dann nicht, wenn es sich nicht um einen urologischen Eingriff handelt. Dagegen ist der urologische Patient mit einer kranken Restniere nicht allein wegen des operativen Eingriffs, sondern vielmehr durch die Narkose als solche, potentiell gefährdet.

Der Anwendung der Narkosepharmaka sind hier Grenzen gesetzt, da
1. alle Narkosepharmaka primär oder sekundär die Nierenfunktion beeinflussen und
2. durch Anurie und Urämie bedingte Intoxikationen, die gesamten Vitalfunktionen in Mitleidenschaft ziehen und somit das Narkoserisiko erheblich erhöhen.

Vor allem folgende Risikofaktoren können die Wahl der Anästhesie erschweren:
1. Die psychische Belastung durch häufige Narkosen in kürzeren Abständen und die Sorge um den evtl. Verlust der Restniere.
2. Polimorbidität, vor allem kardiovaskuläre Erkrankungen und Stoffwechselstörungen.
3. Kurz- oder langfristig eingeleitete Therapien mit Analgetika, Diuretika, Antibiotika, Kardiaka, Antihypertensiva und Psychopharmaka.
4. Fieber bei septischer Niere, toxische Anämie und Flüssigkeitsansammlungen in den Hohlräumen.
5. Oligo-Anurie und deren Folgeerscheinungen sowie
6. hämodynamische Änderungen bei urologischen Operationslagerungen.

Eigene Erfahrungen

In den letzten 15 Jahren wurden an der Urologischen Klinik der RWTH Aachen 920 Anästhesien bei 300 Patienten mit Restniere in urämischem Zustand durchgeführt. Dabei entfielen 615 Anästhesien auf diagnostische und 305 auf große urologische Eingriffe (Tabelle 1). Die Restnierenfunktion war bei allen Patienten gestört und in mehr als 2/3 der Fälle total aufgehoben. 120 Patienten litten an einer septischen Restniere und mußten im septischen Schock operiert werden.

Anästhesie-Methodik

Prämedikation: In Anbetracht der Schwere der Erkrankung wurde bewußt auf die übliche Prämedikation mit Sedativa oder Psychopharmaka verzichtet. Unmittelbar vor Anästhesie-

Tabelle 1. Anästhesiemethoden bei 615 diagnostischen und 305 urologischen Operationen an der Restniere

Operationen	Anzahl der Anästhesien		
	NLA	Allgemein	Spinal
Diagnos. Eingriffe	50	195	370 = 615
Temporäre Nephrostomie	100	20	− = 120
Lithotomie	80	20	10 = 110
Nierenteilresektion	20	5	− = 25
Blasentumoroperation	15	−	10 = 25
Prostatektomie	5	−	15 = 20
Restnephrektomie	5	−	− = 5
Gesamt:	275	240	405 = 920

beginn, nach Kontrolle von Puls, Blutdruck und EKG (Monitoring) wurde bis zu 0,5 mg Atropin i.v. injiziert. Bei 50 Patienten wurde aufgrund der Tachykardie und schweren Herzrhythmusstörungen auf Anraten der Internisten auf Atropin verzichtet oder nur bei Absinken der Pulsfrequenz unter 50/min. verabreicht.

Unsere Anästhesien bei der Restniere unterteilen sich in zwei Gruppen:

Gruppe I: Die Anästhesie bei diagnostischen Eingriffen (Tabelle 2). 370 von 615 diagnostischen Eingriffen wurden in Spinalanästhesie, 50 in NLA und 195 in Allgemeinanästhesie durchgeführt. Die *Allgemeinanästhesie* wurde mit Penthobarbital (100−300 mg) oder mit Diazepam (10−20 mg) eingeleitet und anschließend mit Halothan (0,3−1,0 %) und N_2O/O_2 (6:3) fortgeführt. Die Atmung wurde spontan gehalten oder manuell unterstützt. Die Eingriffe dauerten zwischen 15 bis 40 Minuten. Die *Spinalanästhesie* wurde mit 2 ml Lidocain 5% hyperbar bei 140 diagnostischen Eingriffen vorgenommen und zwar bei Patienten, bei denen entweder eine Allgemeinanästhesie nicht zumutbar erschien oder bei denen der geplante Eingriff vermutlich länger als eine Stunde gedauert hätte. Die *Neuroleptanalgesien* fanden zwischen 1964 bis 1966 statt. Sie wurden ohne Muskelrelaxantien in Maskenbeatmung mit Droperidol (5−15 mg), Fentanyl (0,1−0,3 mg) und N_2O/O_2 durchgeführt.

Tabelle 2. Komplikationen nach diagnostischen Eingriffen an der Restniere (n = 615)

Komplikationen	Anästhesiemethoden		
	NLA (n = 50)	Allgemein (n = 195)	Spinal (n = 370)
Blutdruckabfall	10	25	130 = 165
Erbrechen	5	35	10 = 50
Ateminsuffizienz	2	5	− = 7
Verl. Aufwachphase	5	15	− = 20
Gesamt:	22	80	140 = 242

Tabelle 3. Komplikationen nach großen urologischen Eingriffen an der Restniere (n = 305)

Komplikationen	Anästhesiemethoden		
	NLA (n = 225)	Allgemein (n = 45)	Spinal (n = 35)
Kreislaufstillstand	9	2	– = 11
Postop. Ateminsuffizienz	20	5	– = 25
Lungenödem	2	–	– = 2
Gesamt:	31	7	– = 38

Gruppe II: Die Anästhesie bei großen urologischen Operationen (Tabelle 3). Sie umfassen 305 Eingriffe, die jeweils zwischen 90 und 300 Minuten dauerten. Dabei wurden die meisten Patienten (225) in NLA (Typ II), 45 in Allgemeinanästhesie und 35 in Spinalanästhesie operiert. Die Allgemeinanästhesie erfolgte mit Penthobarbital-Succinylcholin. Alloferin-Halothan und N_2O/O_2, die NLA wurde mit Droperidol-Fentanyl-Pancuroniumbromid und N_2O/O_2 durchgeführt. Sowohl die Patientengruppe der Allgemeinanästhesie als auch die der NLA wurde in mäßiger Hyperventilation kontrolliert mit Pulmonat der Firma Dräger beatmet. Die Spinalanästhesie erfolgte, wie oben, mit Lidocain 5% hyperbar.

Ergebnisse

Die diagnostischen Eingriffe verliefen ohne wesentliche Zwischenfälle. Intra- und postoperative Störungen wie Blutdruckabfall, Erbrechen, Atemstörungen oder verlängerte Aufwachphase traten in 242 Fällen (39,3%) auf, die nur zum Teil anästhesiebedingt waren. Sie konnten alle durch Gegenmaßnahmen (Volumensubstitution, Absaugen und O_2-Beatmung leicht behoben werden.

Bei den in Spinalanästhesie operierten Kranken in Gruppe II traten intra- und postoperativ, abgesehen von der zu erwartenden Hypotension, die durch rechtzeitige Volumensubstitution behoben werden konnte, keinerlei anästhesiebedingte Komplikationen auf, dagegen wurden bei 38 in NLA und Allgemeinanästhesie operierten Patienten ernsthafte Komplikationen registriert (Tabelle 3), die in 11 Fällen letal endeten. Als Ursache der Komplikationen kommen direkte Einwirkungen der Narkosepharmaka auf den Kreislauf und die Herzfunktion in Frage und zwar trat der Tod ein:
3 mal infolge Succinylcholinwirkung bei Serumkaliumwerten von 6–7,5 mval,
2 mal nach massiver Aspiration bei der Narkoseeinleitung und
6 mal postoperativ wegen septischen Schocks bei septischer Restniere.

Diskussion

Die Anästhesie bei Patienten mit Restniere in urämischem Zustand gehört zu den risikoreichsten Narkosen. Dies trifft vor allem dann zu, wenn es sich dabei um Eingriffe am Nierenparenchym handelt. Das Narkoserisiko ist umso höher, wenn die Patienten mit septischer Niere im septischen Schock operiert werden müssen.

Das Krankheitsbild der „septischen Niere" ist gekennzeichnet durch eine schwere Einschränkung des Allgemeinzustandes mit Zeichen des generalisierten Schocks. Ihren Ausgang nimmt die septische Niere häufig von einer infizierten Harnstauungsniere. Durch Urinstau kommt es zu einer Verminderung der Nierendurchblutung und zugleich zu einer explosionsartigen Vermehrung der virulenten Keime im Hohlsystem. Während des Eingriffs kommt es oft zur Ausschwemmung von Eiter und Endotoxin aus dem infektiösen Herd in die Blutbahn. Bakteriämie, miliare bakterielle Abzedierungen in andere Organe sind die Folge. Schon Manipulationen an der Niere während des Eingriffs können zum plötzlichen Kreislaufzusammenbruch führen.

Unsere Narkoseergebnisse zeigen, daß bei Kontraindikationen für die Regionalanästhesie **bei diagnostischen Eingriffen**, die kombinierte Diazepam- und Lachgas/Sauerstoff-Narkose und für große urologische Operationen, die NLA mit geringeren Risiken belastet sind. Besonders bei urologischen Eingriffen an der Restniere ließe sich das Narkoserisiko erheblich senken, wenn man bei der Anästhesie folgende Kriterien berücksichtigt:

1. Trotz gegebener Dringlichkeit sollte vor Beginn der Narkose der Säure-Basen-Haushalt reguliert und intra- und postoperativ überwacht werden.

2. Wegen Hyperkaliämie sollte auf Succinylcholin verzichtet und zur Relaxierung ausschließlich Pancuronium benutzt werden.

3. Bei Gebrauch von nicht-depolarisierenden Substanzen ist oft mit verlängerter Relaxationsdauer zu rechnen. Trotz ausreichender Spontanatmung nach vorheriger Antagonisierung kann es zur Abflachung der Spontanatmung oder Apnoe (Recurarisierung) kommen. Daher ist die intensive postoperative Überwachung mit oder ohne Beatmung dringend geboten.

4. Eine gleichzeitig ausgewogene Volumensubstitution und Diuresetherapie sollte durchgeführt werden.

5. Um hämodynamische Änderungen und damit einen zusätzlichen Risikofaktor zu vermeiden, sollte nach Möglichkeit der Eingriff in Rückenlage des Patienten vorgenommen werden, **wenn auch dies für den Operateur technisch schwierig ist (Abb. 1 und Tabelle 4).**

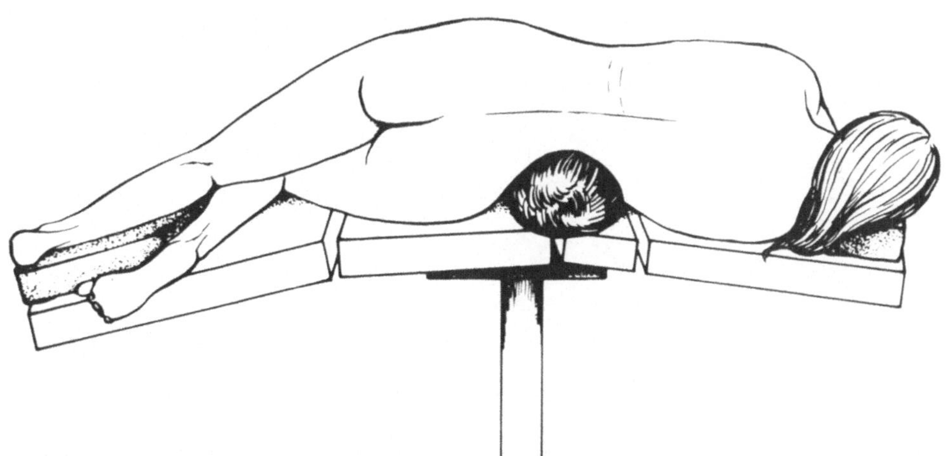

Abb. 1. Die geknickte Seitenlagerung zur Nephrektomie. Sie ist ausgesprochen kreislaufunfreundlich und bedeutet für poor-risk Patienten einen zusätzlichen Risikofaktor

Tabelle 4. Hämodynamische und respiratorische Änderungen während der Narkose bei der Nierenlagerung

 1. Der untere Hemithorax wird komprimiert und in seiner Motilität eingeschränkt
 2. Die kaudalen Rippen werden gegen die Wirbelsäule gedrückt
 3. Es kommt zum Hochstand und zur Behinderung der Beweglichkeit des Zwerchfells
 4. Die funktionelle Residualkapazität des unten liegenden Lungenflügels nimmt ab
 5. Das Atemzug- und Atemminutenvolumen nimmt bis zu 30% ab
 6. In der unteren Thoraxhälfte kommt es zu einem Mißverhältnis zwischen Ventilation und Zirkulation
 7. Die unteren Hohlvenen werden verzogen und angedrückt; es kommt zum Versacken von Blut in den unteren Extremitäten
 8. Der kompensierende Regulationsmechanismus des Sympathikus ist unterdrückt oder vollständig aufgehoben
 9. Die Verminderung des venösen Rückflusses und des Herzminutenvolumens führt zur Hypotonie
10. Diese Nachteile der Nierenlagerung sind dem ansonsten gesunden Organismus durchaus zuzumuten, haben aber schwerwiegende Folgen, wenn der Patient herz- oder lungenkrank ist

Zusammenfassung

Ebenso wie der urologische Eingriff an Patienten mit Restniere zu den Risiko-Operationen gehört, zählt auch die Anästhesie an diesen Patienten zu den Risiko-Narkosen. Dies hat vor allem Gültigkeit, wenn es sich dabei um Eingriffe am Nierenparenchym handelt. Das Risiko der Narkose ist hierbei noch höher, wenn die Patienten mit septischer Restniere in einem septischen Schock operiert werden müssen.

Es wird über die gewonnenen Erfahrungen bei 920 Anästhesien an 300 Patienten mit eingeschränkter oder aufgehobener Restnierenfunktion berichtet. Auf die Problematik der Anästhesie bei septischer Restniere und die zu erwartenden Komplikationen wird hingewiesen.

Combined Hypothermia and Barbiturate Therapy for Cerebrovascular Surgery

M. Belopavlovic and A. Buchthal

Introduction

The beneficial effect of high doses of barbiturates in cerebral ischaemia is well documented in experimental animals [1, 2, 3, 4]. Their action is dose-related and early administration after an ischaemic episode is clearly crucial. The best results might therefore be expected if barbiturate therapy precedes the ischaemic episode. There are now a few clinical reports of barbiturate therapy instituted after resuscitation from cardiac arrest [5], in head injury patients [6], and in metabolic coma [7]. Prompt administration under these conditions is often difficult and the clinical results difficult to interpret.

Fifty one patients have undergone surgery for cerebral artery aneurysms under moderate hypothermia ($27\,^\circ - 29\,^\circ$C) with or without controlled hypotension in the Neurosurgical unit in Groningen in the last 5 years (1974–1978). Cerebral ischaemia, often associated with intraoperative vasospasm and followed by cerebral oedema appeared to be a persistent problem postoperatively so that preventive measures were felt to be indicated. Cerebral protection by barbiturates is thought to be synergistic with that afforded by hypothermia [8, 9, 10], although they have not commonly been used together.

In this preliminary study, nine patients were given thiopentone or pentobarbitone before the start of cerebral aneurysm surgery, which was carried out under moderate hypothermia as before. The results are compared with a retrospective study of the earlier group of 51 patients.

Method

All patients were premedicated with atropine, pethidine, promethazine and chlorpromazine. Hypothermia was induced in all patients by surface cooling.

a) In the first group of 51 patients endotracheal anaesthesia was induced with thiopentone and continued with pethidine, pancuronium and ventilation with 33% O_2, 65% N_2O and 2% CO_2. The E.C.G., arterial pressure via a radial cannula, central venous pressure, end-tidal CO_2 concentration and nasopharyngeal, oesophageal, skin and bath water temperatures were monitored. Arterial blood was taken for intermittent gas, acidbase and electrolyte estimation. 120 ml C.S.F. were drained via a lumbar puncture needle after the dura was open to facilitate surgery. Trimetaphan or sodium nitroprusside was usually needed to control the arterial pressure during dissection and clipping of the aneurysm. After clipping, rewarming with water at 40 °C was begun; the patients were rewarmed to 36 °C before they were extubated and transferred to the intensive care unit. An epidural pressure transducer (Philips) was placed in one of the craniotomy burr holes for continuous postoperative intracranial pressure monitoring.

In both groups B and C cerebral activity was monitored with a Cerebral Function Monitor (Devices) (C.F.M.). A signal is obtained from biparietal scalp electrodes and displayed as a single trace at a slow speed on a chart recorder after heavy filtering and logarithmic amplitude compression. This can be recorded continuously for long periods of time. Cerebral activity is indicated by the level and width of the trace [11].

b) Patients 1–5 were loaded with 50 mg/kg thiopentone in a 2 1/2% infusion over 30–40 minutes beginning at induction. Cooling was begun after the full dose was given.

c) Anaesthesia was induced in patients 6–9 with etomidate in order to avoid tolerance effects as far as possible and to reduce the time interval from barbiturate loading to clipping of the aneurysm. About 20 mg/kg pentobarbitone were given as a 1% infusion beginning with a bolus of 200–400 mg. The infusion was continued at 5–6 mg/minute until after the clip was placed in order to keep the Cerebral Function Monitor trace as nearly isoelectric as possible during dissection and clipping of the aneurysm.

Further hypotensive agents were used. Postoperatively, controlled ventilation and all monitoring were continued for as long as necessary. Anaesthetic management in groups B and C was otherwise the same as in group A.

Results

a) In the control group clips were placed in 35 out of 51 patients. 16 aneurysms ruptured during surgery; this was invariably associated with a hypertensive response to brain retraction which was seen in 37 cases. 7 patients has a neurological deficit on discharge not present preoperatively with or without a psychological deficit and 6 had a psychological deficit only. 3 died postoperatively; 12 are known to be working.

b) In the thiopentone-loaded group, clips were placed in two out of 5 patients. The aneurysm ruptured in one patient. Cardiovascular depression was little more than usually seen at 28 °C; cardiotonic drugs were not needed. Four patients had no neurological deficit on discharge; one had a dense and persistent hemiplegia, sustained two further subarachnoid haemorrhages and died six weeks postoperatively. Controlled ventilation was required for 3–13 hours postoperatively.

c) A clip was placed in 3 out of 4 patients in the pentobarbitone group. No haemodynamic response to brain retraction was seen. No patient had a neurological deficit on discharge and all were able to leave hospital relatively early. Cardiovascular depression was minimal even while the pentobarbitone infusion was continued at 28 °C. Controlled ventilation was required for a longer time postoperatively than in the thiopentone group: the patients were extubated 18, 31, 44, and 53 hours postoperatively.

Discussion

A retrospective study of 51 aneurysm patients suggests that, in addition to the well known problems of vasospasm, the effects of brain retraction present a special problem so that the anaesthetic technique might be improved in close collaboration with the surgeons. Retraction pressures of over 20 mm Hg are known to result in local cerebral ischaemia [12, 13, 14].

Further, acute hypertension, which accompanied brain retraction in over 70% of patients in group A, is known to perdispose to oedema formation [15, 16, 17].

Experimental evidence indicates that barbiturate-induced metabolic depression is maximal with doses just sufficient to render the E.E.G. isoelectric [18]. This provides the basis for taking an isoelectric-E.E.G. as a criterion for effective cerebral protection in-practice, on the assumption that protection is directly related to metabolic depression. This, however, is not certain. Other anaesthetic agents, such as halothane, cause a similar degree of metabolic depression but without comparable cerebral protection [19, 20]. An independent mechanism has also been inferred from the apparent discrepancy between the small doses of barbiturates observed to cause substantial metabolic depression in rat brain in vitro [21] and the massive doses which offered the best protection of cerebral function after middle cerebral artery (MCA) occlusion in baboons [19].

The latter were over twice the dose needed to produce an isoelectric E.E.G. In rhesus monkeys, also, cooling to 26 °C after experimental MCA occlusion failed to prevent oedema formation, whereas treatment with pentobarbitone, resulting in a similar degree of metabolic depression, was effective [22]. Fig. 1 illustrates how much faster cerebral activity recovers after a thiopentone infusion is stopped than after pentobarbitone. Fig. 2 shows that in the thiopentone group, cerebral activity had already recovered to a large extent before dissection and clipping of the aneurysm, so that cerebral protection is unlikely to have been very effective at this time, if protection is directly related to depression of function. Loading with

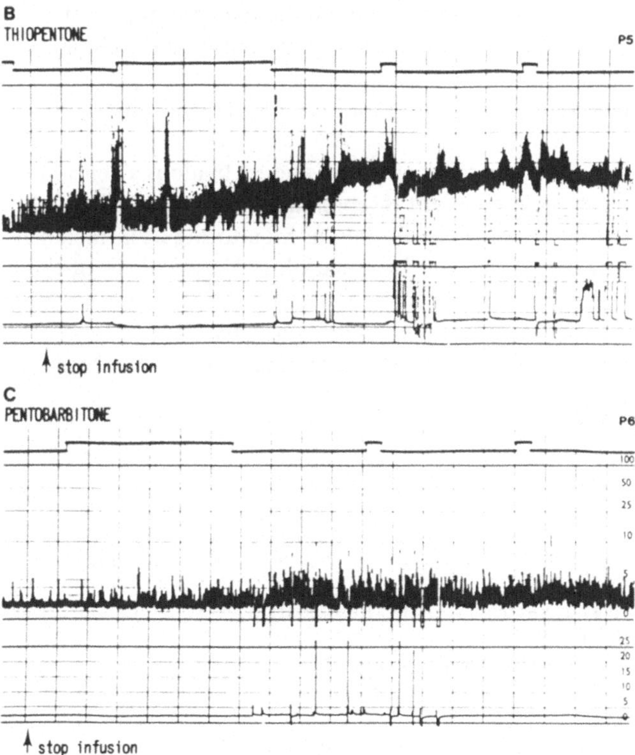

Fig. 1. Recovery of cerebral activity after discontinuing barbiturate infusion

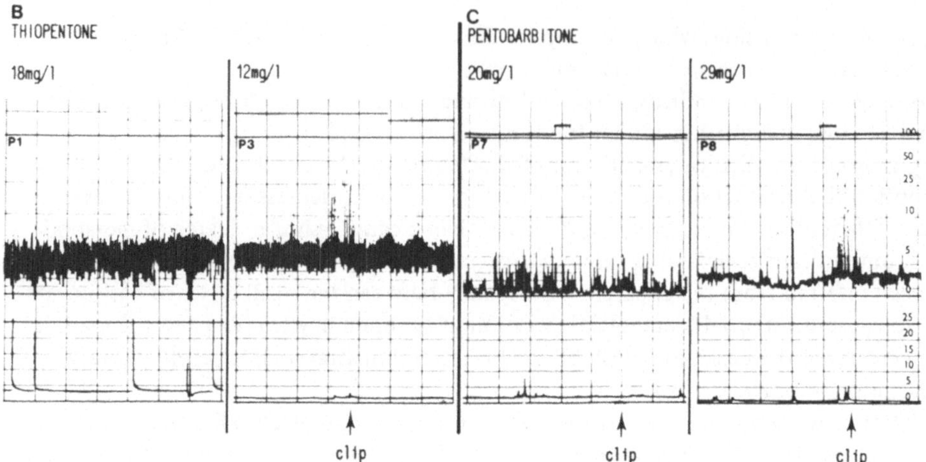

Fig. 2. CFM records and serum barbiturate levels during dissection and clipping of aneurysms

pentobarbitone is associated with little cardiovascular depression while the C.F.M. trace quickly becomes isoelectric or nearly so (Fig. 3). A deep burst-suppression pattern is easily maintained at 28 °C without further hypotension using pentobarbitone (Fig. 4). The hypertensive response to brain retraction is effectively suppressed. This technique also allows the possibility of continuing the pentobarbitone infusion to maintain the required degree of cerebral depression into the postoperative period for as long as may be considered necessary, in the event of severe and persistent vasospasm or occlusion of a vessel during surgery. Pentobarbitone thus appears to be a much more suitable drug for prophylactic use with hypothermia than thiopentone.

The postoperative period can present considerable problems and meticulous attention to the care of a severely depressed and immobile patient is required in order to avoid pulmonary and thrombotic complications in particular [23]. Continuous monitoring of intracranial pressure and cerebral activity are essential postoperatively as neurological assessment of the patient may be difficult.

In conclusion the clinical results of a preliminary study using pentobarbitone prophylactically together with moderate hypothermia are encouraging and we feel that this technique merits more extensive evaluation.

References

1. Smith AL, Hoff JT, Nielsen SL, Larson CP (1974) Barbiturate Protection in acute focal cerebral ischaemia. Stroke 5:1
2. Safar P, Bleyaert A, Nemoto EM, Moossy J, Snyder JV (1978) Resuscitation after global brain ischaemia-anoxia. Critical care Medicine 6:215
3. Smith AL (1977) Barbiturate protection in cerebral hypoxia. Anesthesiology 47:285
4. Belopavlovic M, Buchthal A (1980) Barbiturate therapy in cerebral ischaemia — a review. Anaesthesia, in press.
5. Brievik H, Safar P, Sands P, Fabritius R, Lind B, Lust P, Mullie A, Orr M, Renck H, Snyder JV (1978) Clinical feasibility trials of barbiturate therapy after cardiac arrest. Critical care Medicine 6: 228

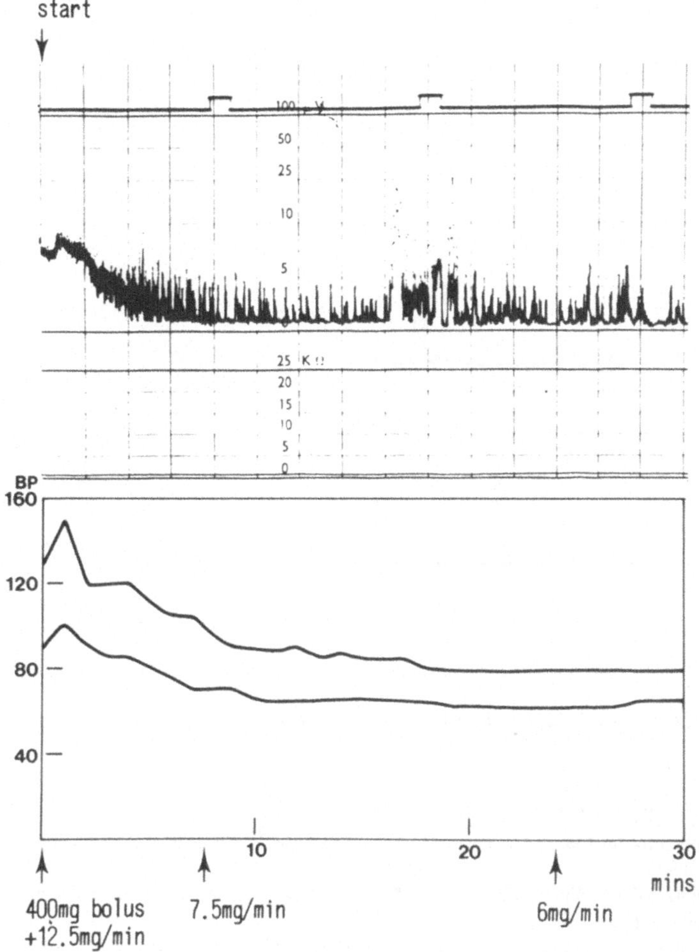

Fig. 3. Loading with 20 mg/kg Pentobarbitone

6. Marshall LF, Smith RW, Shapiro HM (1979) The outcome with aggressive treatment in severe head injuries. Part I, The significance of intracranial pressure monitoring. J Neurosurgery 50:20. Part II, Acute and chronic barbiturate administration in the management of head injury. J Neurosurgery 50:26

7. Marshall LF, Shapiro HM, Rauscher A, Kaufman N (1978) Pentobarbital therapy for intracranial hypertension in metabolic coma. Critical care Medicine 6:1

8. Lafferty JJ, Keykhah MM, Shapiro HM, Van Horn K, Behar MG (1978) Cerebral hypometabolism obtained with deep pentobarbital anaesthesia and hypothermia (30°) Anesthesiology 49:159

9. Hägerdal M, Welsh FA, Keykhah MM, Perez E, Harp JR (1978) Protective effects of combinations of hypothermia and barbiturates in cerebral hypoxia in the rat. Anesthesiology 49:165

10. Hägerdal M, Keykhah M, Perez E, Harp JR (1979) Additive effects of hypothermia and phenobarbital upon cerebral oxygen consumption in the rat. Acta Anaes Scand 23:89

11. Maynard D, Prior PF, Scott DF (1968) Device for continuous monitoring of cerebral activity in resuscitated patients. Brit Med J 4:545

12. Rivano C, Rossi GF, Zattoni J (1972) Variations of intraventricular and local brain pressures during neurosurgical procedures. In: Brock and Dietz (eds) Intracranial Pressure I. Springer Verlag

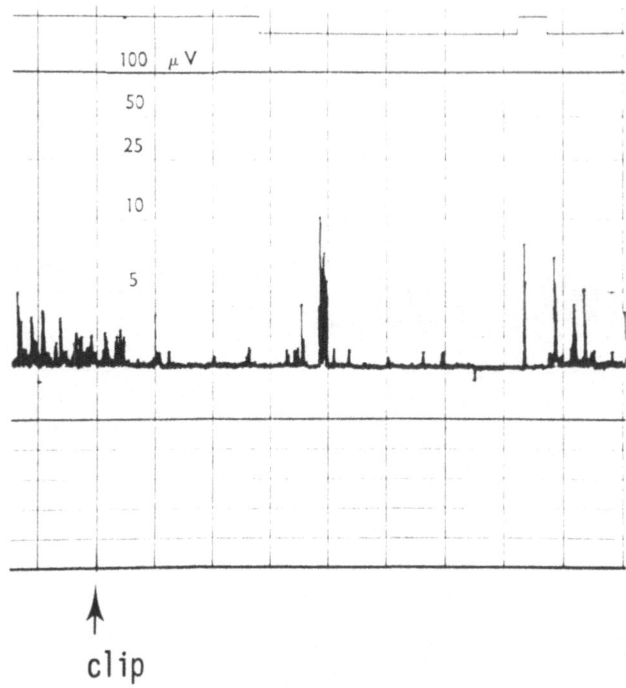

Fig. 4. Clip placed on MCA aneurysm poor filling of MCA branches on angiogram

13. Albin MS, Bunegin L, Helsel P, Marlin A, Babinski MM (1979) Intracranial pressure and cerebral blood flow responses to experimental brain retraction pressure. In: Fourth Symposium on intracranial Pressure, Williamsburg, 1979
14. Miller JD, Stanek AE, Langfitt TW (1973) Cerebral blood flow regulation during experimental brain compression. J Neurosurgery 39:186
15. Forster A, Van Horn K, Marshall LF, Shapiro HM (1978) Anaesthetic effects on blood brain barrier function during acute arterial hypertension. Anesthesiology 49:26
16. Häggendal E, Johansson (1979) On the pathophysiology of the increased cerebrovascular permeability in acute arterial hypertension in cats. Acta Neurol Scand 48:265
17. Schutta HE, Kassess NF, Langfitt TW (1968) Brain swelling produced by injury and aggravated by arterial hypertension. Brain 91:281
18. Michenfelder JD (1974) The interdependency of cerebral functional and metabolic effects following massive doses of thiopental in the dog. Anesthesiology 41:231
19. Hoff JT, Smith AL, Hankinson HL, Nielsen SL (1975) Barbiturate protection from cerebral infarction in primates. Stroke 6:28
20. Michenfelder JD, Theye RA (1975) In vivo toxic effects of halothane on canine metabolic pathways. Am J Physiol 229:1050
21. Crane PD, Braun LD, Cornford EM, Cremer JE, Glass JM, Oldendorf WH (1978) Dose dependent reduction of glucose utilisation by pentobarbital in rat brain. Stroke 9:12
22. Simeone FA, Frazer G, Lawner P (1979) Ischaemic brain edema: Comparative effects of barbiturates and hypothermia. Stroke 10:8
23. Belopavlovic M, Buchthal A (1980) Barbiturate therapy in the management of cerebral ischaemia. Anaesthesia, in press

Kombinationsanästhesien mit Flunitrazepam

P. Kurka

Flunitrazepam als Mononarkoticum wird heute praktisch von allen erfahrenen Anästhesisten abgelehnt. Das ist damit zu erklären, daß Rohypnol als Benzodiazepin eine sehr starke anxiolytische und zentral dämpfende Wirkung hat, aber keineswegs jenen zerebralen Globaleffekt zeigt, der die holenzephalen Anästhetica auszeichnet. Da Rohypnol eine stark schlafanstoßende Wirkung besitzt, schläft der Patient nach einmaliger i.v. Verabreichung, solange im Plasma eine Konzentration von etwa 8 ng überschritten ist. In der ersten Stunde nach der Applikation kommt es zu einem starken Konzentrationsabfall, den Amrein [1] mit dem Abfließen der Substanz in die tieferen Kompartimente erklärt, in denen dann allerdings Flunitrazepam sehr lange nachzuweisen ist. Da es außerdem nicht analgetisch wirkt, fehlen ihm die wichtigsten Eigenschaften, die man von einem Mononarkoticum erwarten muß. Dafür besitzt es jene Qualitäten, die es für die Kombinationsanästhesien so wertvoll macht. Neben der stark schlafanstoßenden und anxiolytischen Wirkung sind der vegetativ reflektorisch dämpfende Effekt sowie die Amnesie und additive beziehungsweise supraaddítive Wechselwirkung zu Hypnotica, Neuroleptica und Analgetica bekannt. So konnten Stumpf, Gogolak [6, 7] im Tierversuch echte supraaddítive Wirkungen zwischen den Benzodiazepinen, Diazepam, Flunitrazepam und Medazepam einerseits und Stickoxydul andererseits nachweisen. Kapp [3], der die Wirkung der Kombination Dehydrobenzperidol-Rohypnol untersuchte, spricht in diesem Fall von einer qualitativ neuartigen Wirkung.

Die unter dem Begriff „Allgemeinanästhesie" verstandene temporäre Ausschaltung von Bewußtsein, Schmerz und Reflexen kann also nur im Bereich „Bewußtsein" allein von Flunitrazepam erreicht werden. Die temporäre Ausschaltung des Schmerzes und der Reflexe wird durch die supraaddítive bzw. additive Wirkung der Kombination Flunitrazepam-Stickoxydul bzw. Flunitrazepam-Neurolepticum erreicht. Die für die moderne Allgemeinanästhesie notwendige Muskelrelaxation bleibt weiterhin die Domäne der Muskelrelaxantien. Ihre Dosierung liegt bei der Flunitrazepam-Kombinationsnarkose nach meiner Erfahrung sogar etwas höher. Wohl wirkt das in dieser Kombination verwendete Rohypnol wie alle Benzodiazepine leicht muskelrelaxierend, jedoch nicht in der hier angewandten Dosierung.

Flunitrazepam kann aber nicht nur mit Stickoxydul oder Dehydrobenzperidol kombiniert werden. Im Laufe der Jahre wurden verschiedene Anästhesietechniken entwickelt und es zeigte sich, daß Flunitrazepam mit allen gas- und dampfförmigen sowie intravenös verabreichbaren Mitteln der modernen Anästhesie kombinierbar ist. Dabei wird besonders die stark anxiolytische und schlafanstoßende Wirkung dieses Mittels geschätzt. Die anxiolytische Wirkung gewinnt besondere Bedeutung in der präoperativen Vorbereitung, während die schlafanstoßende Wirkung von jenen Autoren geschätzt wird, die eine Supplementierung mit Fentanyl oder Fortral bevorzugen (Milewski, Dick [5] und Vontin et al. [8]).

Als besonders günstig hat sich die Kombination von Rohypnol und Ketalar erwiesen (Kurka [4], Vontin [8]). Die bekannten Nachteile des Ketamine, nämlich die psychomimetischen Reaktionen nach dem Eingriff, aber auch die durch Ketamine bedingte kardiovaskuläre Stimulation werden von Rohypnol weitgehend aufgehoben [9], während die hypnotische Wirkung verstärkt wird. Dies ermöglicht eine stark verminderte Dosierung beider Substanzen.

Aufgrund meiner Erfahrung, die ich bei über 2500 Anästhesien gewonnen habe, glaube ich jedoch, daß die meisten Kombinationen mit Flunitrazepam, außer der mit Ketamine, kaum nötig sind. Mit Dehydrobenzperidol in der präoperativen Vorbereitung, Rohypnol für die Einleitung der Anästhesie und Stickoxydul als Analgeticum und zur Aufrechterhaltung der Anästhesie kann man auch stundenlange Narkosen anstandslos durchführen. Die Erklärung dafür dürfte darin liegen, daß einerseits das Neurolepticum und das Benzodiazepin synergistisch im Bereich der Formatio reticularis und im Limbischen System wirken und daß andererseits die stark analgetische Wirkung des Stickoxyduls (Barth [2]) durch das Rohypnol additiv gesteigert wird.

Präoperativ verabreiche ich 5–7,5 mg Dehydrobenzperidol mit Atropin. Nach Anlegen der Infusion nochmals 2,5 mg DHB mit 2,5 mg Alloferin. Die Gesamtdosis an DHB übersteigt nur ganz selten 10 mg. Nach etwa 1 Minute beginnt die Anästhesieeinleitung mit 0,3– 0,4 mg Rohypnol. Um diese kleine Menge genau verabreichen zu können, verdünne ich das Präparat mit physiologischer Kochsalzlösung, sodaß sich in einer 10 ml Spritze 1 mg Rohypnol befindet. Sobald der Patient schläft – man erkennt dies an den meist engen bis mittelweiten Pupillen – wird intubiert. Für die Aufrechterhaltung der Anästhesie ist es im allgemeinen notwendig, die empfohlene Stickoxydulkonzentration (3 l Stickoxydul : 1 l Sauerstoff) aufrechtzuerhalten und für eine ausreichende Relaxation zu sorgen. Sollte es in seltenen Fällen erforderlich sein, kann die Rohypnoldosis ohne Sorge auf 1 mg erhöht werden. Dies kann auch bei Anzeichen einer zu seichten Anästhesie gemacht werden (1–2 % der Anästhesien). Die Anästhesie wird dadurch beendet, daß die Relaxation aufgehoben und das Stickoxydul abgesetzt wird. Nach kürzester Zeit ist der Patient wieder ansprechbar. Die Technik hat sich bei mir seit sieben Jahren bestens bewährt.

Literatur

1. Amrein R (1978) Zur Pharmakokinetik und zum Metabolismus von Flunitrazepam. Klinische Anästhesiologie und Intensivtherapie 17:8–24, Springer Verlag
2. Barth L, Büchel CG (1975) Klinische Untersuchungen über die narkotische Wirkung von Stickoxydul. Anästhesist 24:49–55
3. Kapp W (1978) Zur Pharmakologie von Flunitrazepam. Klin Anästh und Intensivther 17:1–7, Springer Verlag
4. Kurka P (1975) Klinische Erfahrungen mit Flunitrazepam. 7. Internat. Fortbildungskurs für klinische Anästhesiologie 9–13/6/1975 Wien
5. Milewski P, Dick W (1978) Anwendung und Dosierung von Flunitrazepam in Kombination mit Analgetika. Klin Anästh und Intensivth 17:148–162, Springer Verlag
6. Stumpf Ch, Gogolak G (1975) Wirkung zentral dämpfender Pharmaka auf die Stickoxydul-Narkose. Anästhesist 24:264–268
7. Stumpf Ch, Jinra R, Huck S, Ewers H (1979) Wechselwirkung zwischen Stickoxydul und zentral dämpfenden Pharmaka. Anästhesist 1:3
8. Vontin H, Heller W, Schorer R (1976) Analgosedierung und Ataranalgesie: Untersuchungen über Rohypnol und Kombination mit Analgetica. Aus: Bisherige Erfahrungen mit Rohypnol (Flunitrazepam) in der Anästhesiologie und Intensivtherapie. „Editiones Roche" Basel, S 149–159
9. Tarnow J, Hess W, Schmidt D, Eberlein HJ (1979) Narkoseeinleitung bei Patienten mit koronaren Herzkrankheiten: Flunitrazepam, Diazepam, Detamin, Fentanyl. Eine hämodynamische Untersuchung. Anästhesist 1:9

Freie Themen
Postoperative Nachsorge

Vorsitz: P. Günter und J.M. Kapferer

Tramadol bei postoperativem Patientengut

D. Paravicini, C. Baus und P. Lawin

Mit dem Tramadol wurde ein neues, synthetisches Morphinderivat mit morphinagonistischer Wirkung in die klinische Therapie des Schmerzes eingeführt. Wir untersuchten Tramadol bei insgesamt 42 Patienten in der frühen postoperativen Phase nach Eingriffen im Oberbauch (z.B. Cholecystektomie, Magenoperationen, Splenektomie, Hiatushernie). Unser besonderes Interesse galt dabei der Wirkung auf Atmung und Kreislauf, insbesondere bei Patienten mit bereits präoperativ eingeschränkter Lungenfunktion.

Am Vorabend des Operationstages wurde der Patient im Rahmen der Prämedikationsvisite über den Ablauf der Studie orientiert. Es wurden die präoperativen Ausgangswerte von Herzfrequenz, Blutdruck, Atemfrequenz, Atemminutenvolumen und Lungenfunktion bestimmt. Die Messung des Atemminutenvolumens erfolgte mit einem an ein Mundstück angeschlossenen Wright-Spirometer, die Werte der Lungenfunktion wurden in liegender Position mit dem elektronischen Digitalspirometer „Spirotron" der Firma Dräger, Lübeck, bestimmt. Lag die forcierte Vitalkapazität (FVC) über 80% des Soll-Wertes, so wurde der Patient als im wesentlichen „lungengesund" der Gruppe 1 zugeordnet, Patienten mit FVC-Werten unter 80% wurden in Gruppe 2 eingereiht (Tabelle 1).

Tabelle 1. Tramadol in der postoperativen Phase. Einteilung in Patientengruppen

Bestimmung der präop. Lungenfunktion:	
	FVC $\geqslant$ 80% des Sollwerts $\rightarrow$ Gruppe 1
	FVC $\leqslant$ 80% des Sollwerts $\rightarrow$ Gruppe 2
Gruppe 1 (n = 24):	9 Patienten nach Enflurane/N_2O/O_2 (mittleres Alter 45,3 ± 8,4 Jahre) (mittlere Narkosedauer 137,2 ± 73 min)
	15 Patienten nach NLA (mittleres Alter 49 ± 8,6 Jahre) (mittlere Narkosedauer 139,7 ± 51,1 min)
Gruppe 2 (n = 18):	9 Patienten nach Enflurane/N_2O/O_2 (mittleres Alter 42,7 ± 12,6 Jahre) (mittlere Narkosedauer 118,9 ± 38,6 min)
	9 Patienten nach NLA (mittleres Alter 50,4 ± 9,9 Jahre) (mittlere Narkosedauer 143,5 ± 51,9 min)

Entsprechend der klinischen Indikationsstellung erhielten die Patienten eine Enflurane/ N_2O/O_2-Narkose bzw. eine Neuroleptanalgesie (Tabelle 1). Nach erfolgter Extubation und Verlegung in den Aufwachraum wurde mit einer Teflon-Verweilkanüle 20 G nach vorheriger Bestimmung des Allen-Tests die A. radialis kanüliert, um arterielle Blutproben entnehmen und den arteriellen Blutdruck über ein Statham-Element P 23 Db registrieren zu können. Wenn im weiteren Verlauf die Patienten über Schmerzen klagten (nach Enflurane-Narkose im Mittel nach 53 Minuten, nach NLA im Mittel nach 85 Minuten), wurde nach Bestimmung der Herzfrequenz und der Blutdruckwerte arterielles Blut für die Blutgasanalyse entnommen, anschließend wurden, wiederum in liegender Stellung, die Werte der Lungenfunktion ermittelt (Tabelle 2). Unmittelbar darauf erhielt der Patient 1 mg/kg KG Tramadol i.v. verabreicht. In 5minütigen Abständen erfolgten die Messungen von Herzfrequenz und Blutdruck, nach 10, 30 und 60 Minuten nach Tramadol-Gabe wurden zusätzlich Blutgasanalyse, Atemparameter und Lungenfunktion bestimmt.

Tabelle 2. Tramadol in der postoperativen Phase. Methodik

präop. Ausgangswert	Anästhesie	0	Tramadol 1 mg/kg KG i.v.	Aufwachraum							
				5	10	15	20	25	30	35...	60 min
HF		HF		HF	HF	HF	HF	HF	HF	HF	HF
P_{art}		P_{art}		P_{art}	P_{art}	P_{art}	P_{art}	P_{art}	P_{art}	P_{art}	P_{art}
AF		AF			AF					AF	AF
V_T		V_T			V_T					V_T	V_T
AMV		AMV			AMV					AMV	AMV
FVC		FVC			FVC					FVC	FVC
FEV_1		FEV_1			FEV_1					FEV_1	FEV_1
		BGA art.			BGA art.					BGA art.	BGA art.
		pH			pH					pH	pH
		pCO_2			pCO_2					pCO_2	pCO_2
		pO_2			pO_2					pO_2	pO_2
		HCO_3^-			HCO_3^-					HCO_3^-	HCO_3^-
		BE			BE					BE	BE
		SO_2			SO_2					SO_2	SO_2

Die Tramadol-Gabe führte nach Enflurane-Narkose in 2/3 der Fälle zu einer sehr guten bzw. guten Analgesie, bei 6 Patienten reichte die Schmerzfreiheit nicht aus. Nach Neuroleptanalgesie gaben mehr als 3/4 der Fälle eine sehr gute bzw. gute Schmerzfreiheit an, nur 4 Patienten wurden durch die Tramadol-Gabe nicht ausreichend schmerzfrei (Tabelle 3). Der Wirkungseintritt der Schmerzfreiheit setzte in aller Regel 5–10 Minuten nach intravenöser Tramadol-Gabe ein und hielt für etwa 4 Stunden an. Auffallend starke Sedierung hatte Tramadol bei 10 Patienten nach Neuroleptanalgesie, aber bei nur 3 Patienten nach Enflurane-Narkose. Starkes Schwitzen wurde nach Enflurane-Narkose einmal, nach NLA dreimal beobachtet. Eine mäßige Übelkeit, jedoch ohne Erbrechen, trat in einem Fall nach Neuroleptanalgesie auf.

Die Herzfrequenz war postoperativ, als der Patient im Aufwachraum über Schmerzen klagte, gegenüber dem präoperativen Ausgangswert deutlich erhöht. Nach Tramadol-Gabe

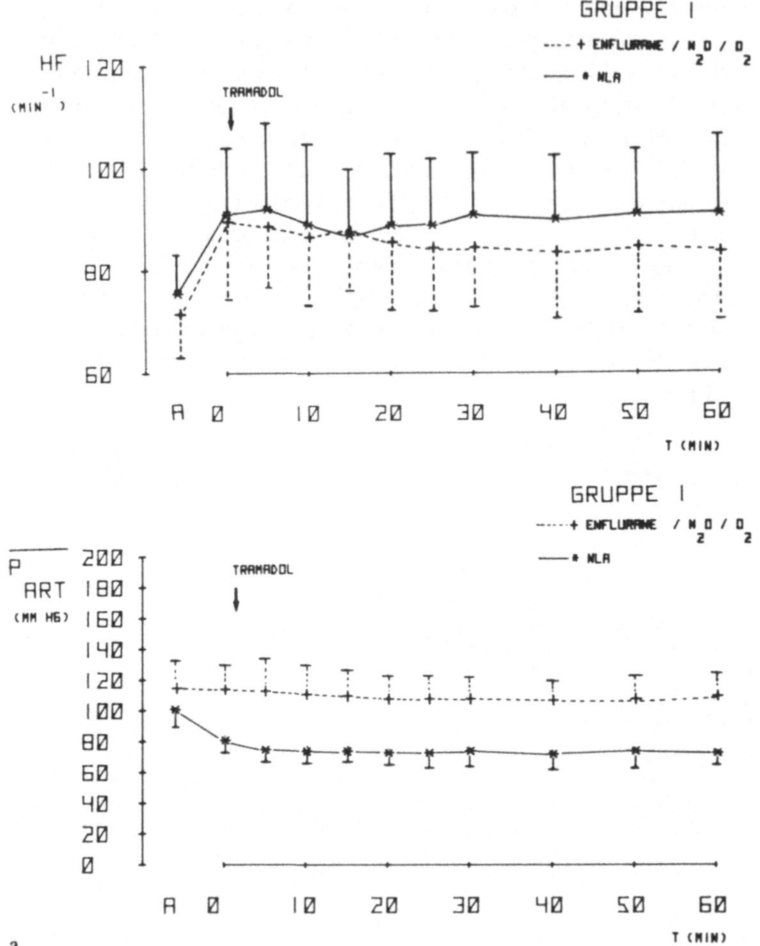

Abb. 1a, b. Herzfrequenz (HF) und partieller Mitteldruck ($\bar{P}_{art}$) von Patienten nach Oberbaucheingriffen und Gabe von Tramadol (1 mg/kg KG i.v.). Gruppe 1: Patienten mit unauffälliger Lungenfunktion nach Enflurane/N_2O/O_2-Narkose (n = 9) bzw. nach Neuroleptanalgesie (n = 15). Gruppe 2: Patienten mit Einschränkung der forcierten Vitalkapazität unter 80% des Soll-Wertes, nach Enflurane/N_2/O_2-Narkose (n = 9) bzw. nach NLA (n = 9)

GRUPPE 2
+ ENFLURANE / N O / O
NLA
HF 120
(MIN)
TRAMADOL
100
80
60
A 0 10 20 30 40 50 60
T (MIN)

GRUPPE 2
+ ENFLURANE / N O / O
NLA
P
ART 200 180 160 140 120 100 80 60 40 20 0
(MM HG)
TRAMADOL
A 0 10 20 30 40 50 60
T (MIN)

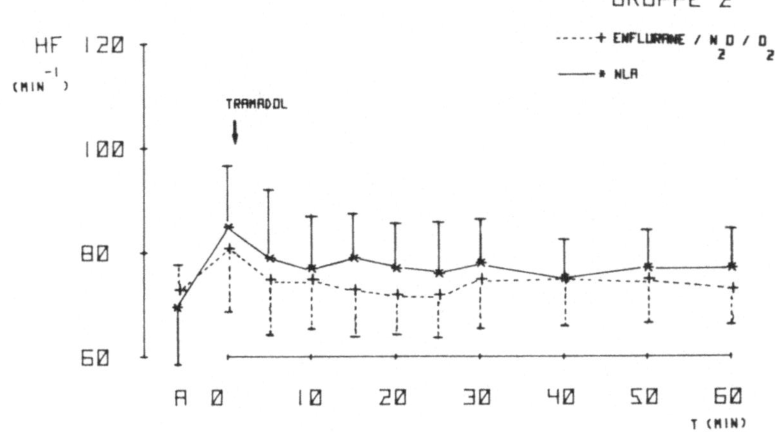

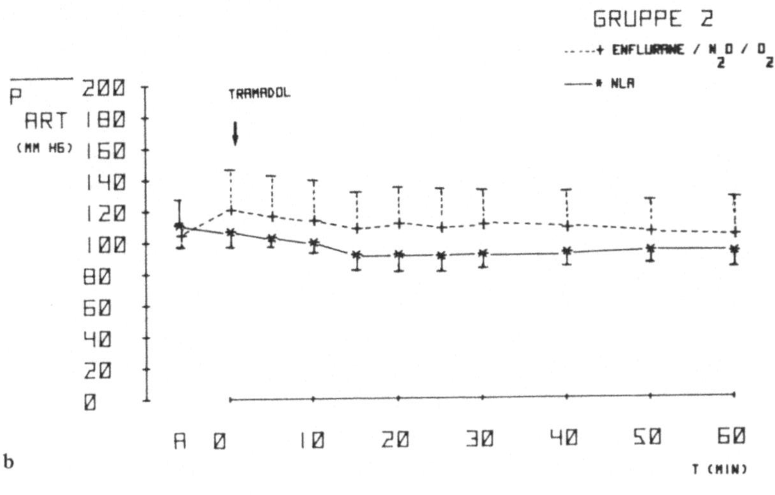

b

                                                                D. Paravicini et al.

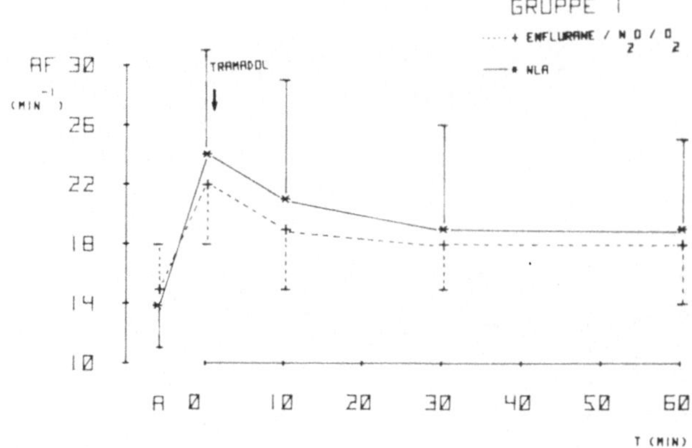

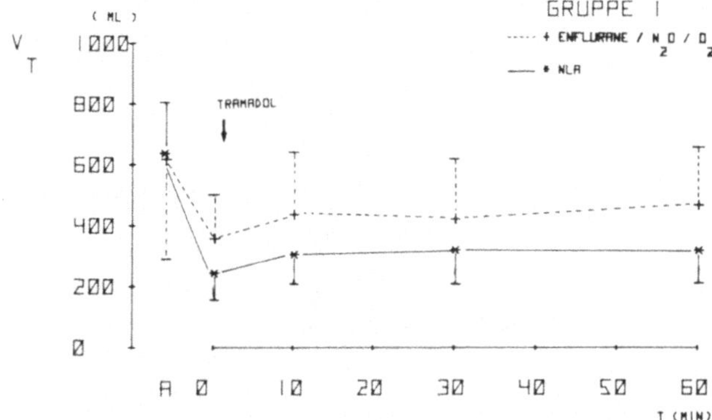

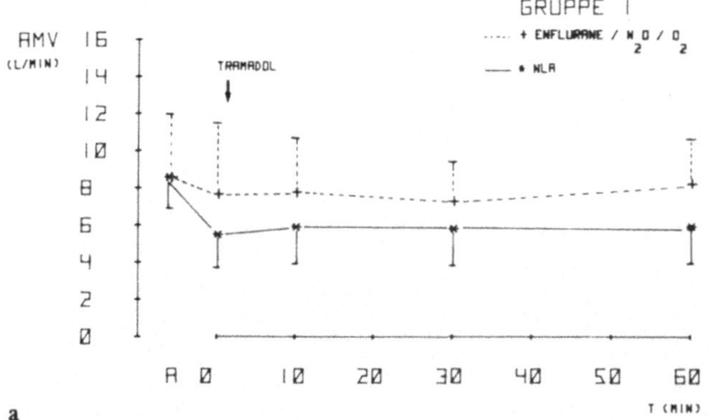

a

Abb. 2a, b. Atemfrequenz (AF), Atemzugvolumen (V_T) und Atemminutenvolumen (AMV) bei Patienten nach Oberbaucheingriffen und Gabe von Tramadol. Weitere Angaben siehe Abbildung 1a und b

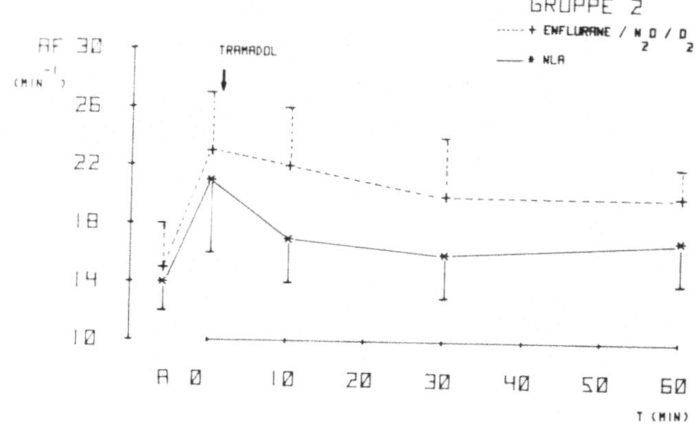

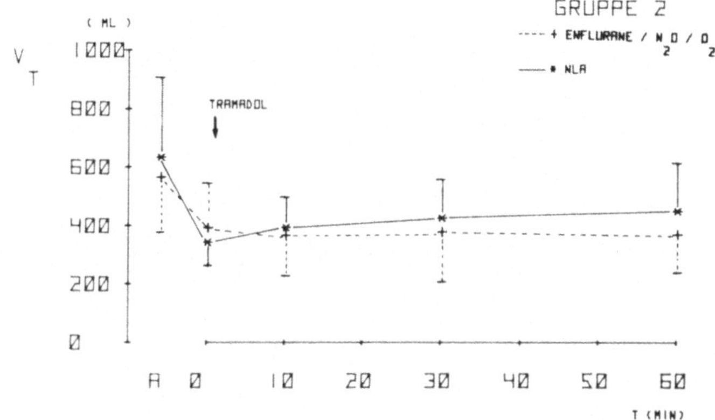

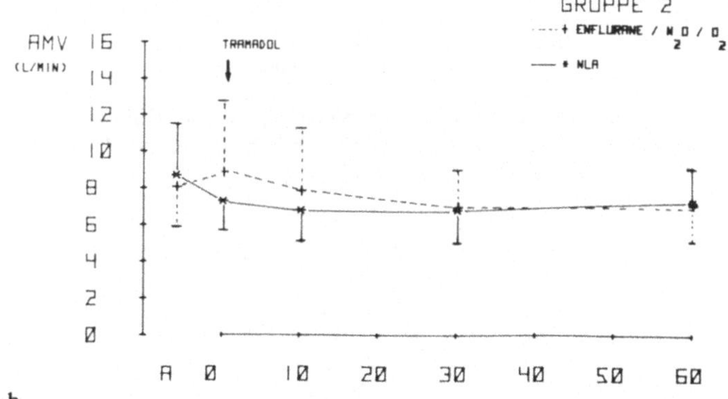

b

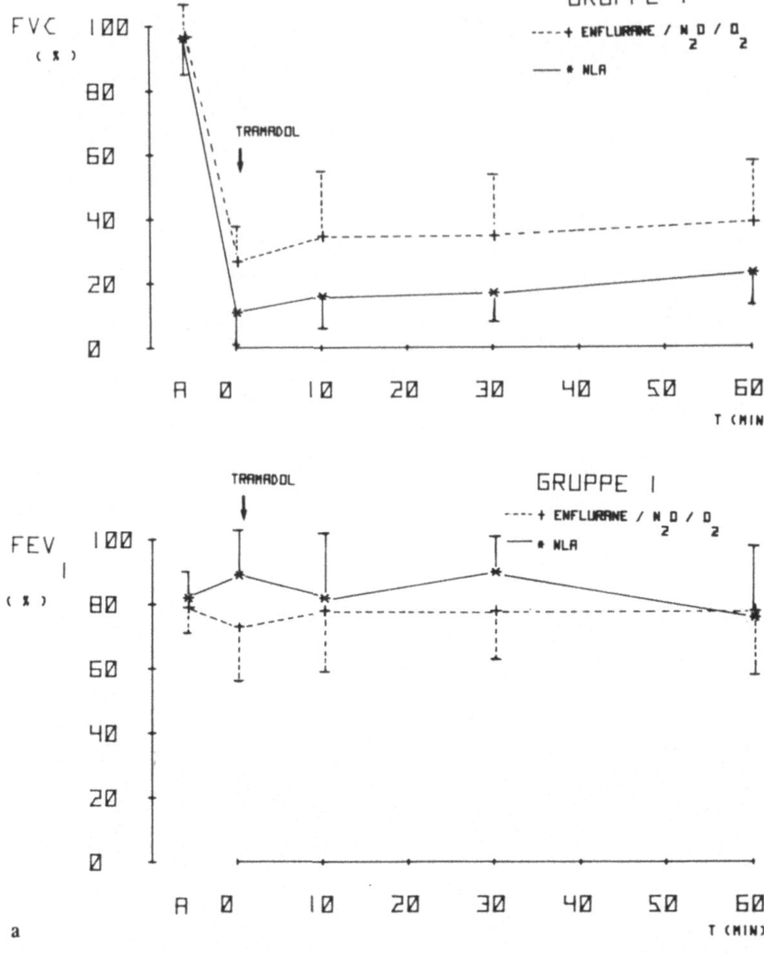

Abb. 3a, b. Forcierte Vitalkapazität (FVC) und forciertes Einsekundenvolumen in Prozent (FEV$_I$) von Patienten nach Oberbaucheingriffen und Gabe von Tramadol. Nähere Angaben siehe Abbildung 1a und b

GRUPPE 2
+ ENFLURANE / N O / O
NLA
FVC
(%)
100
80
60
40
20
0
TRAMADOL
A 0 10 20 30 40 50 60
T (MIN)

TRAMADOL
GRUPPE 2
+ ENFLURANE / N O / O
NLA
FEV
1
(%)
100
80
60
40
20
0
A 0 10 20 30 40 50 60
T (MIN)

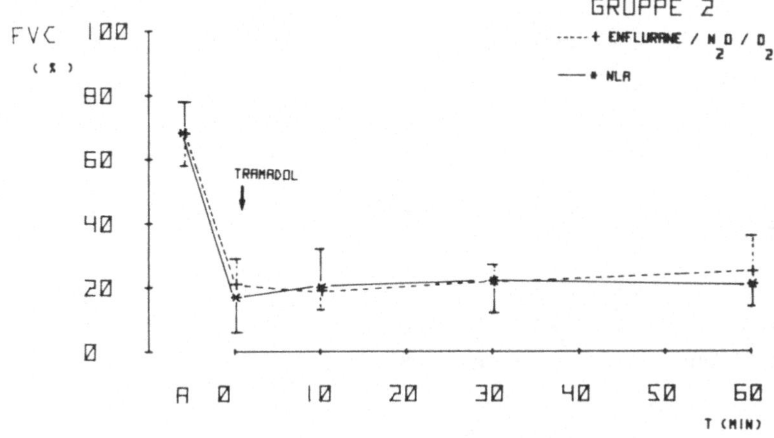

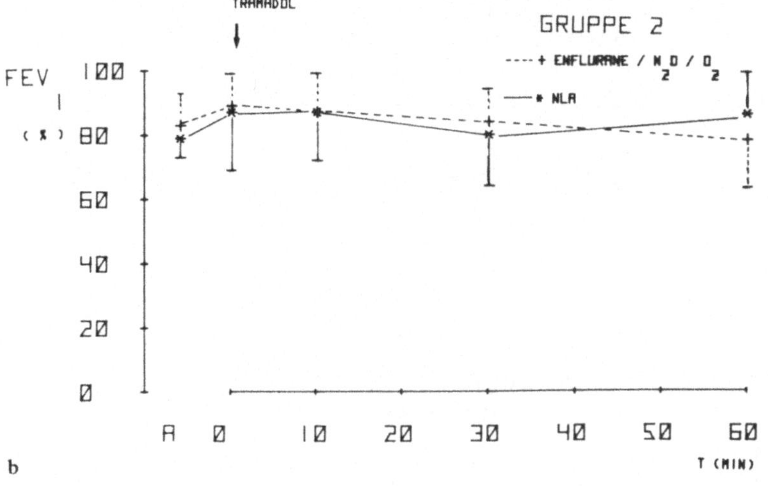

b

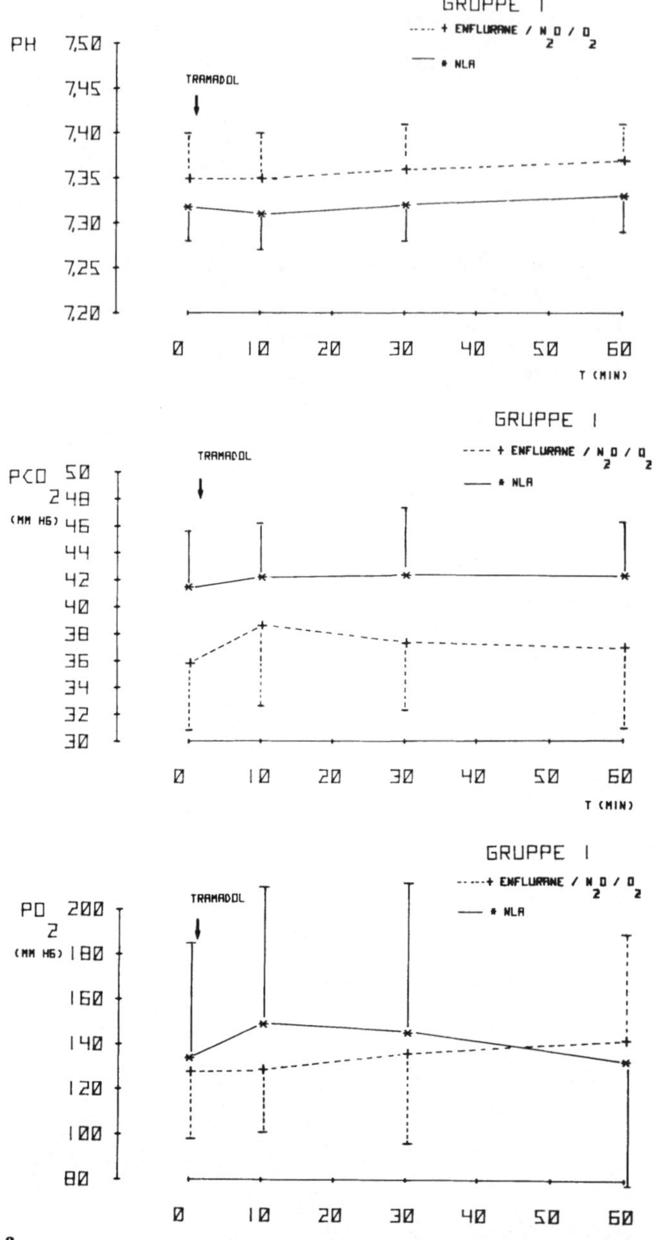

Abb. 4a, b. pH-Wert, CO_2-Partialdruck (pCO_2) und Sauerstoffpartialdruck (pO_2) von Patienten nach Oberbaucheingriffen und Gabe von Tramadol. Nähere Angaben siehe Abbildung 1a und b

GRUPPE 2
+ ENFLURANE / N O / O
2 2
* NLA
PH
7.50
7.45
7.40
7.35
7.30
7.25
7.20
TRAMADOL
0 10 20 30 40 50 60
T (MIN)

GRUPPE 2
+ ENFLURANE / N O / O
2 2
* NLA
PCO
2
(MM HG)
50
48
46
44
42
40
38
36
34
32
30
TRAMADOL
0 10 20 30 40 50 60
T (MIN)

GRUPPE 2
+ ENFLURANE / N O / O
2 2
* NLA
PO
2
(MM HG)
200
180
160
140
120
100
80
TRAMADOL
0 10 20 30 40 50 60
T (MIN)

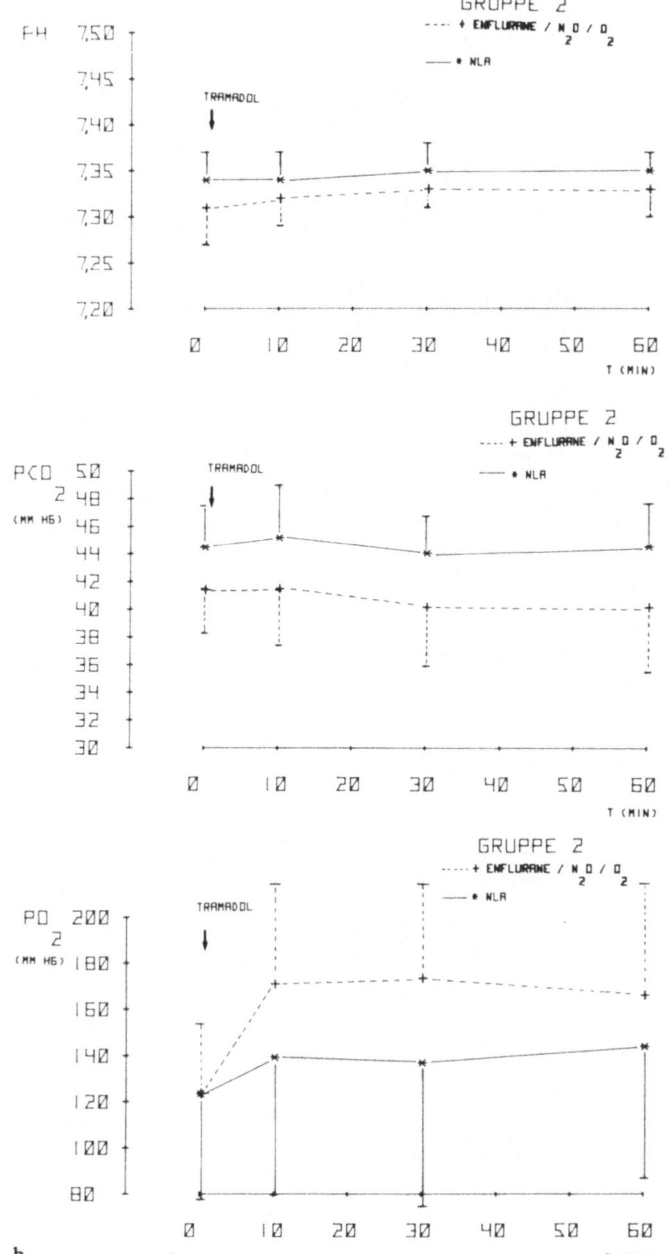

b

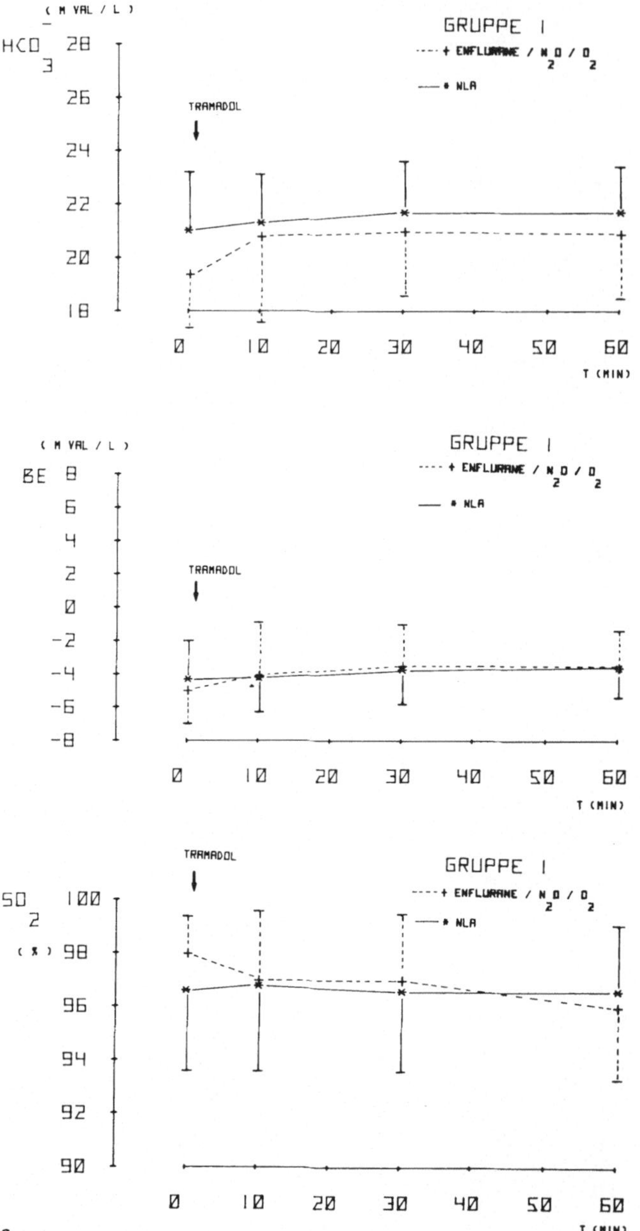

Abb. 5a, b. Bikarbonat (HCO_2), Base exzess (BE) und Sauerstoffsättigung (SO_2) von Patienten nach Oberbaucheingriffen und Gabe von Tramadol. Nähere Angaben siehe Abbildung 1a und b

(M VAL / L)
GRUPPE 2
HCO3 28
TRAMADOL
+ ENFLURANE / N2O / O2
* NLA
26
24
22
20
18
0 10 20 30 40 50 60
T (MIN)

(M VAL / L)
GRUPPE 2
BE 8
+ ENFLURANE / N2O / O2
* NLA
6
4
TRAMADOL
2
0
-2
-4
-6
-8
0 10 20 30 40 50 60
T (MIN)

TRAMADOL
GRUPPE 2
+ ENFLURANE / N2O / O2
SO2 100
* NLA
(%) 98
96
94
92
90
0 10 20 30 40 50 60
T (MIN)

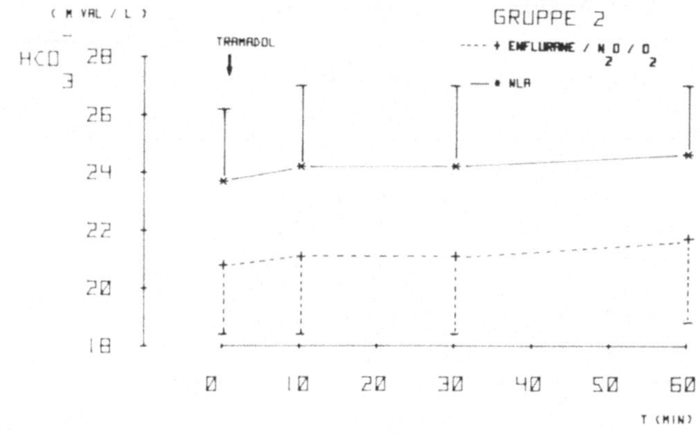

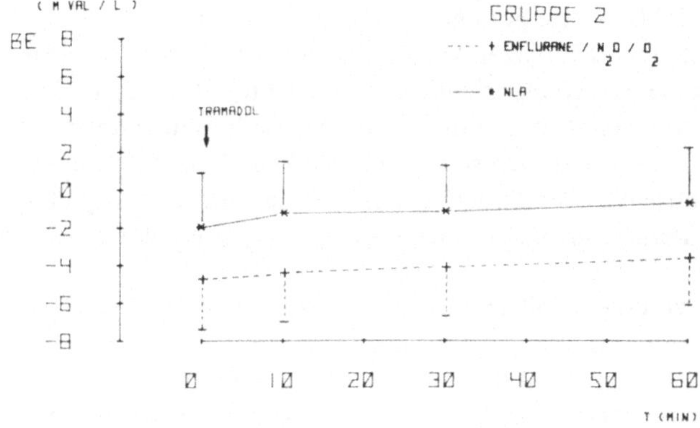

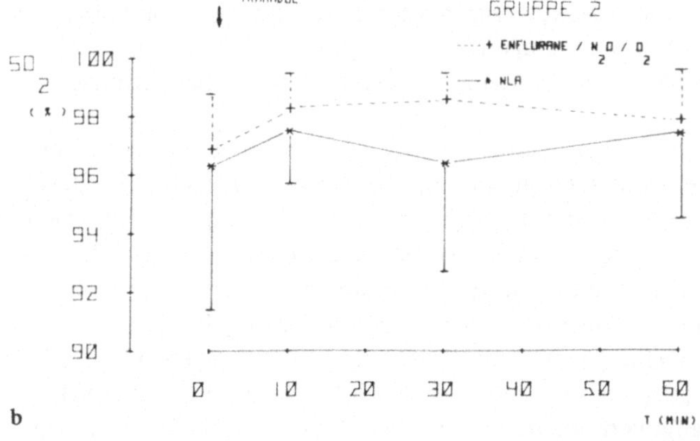

b

Tabelle 3. Tramadol in der postoperativen Phase. Wirkungen und Nebenwirkungen

	nach Enflurane/N_2O/O_2 (n = 18)	nach NLA (n = 24)
Analgesiequalität:		
sehr gut	5 Pat. = 27,8%	13 Pat. = 54,2%
gut	7 Pat. = 38,9%	7 Pat. = 29,2%
nicht befriedigend	6 Pat. = 33,5%	4 Pat. = 16,6%
Starke Sedierung	3 Pat. = 16,7%	10 Pat. = 41,7%
Schwitzen	1 Pat. = 5,6%	3 Pat. = 12,5%
Übelkeit (ohne Erbrechen)	/ = 0%	1 Pat. = 4,2%

zeigte sie fallende Tendenz, der Ausgangswert wurde jedoch nicht wieder erreicht. Der arterielle Mitteldruck fiel nach Tramadol-Gabe nur geringfügig ab (Abb. 1 a und b).

Als der Patient im Aufwachraum über Schmerzen klagte (Zeitpunkt 0), wurde bei allen Patienten eine deutliche Einschränkung des Atemzugvolumens beobachtet (Abb. 2a und b). Gleichzeitig war die Atemfrequenz kompensatorisch erhöht. Das Atemminutenvolumen war in beiden Gruppen nach Neuroleptanalgesie deutlich stärker abgesunken als nach Enflurane-Narkose. Die Gabe von Tramadol führte bei allen Patienten zum Anstieg des Atemzugvolumens bei gleichzeitigem Abfall der Atemfrequenz, die Ausgangswerte wurden jedoch nicht wieder erreicht.

Durch Eingriffe im Oberbauch wird die Vitalkapazität besonders stark eingeschränkt, der von uns beobachtete Abfall der FVC auf ca. 20% des Ausgangswertes stimmt mit der Literatur überein [2, 3, 4] (Abb. 3a und b). Die flache, frequente Atmung mit Einschränkung des Atemzugvolumens und der forcierten Vitalkapazität ist verursacht durch postoperative Schmerzen, möglicherweise auch durch beengenden Verband und das Auftreten eines Pneumoperitoneums [4, 6]. Nach Tramadol-Gabe zeigt die forcierte Vitalkapazität einen leichten Anstieg, möglicherweise als Folge der eingetretenen Schmerzlinderung. Auf die Bedeutung der FVC-Bestimmung als Maß für die Analgesie-Qualität hat erstmals Bromage 1955 hingewiesen [1].

In der postoperativen Phase konnten nach Gabe von Tramadol keine wesentlichen Veränderungen der Blutgase beobachtet werden (Abb. 4a und b, 5a und b). Metabolische Veränderungen mit pH-Verschiebung traten nicht auf. Die in der Literatur vielfach beschriebene Hypoxie nach Oberbaucheingriffen als Folge intrapulmonaler Shunt-Erhöhung durch Mikroatelektasen [4] sahen wir nicht, da alle Patienten im Aufwachraum 4 l Sauerstoff/min über eine Gesichtsmaske erhielten. Besondere Aufmerksamkeit verdient der CO_2-Partialdruck als Maß für eine medikamentbedingte Atemdepression mit Einschränkung der alveolären Ventilation. In unseren Untersuchungen stieg der pCO_2 nach Tramadol-Gabe um max. 2 mmHg an, um dann sogar unter den Ausgangswert abzufallen. Wie bereits von Vogel [5] angegeben, kann somit für Tramadol eine atemdepressive Wirkung ausgeschlossen werden. Dies gilt nach unseren Untersuchungen insbesondere auch für Patienten mit präoperativ eingeschränkter Lungenfunktion (restriktive Ventilationsstörungen).

Zusammenfassend bleibt festzustellen, daß mit Tramadol eine neue Substanz in die Schmerztherapie eingeführt wurde, die nicht zu nennenswerten Veränderungen von Atem- und Kreislaufparametern führt, auch nicht bei Patienten mit präoperativ bestehender Einschränkung der Lungenfunktion. Die analgetische Wirkung des Tramadol ist etwa den bereits bekannten Morphinderivaten vergleichbar, die Versagerquote, insbesondere nach Enflurane-Narkose, könnte möglicherweise dosisbedingt sein. Die gelegentlich beobachtete, auffällig starke Sedierung — die Patienten waren jedoch jederzeit erweckbar — halten wir in der frühen postoperativen Phase für eher günstig, zumal da sie nicht mit einer gleichzeitigen Atemdepression verbunden ist. Insgesamt scheint Tramadol zur Schmerzbekämpfung in der frühen postoperativen Phase nach Enflurane-Narkose wie nach Neurolept-Analgesie gleichermaßen geeignet zu sein.

Literatur

1. Bromage PR (1955) Spirometry in assessment of analgesia after abdominal surgery. A method of comparing analgesic drugs. Brit Med J 3:589–593
2. Churchill ED, McNeil D (1927) The reduction in vital capacity following operation. Surg Gynecol Obstet 44:483–488
3. Egbert LD, Bendixen HH (1964) Effect of morphine on breathing pattern. A possible factor in atelectasis. JAMA 188:113–116
4. Klose R, Osswald P, Lutz H (1977) Präoperative spirometrische Beurteilung der Lungenfunktion und postoperativer Verlauf. Z Prakt Anästh 12:297–306
5. Vogel W, Burchardi H, Sihler K, Valič L (1978) Über die Wirkung von Tramadol auf Atmung und Kreislauf. Arzneim Forsch Drug Res 28:183–186
6. Wallace PGM, Norris W (1975) The management of postoperative pain. Brit J Anaesth 47:113–120

Clinical Experience with Epidural Pressure Monitoring: The Relevance of Transducer Location

M. Belopavlovic and A. Buchthal

Introduction

Continuous intracranial pressure monitoring is increasingly being employed postoperatively in neurosurgical practice. It is anticipated that this may allow earlier recognition of complications requiring active treatment than is possible by clinical observation alone. Use of an epidural technique is of practical interest as it is essentially non-invasive and because the transducer can be placed near the site of surgery and of pathology.

During the last five years continuous epidural pressure measurements have been made in 300 patients in the Neurosurgical Unit in Groningen. These include 253 postoperative craniotomy patients, comprising 115 cerebral tumours, 59 pituitary tumours, 59 cerebral aneurysms, 11 AV malformations and 9 posterior fossas. In this paper we present a retrospective study of epidural pressure measurements in the cerebral tumour group only.

Method

An epidural pressure transducer (Philips) [1] was placed in one of the craniotomy burr holes during closure. Great care is required to ensure that the transducer is securely fixed, is coplanar with the dura and that there is no blood between the transducer and the dura [2, 3]. A Queckenstedt test was performed to test the transducer in situ. Epidural pressure (EDP) was recorded automatically at 6 minute intervals on a trend recorder for up to five days postoperatively. Trend records of the first 72 hours were smoothed and digitised by hand with a bias towards lower values of EDP.

The cases were classified according to:
1. Pathology of the tumour.
2. Location of the transducer: Frontal, parietal and temporal, and occipital and parieto-occipital.
3. Clinical postoperative course.
4. The use of diuretics during induction of anaesthesia.

Only clinically uncomplicated cases were subjected to statistical analysis.

Results

Of 115 cases, measurement was technically unsatisfactory in 34 (29.5%). Of 81 remaining cases, 29 were clinically complicated (36%) and 52 uncomplicated (64%). The uncomplicated group consisted of 29 gliomas, 10 meningiomas and 13 metastases.

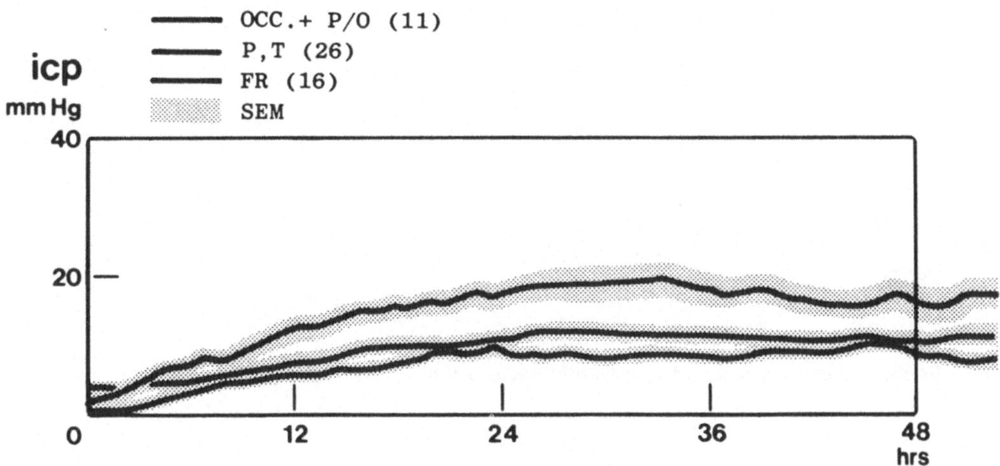

Fig. 1. Relation between epidural pressure measurement and transducer location

In the clinically uncomplicated cases the location of the transducer was found to be the most striking factor (Fig. 1). The difference between the mean pressures in the frontal and occipital groups is highly significant. For example, 24 hours postoperatively the mean pressure in the frontal group was 10 mmHg while that in the occipital group was 17 mmHg with standard errors of 1.2 and 1.7 mmHg respectively; $p < 0.001$. 36 hours postoperatively $p < 0.0025$. There is considerable overlap between the three populations when no other factors are taken into account, the standard deviations being 4, 5 and 6 mmHg respectively 24 hours postoperatively in the frontal, parietal/temporal and occipital/parieto-occipital groups.

Clinically complicated cases are usually easily distinguished from uncomplicated cases. For example, patient 78 developed clinical signs of very high intracranial pressure preoperatively and had obvious cerebral oedema at operation where a frontal glioma was removed. Fig. 2 shows his EDP's recorded postoperatively superimposed on those of uncomplicated frontal cases. Patient 229 underwent a frontal craniotomy for subtotal excision of a falx meningioma (Fig. 3). The EDP immediately postoperatively was in the normal range but af-

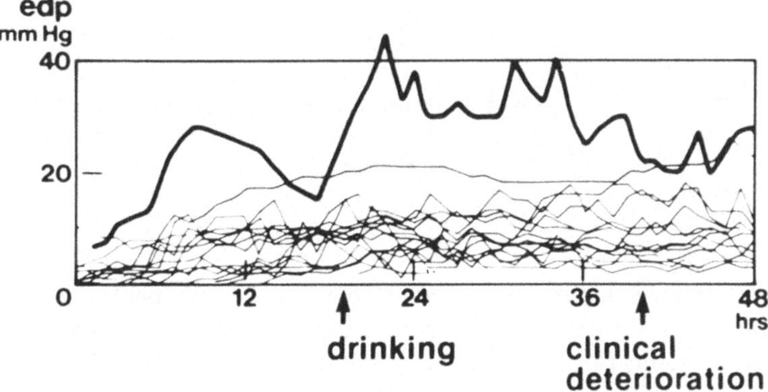

Fig. 2. Frontal craniotomy large glioma preoperative cushing response intra operative cerebral oedema

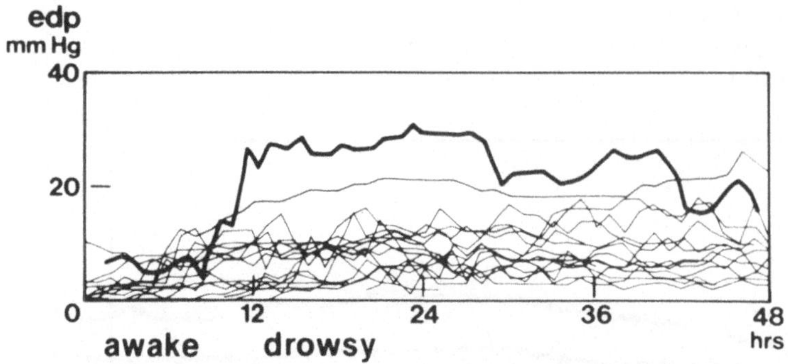

Fig. 3. Frontal craniotomy falx meningioma subtotal excision

ter 12 hours it rose well above pressures recorded in uncomplicated cases. At the same time, his level of consciousness deteriorated. There was no hypoxia or hypercarbia.

The value of epidural pressure recorded depends on the relationship between the location of the transducer and the posture of the patient (Fig. 4). In this patient with a left parietal transducer the measured EDP fell by about 10 mmHg when he turned from his left side on-to his right side.

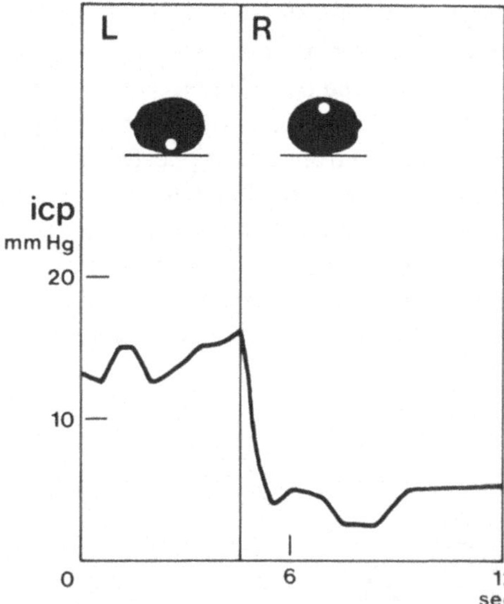

Fig. 4. Influence of posture and transducer location on epidural pressure measurement. Left parietal epidural transducer

Discussion

Since the development of epidural techniques for intracranial pressure measurement, there has been much interest in their clinical validation by comparing simultaneous epidural and intraventricular pressure measurements [4, 5, 6, 7]. Little attention has been paid in these comparisons to the relative locations of the epidural and ventricular transducers or to the vertical distance between them, which may vary with the posture of the patient (Fig. 5).

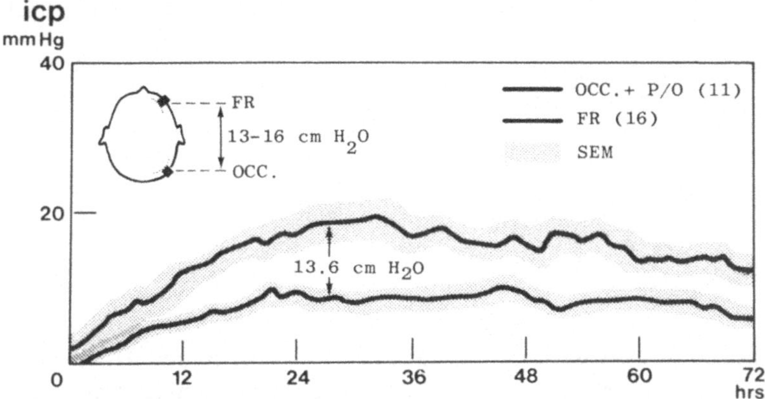

Fig. 5. Influence of epidural transducer location on pressure measurement

The difference between the mean frontal and parieto-occipital pressures between 12 and 48 hours postoperatively is around 13 to 16 cm water. This is similar to the vertical distance between two transducer locations in the supine patient so that it can be explained on the basis of a hydrostatic model. Unless a correction is first made for any hydrostatic difference, the influence of other factors, which may be smaller, is unlikely to be seen clearly.

The effect of postural changes will be reduced by placing the transducer as near to the midline as possible and near the midparietal region. At the same time, however, the transducer should lie over or near the site of operation for maximal sensitivity to local changes.

In conclusion a careful note be made of transducer location and posture of the patient and of all the other factors which are well known to affect intracranial pressure. These all tend to raise intracranial pressure and include coughing, vomiting, convulsions, respiratory depression, physiotherapy and other activities of the patient. Epidural pressure measurements can only be interpreted if all these factors as well as the clinical condition of the patient are taken into account.

References

1. Gieles ACM, Somers GHJ (1973) Miniature pressure transducers with a silicon diaphragm. Philips technical review 33:14
2. Dorsch NWC, Symon L (1975) The validity of extradural measurement of intracranial pressure. In: Lundberg, Ponten and Brock (ed) Intracranial pressure II. Springer Verlag, p 403
3. Schettini A, Walsh E (1975) Simultaneous pressure-depth measurement of the intracranial system made epidurally. In: Lundberg, Ponten and Brock (ed) Intracranial pressure II. Springer Verlag, p 409
4. Schettini A, McKay L, Majors R, Mahig J, Nevis A (1971) Experimental approach for monitoring surface brain pressure. J Neurosurgery 34:38
5. McGraw CP (1975) Epidural Intracranial Pressure monitoring. In: Lundberg, Ponten and Brock (ed) Intracranial pressure II. Springer Verlag, p 394
6. Coroneos NJ, McDowall DG, Gibson RM, Pickerodt V, Keaney NP (1972) A comparison of extradural pressure with cerebrospinal fluid pressure. In: Fleschi C (ed) Cerebral Blood Flow and Intracranial pressure. S. Karger, Basel, p 79
7. Sundbärg G, Nornes H (1972) Simultaneous recordings of epidural and ventricular fluid pressure. In: Brock and Dietz (ed) Intracranial pressure I. p 46

Postoperative Hypertension nach Neuroleptanästhesie

U. Brenken, G. Karliczek und D. Birks

In der unmittelbar postoperativen Phase kommt es häufig zu Vasokonstriktion, Hypertension und Kältezittern. In besonderem Maße ist dies der Fall nach großen und langdauernden Operationen, wie z.B. Koronaroperationen [2, 6]. Es war uns aufgefallen, daß diese Erscheinungen kurz nach Beendigung der Lachgasanästhesie einsetzen und sich kaum durch zusätzliche Gaben von Morphinomimetika verhüten lassen. Der Einfluß der Beendigung der Lachgasanästhesie auf das Zustandekommen der postoperativen Hypertension ist bisher nicht beschrieben worden.

Wir haben daher bei 30 Patienten untersucht, welche hämodynamischen Veränderungen eintreten, wenn nach Beendigung der Operation das Lachgas aus dem Einatmungsgemisch weggelassen wird. Es handelt sich dabei vornehmlich um koronarchirurgische Eingriffe, die in Neuroleptanästhesie durchgeführt wurden.

Methodik

Die Narkose wurde mit Etomidate eingeleitet und mit Fentanyl (gemittelt 1,6 mg), Dehydrobenzperidol (im Durchschnitt 15 mg) und 50% Lachgas bei Relaxierung mit Pavulon unterhalten.

Die Beatmung erfolgte mit dem Servoventilator und wurde mit einem Siemens Elema CO_2-Analysator auf endexpiratorische CO_2-Werte von 5% eingestellt. Dieser CO_2-Analysator lieferte auch kontinuierliche Angaben über die CO_2-Produktion. Thermistorbestückte Swan-Ganz-Katheter vervollständigten das Monitoring. Alle Perfusionen wurden mit einem TMO-Oxygenator und Hämodilutionstechnik bei mittlerer Hypothermie (28–30 °C) durchgeführt.

Nach Beendigung der extrakorporalen Zirkulation bei 37 °C nasopharyngeal wurde kein Muskelrelaxans mehr gegeben, Fentanyl jedoch in zur Analgesie ausreichenden Mengen, insbesondere kurz vor Operationsende beim Sternumverschluß (0,2 mg i.v.). Nach der letzten Hautnaht begannen wir mit unseren Messungen und bestimmten die Nullwerte. Danach wurde das Lachgas im Ventilationsgemisch abgesetzt und gegen Luft ausgetauscht, die Beatmung blieb ansonsten gleich, insbesondere die inspiratorische Sauerstoffkonzentration. Die Messungen wurden bis zu 30 Minuten nach Absetzen des Lachgases wiederholt.

Ergebnisse

Innerhalb dieser halben Stunde erwachten 19 der 30 Patienten (63%), 7 begannen zu zittern (23%) und 2 weitere Patienten wurden so unruhig, daß sie sediert werden mußten. Fast alle

(93%) zeigten deutliche Blutdruckanstiege; 5 Patienten (17%) behandelten wir wegen ihrer Blutdruckanstiege mit Vasodilatatoren. Diese und die wegen Unruhe behandelten Patienten wurden von der statistischen Auswertung der hämodynamischen Ergebnisse ausgeschlossen.

Bei den übrigen 24 Patienten stieg der Blutdruck von gemittelt 120/65 (Standardabweichung $\pm$ 13/11) auf im Mittel 165/77 mmHg ($\pm$ 16/13), p < 0,001; die Herzfrequenz stieg von 95 auf gemittelt 105 Schläge pro Minute (Abb. 1). Der Pulmonalisdruck stieg von 28/14 ($\pm$ 8/6) nach 38/17 mmHg ($\pm$ 16/7), p < 0,01. Der Cardiac Index stieg innerhalb von 10 Minuten von 3,9 ($\pm$ 0,77) auf 4,6 ($\pm$ 1,0) $1 \cdot min^{-1} \cdot m^{-2}$ (p < 0,01); ebenso der Schlagvolumenindex von 41,3 ($\pm$ 9) nach 45 ($\pm$ 11) $ml \cdot m^{-2}$. Rechter und linker Vorhofdruck blieben weitgehend konstant.

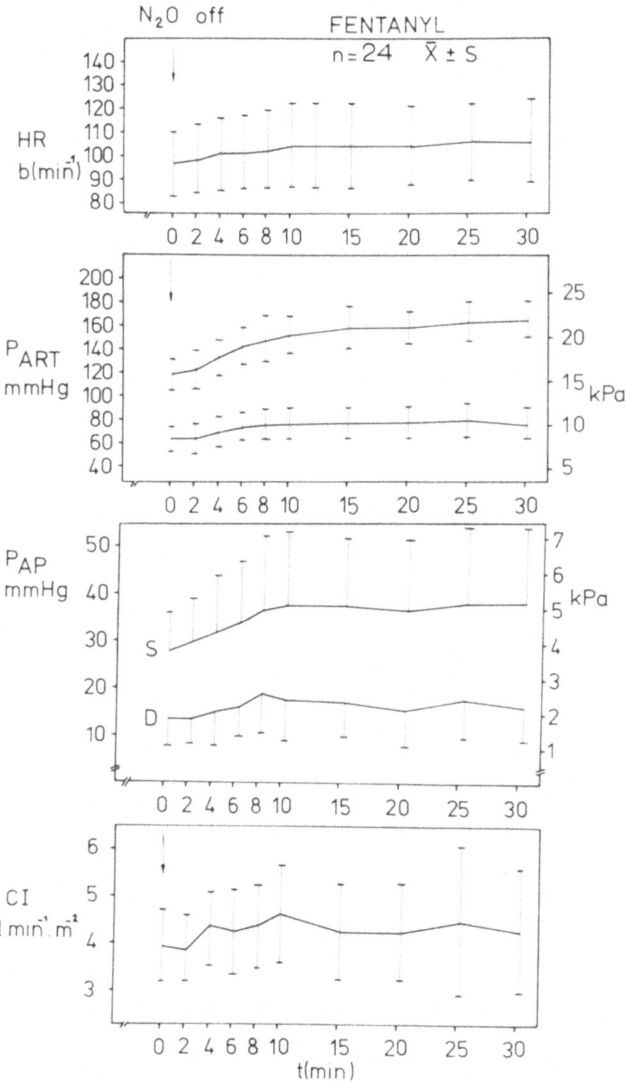

Abb. 1. Darstellung von Pulsfrequenz (HR), systolischem und diastolischem Druck (PART), Pulmonalarteriendruck (PAP) und Herzindex (CI) nach Beendigung der Lachgasanästhesie in Neuroleptnarkose

Es kam zu einer signifikanten Zunahme des peripheren Widerstandes (Abb. 2):
von 89 ($\pm$ 24) nach 112 ($\pm$ 32) m.N. sec $\cdot$ m^{-5}; (p $<$ 0,001). Gleichzeitig sank die Hauttemperatur von 27,7° auf 26,8 °C, wobei Δ t (Differentialtemperatur $T_{NP} - T_H$) von 8,06°
nach 9,42 °C stieg. Die CO_2-Produktion stieg von 125 ($\pm$ 23) nach 144 ($\pm$ 52) ml $\cdot$ min^{-1} $\cdot$ m^{-2}.
Das Produkt aus systolischem Blutdruck und Herzfrequenz als Ausdruck des linksventrikulären myokardialen Sauerstoffbedarfes [4] stieg hochsignifikant.

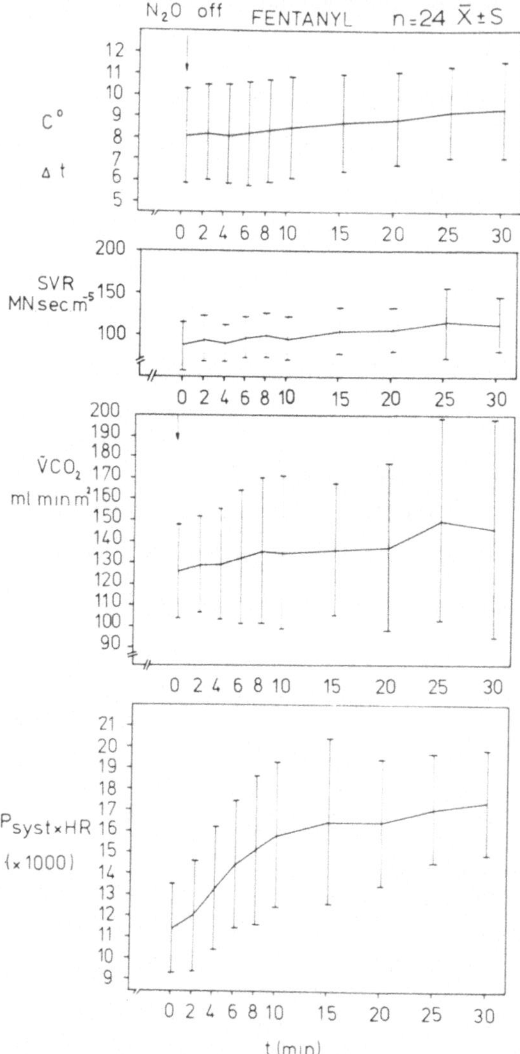

Abb. 2. Darstellung von Δt (Differentialtemperatur Nasopharynx – Haut), Systemgefäßwiderstand (SVR),
CO_2-Produktion (V CO_2) und systolischem Druck-Frequenz-Produkt ($P_{syst} \times$ HR)

Diskussion

Bei fast allen Patienten führt das Absetzen von Lachgas zu einem deutlichen Blutdruckanstieg. Daran sind sowohl Widerstandsanstieg als auch Herzzeitvolumenzunahme beteiligt. Das Ausmaß dieser Drucksteigerungen kann exzessiv sein. Innerhalb von Minuten können systolische Blutdruckwerte von über 200 mmHg erreicht werden.

Für Patienten mit Koronar- oder Herzinsuffizienz stellen solche Druckanstiege ein erhebliches Risiko dar. Das wiegt umso schwerer, da in dem Zeitraum zwischen Operationsende und Intensivbehandlung nur geringe Möglichkeiten für Monitoring und Behandlung gegeben sind.

Wir können an dieser Stelle nicht näher auf die zahlreichen anderen Ursachen für die postoperative Hypertension [1, 3, 5, 6, 7] eingehen.

Wir glauben, daß mangelnde Anästhesie keine wichtige Rolle spielt. Schmerzen äußerte keiner der Patienten und ähnliche Blutdruckanstiege finden wir auch nach Neuroleptanästhesien mit langwirkenden Opiaten wie Morphin, Pethidin oder Dipidolor (Abb. 3). Auch das

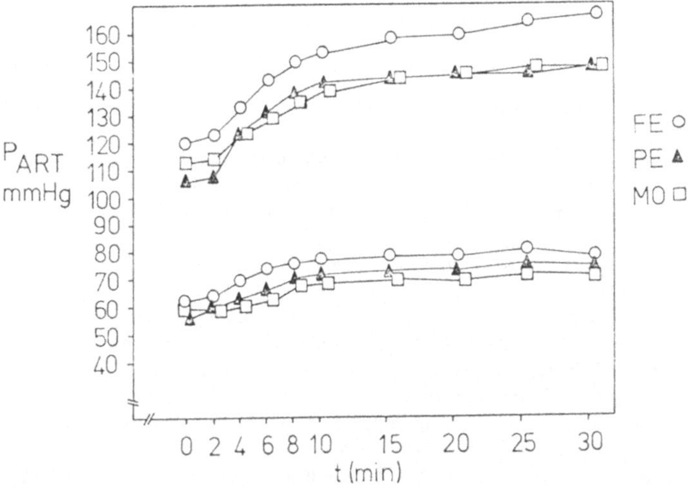

Abb. 3. Anstieg des arteriellen Blutdruckes (P_{ART}) nach Absetzen von Lachgas bei Neuroleptanästhesie mit Fentanyl (FE), Pethidin (PE) und Morphin (MO)

Erwachen an sich spielt keine entscheidende Bedeutung. Denn auch nach Anästhesien mit langer Nachschlafdauer wie z.B. Dipidolor in Kombination mit Rohypnol kommt es nach dem Absetzen von Lachgas noch immer zu Blutdruckanstiegen (Abb. 4).

Diese Untersuchungen machen deutlich, daß das Absetzen von Lachgas unter Umständen zu gefährlichen Hypertensionen führen kann. Eine wirksame Vorbeugung ist uns bisher nicht bekannt. Wir empfehlen daher, Lachgas bei gefährdeten Patienten nur dann abzuschalten, wenn die Möglichkeit einer ausreichenden Blutdrucküberwachung gegeben ist und Vasodilatatoren unverzüglich gegeben werden können.

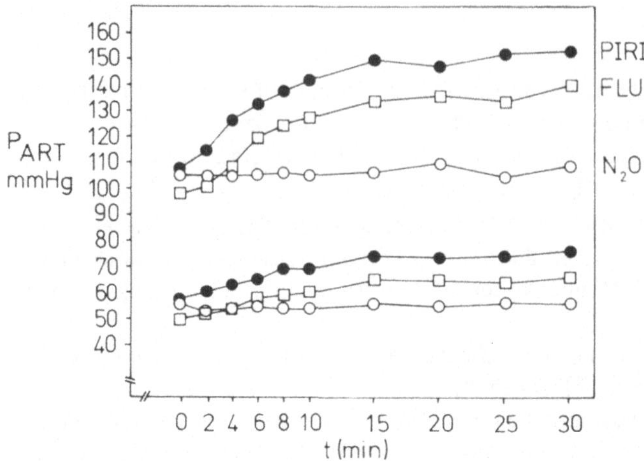

Abb. 4. Das Verhalten des arteriellen Blutdruckes nach Absetzen von Lachgas nach Neuroleptanästhesie
mit Dipidolor (PIRI), und der Kombination von Dipidolor und Rohypnol (FLU). Zum Vergleich
eine Kontrollgruppe mit kontinuierlicher Lachgasapplikation (N_2O)

Literatur

1. Anton AH, Gravenstein JS, Wheat MW Jr (1964) Extracorporeal circulation and endogenous epinephrine and norepinephrine in plasma, atrium and urine in man. Anaesthesiology 25:262
2. Estafanous FG, Tarazi RC, Viljoen JF, El Tawil MY (1973) Systemic hypertension following myocardial revascularization. Am Heart J 85:732
3. James TN, Isobe JH, Urthaler F (1975) Analysis of components in a cardiogenic hypertensive chemo-
   reflex. Circulation 52:179
4. Nelson RR, Gobel FL, Jorgensen ChR, Wang K, Wang Y, Taylor HL (1974) Haemodynamic predic-
   tions of the myocardial oxygen consumption during static and dynamic exercise. Circulation 50:1179
5. Pratilas V, Pratila MG, Vlachakis ND (1978) Hypertension and plasma catecholamines following aorto-
   coronary bypass surgery. (Presentation at V European Congress of Anesthesiology, Paris)
6. Roberts AJ, Niarchos AP, Subremanian VA (1977) Systemic hypertension associated with coronary
   artery bypass surgery. J Thoracic and Cardiovascular Surgery 74:846
7. Taylor KM, Morton IJ, Brown JJ, Bain WH, Caves PK (1977) Hypertension and the renin-angiotensin
   system following open heart surgery. J Thoracic and Cardiovascular Surgery 74:840

Antiplasmin- und Antithrombin-Spiegelveränderungen bei cholecystektomierten Patienten

C.K. Spiss, F. Schulz und L. Fridrich

Einleitung

Das Problem der Klärung der postoperativen Thrombosegefährdung scheint noch immer einigermaßen ungelöst. Bisher wurden zwei Wege, nämlich die Heparinprophylaxe einerseits, sowie die Verabreichung von hochmolekularen Substanzen andererseits, beschritten, um dieses Problem in den Griff zu bekommen. Beide Methoden bergen nicht unbeträchtliche Gefahren in sich, bei Heparin die Blutungsgefahr, bei Dextran allergoide Reaktionen. Es muß daher jeder Weg begrüßenswert erscheinen, der in den ersten 24 Stunden postoperativ die Diagnose „erhöhtes Thromboserisiko" ermöglicht und in der klinischen Praxis gangbar ist. Wir beschritten den Weg der prae-intra- und postoperativen Verfolgung des AP-Spiegels, wobei der Aktivitätsverlauf des von Dollen, Müllertz und Adki (1976) beschriebene alpha$_2$AP untersucht wurde. Als weiterer Parameter wurde auch der Antithrombin-Spiegel verfolgt.

Material und Methodik

Die untersuchten 10 (bzw. 8) Patienten im Alter zwischen 31 und 62 Jahren (Durchschnittsalter: 45 Jahre). Bei allen der Untersuchung zugeführten Patienten konnte außer der Cholelithiasis kein pathologischer Befund erhoben werden. Gerinnungsparameter (Thrombozyten, Fibrinogen, NT, PTT) und Leberfermente (GOT, GPT, YGT und LDH) bewegten sich im physiologischen Bereich. Patienten mit erhöhtem Thromboserisiko infolge organischer Veränderungen (Varizen), oder einer Dauermedikation (Ovulationshemmer) wurden aus der Untersuchung ausgeschlossen, ebenso Patienten, die sich während eines Zeitraumes bis zu einem Jahr einer Narkose mit halogenierten Kohlenwasserstoffen unterziehen hatten müssen. Alle Patienten waren mit der NLA-Technik narkotisiert, intubiert, relaxiert und kontrolliert beatmet. Intraoperativ wurden 1500 ml einer 5%igen Kohlenhydrat-Elektrolytlösung zugeführt. Als Indikator für die Plasmaverdünnung durch parenterale Flüssigkeitsgabe wurde der Serumalbuminspiegel herangezogen. 10 ml Citrat-Vollblut wurden am kontralateralen Infusionsarm:
1. unmittelbar vor der Narkoseeinleitung
2. eine Stunde nach Operationsbeginn
3. unmittelbar postoperativ und
4. 24 Stunden postoperativ
abgenommen, sofort zentrifugiert, das Plasma abpippetiert, schockgefroren und zu einem späteren Zeitpunkt verarbeitet. Die Antiplasmin- bzw. Antithrombinbestimmungen unter Verwendung von chromogenen Substraten (S-2251 bzw. S-2238, Fa. Kabi, Peptide Res.,

Molndal, Schweden) durchgeführt. Die Bestimmung des Serumalbuminspiegels erfolgte elektrophoretisch.

Ergebnisse

Tabelle 1 zeigt die bereits auf den Ausgangswert des Serumalbumins korrigierten AP-Werte zu den verschiedenen Meßzeitpunkten. Man erkennt bei den Patienten 1, 4, 8, 9, 10, einen postoperativ beträchtlich erhöhten AP-Spiegel.
Abb. 1 zeigt die perzentuellen Änderungen der Mittelwerte der AP-Spiegel im Vergleich zum praeoperativen Wert. Intraoperativ kommt es zu einem Abfall von etwa 7%, postoperativ zu einer geringgradigen Steigerung des AP-Spiegels, der jedoch noch immer um 3% niedriger als der Ausgangswert ist. Der Unterschied zwischen Operationswert und 24 Stunden postoperativ beträgt +17%. (Dieser Unterschied läßt sich im gepaarten t-Test mit 2% statistisch sichern.)
Die Antithrombin-Spiegel zeigten in ihrem Verlauf keine signifikante Änderung.

Tabelle 1. Antiplasminwerte zu den verschiedenen Meßzeitpunkten

Patienten	prae-op.	intra-op.	post-op.	24 St. post-op.
1. J.F. 39 a	103	106	98	136
2. E.M. 62 a	100	102	111	106
3. F.S. 41 a	91	78	101	97
4. L.A. 47 a	89	92	90	119
5. M.I. 34 a	124	116	117	123
6. B.M. 32 a	116	94	91	117
7. K.R. 49 a	115	95	86	108
8. G.H. 62 a	86	94	99	102
9. E.I. 31 a	92	67	88	118
10. R.T. 53 a	127	124	129	172
M.W.	104	97	101	120

Diskussion

Das Vorhandensein von Plasmininhibitoren ist seit Norman 1958 [9] bekannt. Seither konzentriert sich das Interesse der Forschung auf die Frage möglicher Zusammenhänge zwischen AP-Aktivität-postoperativer Fibrinolysehemmung und thrombotischen Komplikationen (Ellison und Brown [4], Gallus et al. [5]). Steinbuch [11] beschrieb 1971 fünf recht gut definierte plasmininhibierende Plasmaproteine.
Die allgemein vorherrschende Meinung, daß vor allem L_2-Macroglobulin und L_1-Antitrypsin für die Plasmininhibierung verantwortlich seien, wurde durch verschiedene Untersuchungen der letzten Jahre etwas erschüttert.
Unabhängig voneinander zeigten Aoki, Collen und Müllertz, daß im wesentlichen nur zwei Plasmaproteine, in dem durch Streptokinase bzw. Urokinase aktivierten fibrinolyti-

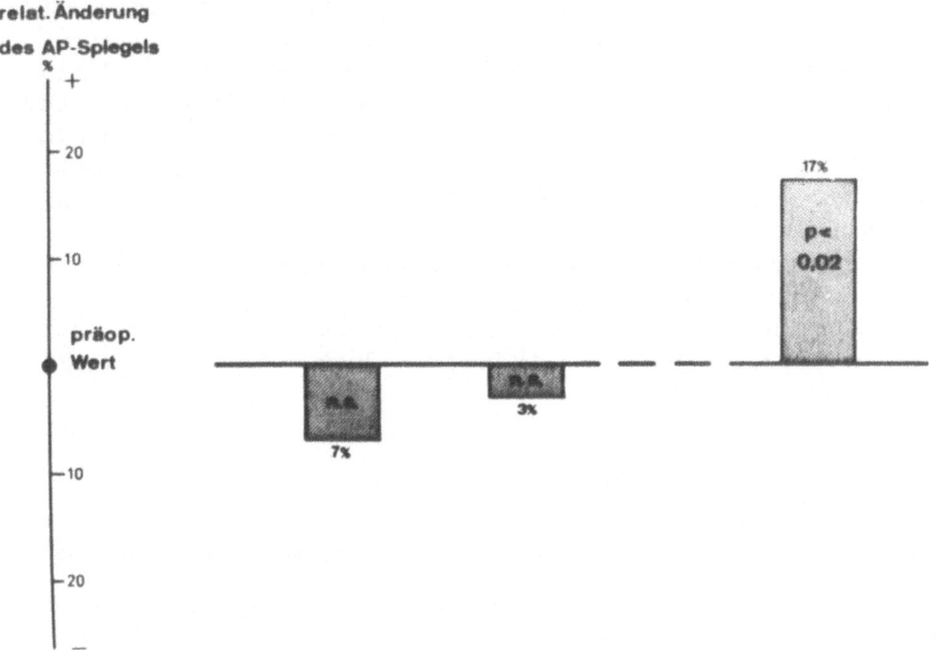

Abb. 1. Perzentuelle Änderung der Mittelwerte der Antiplasminspiegel im Vergleich zum praeoperativen Wert

Tabelle 2. Plasmininhibierende Plasmaproteine (Steinbuch [11])

alpha-2-macroglobulin
alpha-1-antitrypsin
inter-alpha-trypsin inhibitor
antithrombin-3-heparin complex
C-1 esterase-inhibitor

Tabelle 3. Plasmininhibierende Plasmaproteine (Aoki, Collen, Müllertz 1976) – derzeitiger Stand

alpha-2-antiplasmin
alpha-2-macroglobulin

schen System, für die Plasmininhibierung verantwortlich seien; und zwar in erster Linie, daß von diesen Arbeitsgruppen bestimmte L_2-Antiplasmin, das auch in unserer Untersuchungsreihe bestimmt wurde, sowie L_2-Macroglobulin. Hierbei ist L_2-Antiplasmin anscheinend als sofort wirksamer Inhibitor aufzufassen, wobei L_2-Macroglobulin vermutlich die Aufgabe besitzt, das noch verbleibende Plasmin zu neutralisieren. Die Bedeutung der übrigen oben erwähnten Plasmininhibitoren ist heute sehr fraglich. Es liegt nun die Annahme nahe, daß das

L_2-Antiplasmin indirekte Schlüsse auf das Verhalten des fibrinolytischen Systems erlaubt. Intraoperativ scheint es durch den Operationsstreß zu einer gesteigerten Fibrinolyse zu kommen, der dadurch bedingte AP-Verbrauch könnte den intraoperativen Abfall des AP-Spiegels erklären. Die Ursache der Verminderung der fibrinolytischen Aktivität in der postoperativen Periode scheint derzeit nicht völlig geklärt. Allerdings ist die Möglichkeit nicht von der Hand zu weisen, daß es sich bei der postoperativen Erhöhung des AP-Spiegels um ein Rebound-Phänomen, nach erhöhtem intraoperativen Verbrauch (als Akut-Reaktion), handeln könnte.

Im Gegensatz zum AP-Spiegel dürfte sich der Antithrombin-Spiegel erst in der späteren postoperativen Phase verändern.

Zusammenfassend haben wir nachweisen können, daß es bei 80% der von uns untersuchten Fälle zu einem postoperativ erhöhten AP-Spiegel, als Ausdruck eines möglicherweise gesteigerten Thromboserisikos, kommt.

Literatur

1. Aoki N, Moroi M, Matsuda M, Tachiya K (1977) The Behavior of L_2-Plasmin Inhibitor in Fibrinolytic States. J of Clinical Investigation 60:361–369
2. Aoki N, von Kaulla KN (1971) Human serum plasminogen antiactivator: its distinction from antiplasmin. Am J Physiol 220:1137–1145
3. Collen D (1976) Identification and some properties of a new fastreacting plasmin inhibitor in human plasma. Eur J Biochem 69 (1): 209–16, 1. Oct. 1976
4. Ellison RC, Brown J (1965) Fibrinolysis in pulmonary vascular disease. Lancet 1:786
5. Gallus AS, Hirsch J, Gent M (1973) Relevance of preoperative and postoperative blood tests to postoperative leg vein thrombosis. Lancet 2:806
6. Gyzander E, Friberger P, Myrwold H, Olsson R, Teger-Nilsson AC, Wallmo L (1976) Antiplasmin Determination by Means of the Plasmin Specific Substrate S-2251-Methodological Studies and Some Clinical Applications, Proceeding of the Symposium of the Deutsche Gesellschaft für Klinische Chemie, Titisee, Breisgau, West-Germany, July 1976
7. Marciniak E, Gockermann JP (1977) Heparin-induced Decrease in Circulating Antithrombin III. Lancet 2:581
8. Müllertz S, Clemmensen J (1976) The primary inhibitor of plasmin in human plasma. Biochem J 159 (3):545–53, 1 Dec. 1976
9. Norman PS (1958) Studies of the plasmin system; inhibition of plasmin by serum or plasma. J Exp Med 108:53
10. Ødegard OR, Abildgaard U (1978) Antithrombin III: Critical Review of Assay Methods. Significance of Variations in Health and Desease. Haemostasis 7:127
11. Steinbuch M (1971) Rev Fr Transfus 14:61–82

Verlängerung der Aufwachphase durch das Zentral-Anti-Cholingergische Syndrom: ein Vergleich von Atropin und Glycopyrrolate

F.R. Brosch

Einleitung

Anticholinergische Medikamente sind von jeher ein wesentlicher Faktor in der Praxis der Anästhesie. Die unbestreitbaren Vorteile — reduzierte Magen- und Speichelsekretionen, sowie ein gewisser Schutz gegen vagale Reflexe — haben bis vor kurzem nachteilige Nebenwirkungen überschattet.

Neben dem wohlbekannten Scopolamin-Delirium wurde im Zusammenhang mit toxischen Dosen von Belladonna-Alkaloiden auch eine langandauernde Somnolenz beobachtet. Dieser Symptomenkomplex wurde 1966 von Longo [1] als „Zentrales Anticholinergisches Syndrom" (Z.A.S.) beschrieben. Seit 1972 haben verschiedene Autoren [2, 3, 4] darauf hingewiesen, daß diese — oft viele Stunden in die postoperative Phase hinein andauernde — Somnolenz auch nach klinisch üblichen Dosen von Atropin beobachtet werden kann.

Erst nach Erscheinen dieser Berichte haben wir an unserem eigenen Institut eine überraschend hohe Zahl ähnlicher Fälle beobachtet und mit Physostigmin (Eserin) erfolgreich behandelt. Bis dahin wurden diese Symptome entweder nicht erkannt oder auf verschiedene andere Faktoren zurückgeführt z.B. Überempfindlichkeit gegen bzw. verzögerter Abbau von Inhalations-Anästhetika, Narkotika oder Barbituraten. Das neuere Anticholinergikum Glycopyrrolate (Robinul) durchdringt angeblich die Blut-Liquorschranke nicht und wird als frei von zentralen Nebenwirkungen empfohlen [2, 4].

Um die Stichhaltigkeit dieser Theorie nachzuprüfen und die Frequenz des Z.A.S. nach klinisch üblichen Dosen von anticholinergischen Medikamenten zu studieren, wurde die folgende Untersuchung unternommen.

Methodik

41 Patienten in gutem Allgemeinzustand im Alter von 13—55 Jahren waren zur Allgemein-Narkose vorgesehen. Alle hatten ein ungetrübtes Sensorium und waren frei von psychotropen Medikamenten wie z.B. Sedativa, Tranquilizer, Anti-Depressiva etc. Patienten und Operationen, die postoperative Beatmung erwarten ließen, wurden von der Untersuchung ausgeschlossen.

Im Doppel-Blindverfahren erhielten 20 Patienten Atropin und 21 Patienten Glycopyrrolate als prä- und intra-operatives Anticholinergikum in einer Konzentration von 0,4 mg/ml für Atropin und 0,2 mg/ml für Glycopyrrolate. Diese Dosis wird von den meisten Autoren als equipotent angesehen und entspricht im wesentlichen den Praxisgepflogenheiten. Die Prämedikation bestand aus 8—10 mg Morphin i.m. etwa eine Stunde präoperativ. Keiner der Patienten zeigte mehr als eine minimale Sedierung.

Ein ml der Testsubstanz wurde unmittelbar vor der Narkose-Einleitung i.v. verabreicht. Die Narkose-Führung wurde weitgehend standardisiert und bestand aus einer Thiopental-Einleitung (4–6 mg/kg), kontrollierter Beatmung mit N_2O/O_2 im Verhältnis 2:1 und zusätzlicher Analgesie mit Fentanyl in Dosen von 0,05–0,1 mg nach klinischem Bedarf. Zur Intubation und Relaxation wurde Pancuronium in klinisch üblichen Dosen verwendet (0,08 mg/kg zur Intubation und 1–2 mg als Zusatzdosis nach Bedarf).

Wir nahmen darauf Bedacht, die Narkotika besonders gegen Ende der Operation konservativ zu dosieren, um die Notwendigkeit einer Antagonisierung mit Naloxon zu vermeiden. Die Relaxantien wurden mit einer Standard-Dosis von 10–15 mg Pyridostigmin antagonisiert, zusammen mit 3 ml des anticholinergischen Präparats (1,2 mg Atropin bzw. 0,6 mg Glycopyrrolate).

Unmittelbar nach der Extubation und in 15minütigen Abständen danach wurde das Sensorium des Patienten an Hand einer Tabelle nach Punkten bewertet (Tabelle 1). Alle Auswertungen erfolgten durch denselben Beobachter.

Tabelle 1. Punkte-Bewertung

Patient unansprechbar, reagiert auf keine Stimulation	0
Patient unansprechbar, reagiert nur auf mechanische Stimulation	1
Patient reagiert auf variable Stimulation	2
Patient reagiert auf Fragen und Kommandos	3
Patient reagiert mit Grunzen bzw. einsilbigen Lauten	4
Patient antwortet schläfrig, doch zusammenhängend	5
Patient antwortet klar und zusammenhängend, doch döst ohne Stimulation	6
Patient spricht spontan, zeigt Interesse an seiner Umgebung	7

In allen Fällen von prolongierter Somnolenz wurden außerdem Körpertemperatur und Blutgase bestimmt.

Ergebnisse

In der Atropin-Gruppe zeigten 3 Patienten eine dem Z.A.S. ähnliche Symptomatik. (Fall No. 12 reagierte zu früh und erhielt 0,1 mg Fentanyl + 100 mg Thiopental unmittelbar bevor Operationsende, war aber nach 15 Minuten voll ansprechbar.)

Die Z.A.S. Patienten wurden 1–2 Stunden auf der Wachstation beobachtet, um einen eventuellen Fentanyl-Effekt abklingen zu lassen. Das Sensorium blieb in typischer Weise über längere Zeit unverändert, doch gaben die Patienten nach kurzer Zeit auf Befragen an, Schmerzen zu haben. Zu diesem Zeitpunkt, wenn das Syndrom wohl-etabliert erschien und eine spontane Besserung nicht beobachtet werden konnte, gaben wir das Antidot Physostigmin (Eserin) in der üblichen Dosis von 2 mg langsam i.v. [3, 5].

Der Effekt war in jedem Falle klassisch. Wir vermieden jede Stimulation des dösenden Patienten und nach 4–5 Minuten wurde die mimische Muskulatur abrupt wieder aktiv, die Augen öffneten sich spontan und der Patient blickte um sich, versuchte sich aufzurichten und begann zu sprechen. Gelegentlich bestand eine retrograde Amnesie für die Wachstation-

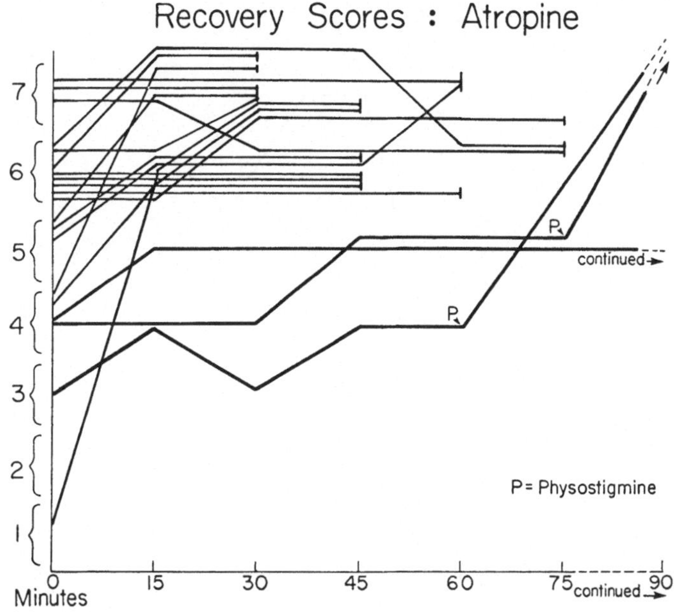

Abb. 1

Phase, obwohl der Patient auf Ansprache und Kommandos reagiert hatte bzw. informiert worden war, wo er sich befand.

Andere Medikamente mit einem gewissen anticholinergischen Effekt, wie Phenothiazine und Anti-Depressiva; sowie Butyrophenon- und Benzodiazepin-Derivate, die gelegentlich mit einem „unspezifischen Aufwach-Effekt" in Zusammenhang gebracht wurden, waren durch das Versuchsprotokoll ausgeschlossen [3, 4].

Fall No. 35 demonstrierte die vielfach beschriebene Tendenz zum Rezidiv nach augenscheinlich vollständiger Antagonisierung mit Physostigmin (Abbauzeit 60—120 Minuten). Nachdem Glycopyrrolate als quarternäre Ammoniumverbindung die Blut-Liquorschranke nach bisherigen Berichten nicht in signifikanten Konzentrationen passiert, erwarteten wir in der Kontrollgruppe keine derartige Symptomatik [6, 7].

Alle Patienten waren auch sofort oder innerhalb von 15 Minuten völlig ansprechbar, inklusive Fall No. 29, der kurz nach Eintreffen in der Wachstation kurzfristig unansprechbar und cyanotisch wurde. Die Atemdepression konnte mittels manueller Beatmung prompt behoben werden.

Mit einer Ausnahme. Fall No. 17 zeigte völlig überraschend das typische Bild des Z.A.S., reagierte in typischer Weise auf Physostigmin, zeigte den typischen Rückfall nach ca. 45 Minuten und erforderte eine zweite Dosis bevor Überstellung auf die Station. 2 Stunden später bekamen wir einen besorgten Anruf von der Station, da die Patientin nur schwer ansprechbar war. Analyse der Testsubstanz No. 17 schloß einen Irrtum aus.

Die Annahme, daß Glycopyrrolate die Blut-Liquorschranke nicht in nennenswerten Konzentrationen passiert, scheint damit unhaltbar, obwohl bisher weder in der Fachliteratur noch in unserer eigenen Praxis ein ähnlicher Fall beobachtet worden war. Im Zuge der weite-

F.R. Brosch

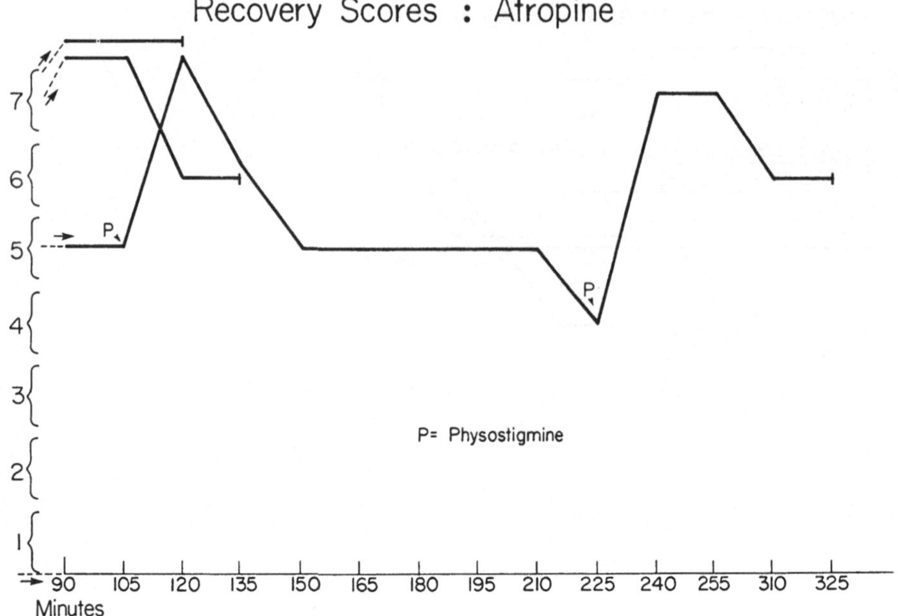

Abb. 2

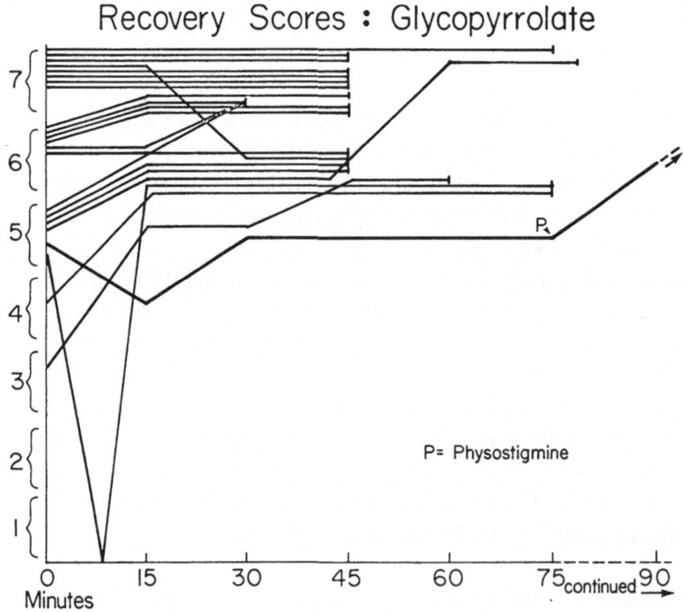

Abb. 3

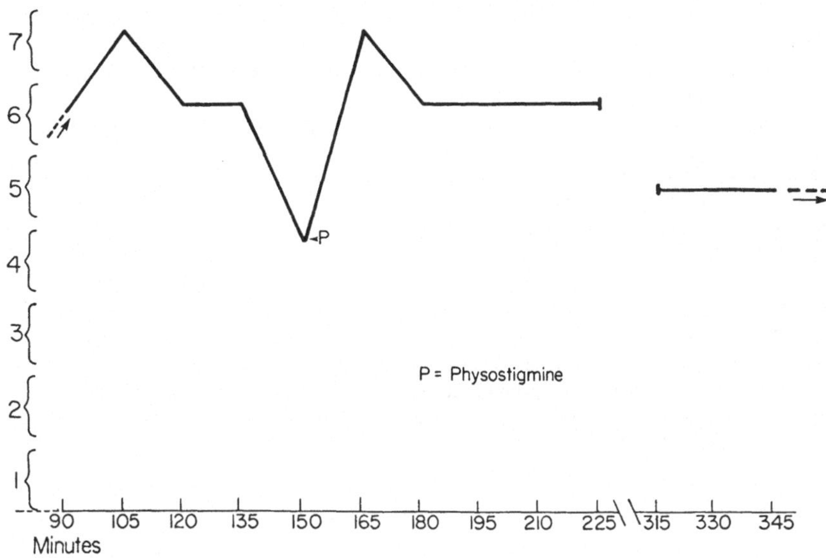

Abb. 4

ren Analyse dieses Falles fanden wir, daß die Patientin zur Zeit der Operation über einen postspinalen Kopfschmerz als Folge einer vorangegangenen P.E. der Zervix klagte. Sie zeigte überdies eine zwei Tage prä-operativ andauernde Übelkeit mit gelegentlichem Erbrechen. Andere Symptome meningealer Irritation ließen sich nicht eruieren.

Nachdem verschiedene Autoren [8, 9] gezeigt haben, daß gewisse Antibiotika nur in der Gegenwart von meningealer Irritation die Blut-Liquorschranke in effektiver Konzentration passieren, ist es denkbar, daß in diesem Falle Glycopyrrolate auf ähnliche Weise eine sonst nicht beobachtete Z.N.S. Wirkung ausübte.

Schlußfolgerungen

Auf der Basis unserer Untersuchungen können wir daher schließen:
1. daß das Z.A.S. auch nach Atropin und Glycopyrrolate auftreten kann,
2. daß es dazu nicht notwendig ist, klinisch übliche Dosen zu überschreiten,
3. daß das Z.A.S. anscheinend häufiger auftritt als bisher angenommen (ca. 10%; bzw. für Atropin allein 15%),
4. daß die Symptome durch den Antagonisten Physostigmin weitgehend behoben werden können,
5. daß der zentrale Belladonna-Effekt oft die Wirkung des Physostigmins überdauert, und
6. daß — entgegen bisherigen Berichten — Glycopyrrolate ebenfalls Nebenwirkungen im Sinne des Z.A.S. zeigen kann, wenn auch möglicherweise nur unter Bedingungen einer kompromittierten Blut-Liquorschranke.

Literatur

1. Longo VG (1966) Behavioral and electro-encephalographic effects of atropin and related compounds. Pharm Rev 18:965–991
2. Ramamurthy S, Shaker MH, Winnie AP (1972) Glycopyrrolate as a substitute for atropine in neostigmine reversal of muscle relaxant drugs. Can Anaesth Soc J 19:399–411
3. Bernards WC (1973) The central anticholinergic syndrome and its reversal with physostigmine. 20th Annual Anesthesiology Review Course, June 11–15, 1973, San Antonio, Texas
4. Winnie AP, et al. (1975) Anticholinergic differences: A matter of safety. A scientific exhibit, presented at the 1975 ASA Annual Meeting, Chicago, Illinois
5. Greene LT (1971) Physostigmine treatment of anticholinergic drug depression in postoperative patients. Anesth and Analg (Cleve) 50:222–226
6. Franko BV, Alphin RS, Ward JW, Lunceford CD (1962) Pharmacodynamic evaluation of glycopyrrolate in animals. Ann NY Acad Sci 99:131–149
7. Proakis AG, Harris GB (1978) Comparative penetration of glycopyrrolate and atropine across the bloodbrain and placental barriers in anesthetized dogs. Anesthesiology 48:339–344
8. Hoeprich PD (ed) (!977) Infectious Diseases, 2nd edn. Harper and Row, New York, pp 158, 897
9. Kane JG, et al. (1977) Nafcillin concentration in cerebrospinal fluid during treatment of staphylococcal infections. Ann Intern Med 87:309–311

Postoperative Reaktionsfähigkeit nach Ethrane- bzw. Halothan-Kurznarkosen

G. Scheible, P. Milewski, A. Driessen und W. Dick

Verschiedenen klinischen und klinisch-experimentellen Untersuchungen zufolge soll ein entscheidender Vorteil der Anwendung von Ethrane, insbesondere im Hinblick auf Kurznarkosen, darin liegen, daß die Elimination von Ethrane gegenüber Halothan schneller erfolgt und dadurch die postnarkotische Aufwachphase gegenüber Halothan verkürzt ist. Da teilweise unterschiedliche Beurteilungskriterien herangezogen wurden bzw. die verwendeten Untersuchungsbedingungen nicht oder nur schwer vergleichbar sind, kommen die verschiedenen Untersuchungen zu keiner einheitlichen Aussage.

Um subjektive Kriterien bei der Beurteilung beider Anästhetika im Hinblick auf die postnarkotische Erholung weitgehend auszuschalten, wurden folgende Untersuchungsbedingungen hergestellt (Abb. 1):

1. Strenge Randomisierung der insgesamt 50 Patienten im Alter von 18 bis 60 Jahren, bei denen kurzdauernde urologische bzw. gynäkologische Eingriffe durchgeführt wurden (Narkosedauer 42 bzw. 35 min).

2. Untersucher und der die Narkose durchführende Anästhesist waren verschieden; der jeweilige Prüfer war über die Art des eingesetzten Anästhetikums nicht orientiert.

3. Prämedikation und Kombination der jeweiligen Narkose waren bis auf die Inhalationsanästhetika — Halothan oder Ethrane — identisch.

```
                    PRÄMEDIKATION

                      NARKOSE


    HALOTHAN              -          ETHRANE
    BIS 1,0 VOL.%                    BIS 1,5 VOL.%


        ANÄSTHESIEENDE    -     BEWUSSTSEINSLAGE

                                       +

        30 MIN.
                          -      REAKTIONSZEIT
        60 MIN.

                                       +

        120 MIN.
                          -      BELASTUNGSTEST
        240 MIN.

            BLUTSPIEGELBESTIMMUNG
```

Abb. 1. Untersuchungsablauf (zu allen Zeitpunkten wurde die Blutspiegelbestimmung durchgeführt)

4. Am Ende der Anästhesie wurde die Bewußtseinslage nach den Kriterien
D — bewußtlos, reagiert nur auf starke Schmerzreize,
C — bewußtlos, reagiert auf leichte Reize,
B — benommen, aber ansprechbar und
A — wach
beurteilt sowie die jeweiligen Blutkonzentrationen im venösen Blut bestimmt.

30 und 60 Minuten nach Anästhesieende wurden zusätzlich die Reaktionszeiten auf optische und akustische Reize geprüft, nachdem am Vortag des operativen Eingriffs die Patienten jeweils mit der zugrunde liegenden Methodik vertraut gemacht und die Ausgangswerte erhoben worden waren.

120 und 240 Minuten nach Anästhesieende wurden die Patienten schließlich zusätzlich einem Buchstaben-Anstreichtest nach Brickenkamp (d2-Test) unterzogen, der die Reaktionslage in Bezug auf Reaktionsgeschwindigkeit, Leistungsfähigkeit und Fehlerhäufigkeit überprüft.

Unabhängig davon wurden die klinisch üblichen Kreislaufparameter registriert.

Ergebnisse

Die Bewußtseinslage am Ende der Anästhesie sowie zu den einzelnen Meßzeitpunkten wurde nach rein klinischen Kriterien überprüft. Dabei zeigte sich, daß bei Narkoseende in der Ethrane-Gruppe bereits 64% der Patienten ansprechbar waren gegenüber nur 40% in der Halothan-Gruppe. 30 Minuten nach Narkoseende waren in der Ethrane-Gruppe doppelt so viel Patienten wach und voll orientiert wie in der Halothan-Gruppe. Ähnliche Relationen ließen sich bis zu zwei Stunden nach Narkoseende nachweisen.

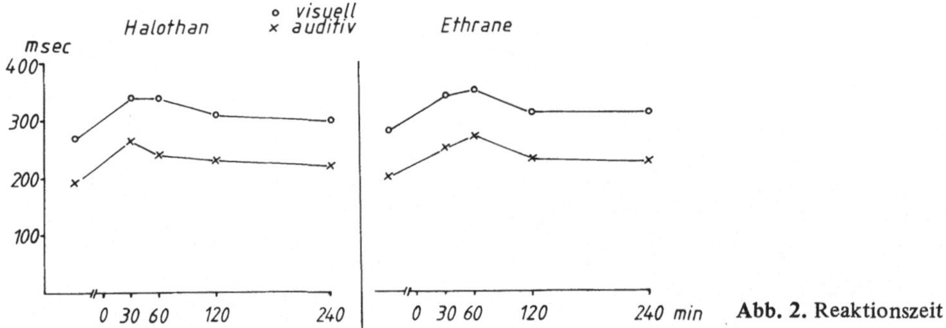

Abb. 2. Reaktionszeit

Abb. 2 zeigt die Reaktionszeiten der jeweiligen Patienten unter dem Einfluß von Halothan oder Ethrane, wobei die Kreise die Reaktionszeiten auf visuelle Reize, die Kreuze die Reaktionszeiten auf auditive Reize markieren. Man sieht, daß in beiden Kollektiven die Reaktionszeiten auf auditive Reize deutlich unter denen auf visuelle Reize liegen. Man erkennt aber auch, daß beide Kollektive sich in den Reaktionszeiten auf beide Reizformen nicht unterscheiden. (Aus Gründen der Übersichtlichkeit wurden lediglich die Mittelwerte, nicht aber die Standardabweichungen aufgetragen.)

Abb. 3 gibt die Ergebnisse des Aufmerksamkeits-Belastungstestes wieder. Auf der Ordinate ist die insgesamt erreichte Zahl angestrichener Buchstaben mit GZ bezeichnet, die Fehlerquote mit F. Die weißen Quadrate geben die Anzahl angestrichener Buchstaben in Prozent wieder, wobei der erste Wert als Ausgangswert = 100% gesetzt worden ist; die ausgefüllten Kreise geben die Fehlerquote in Prozent der angestrichenen Buchstabenzahl wieder.

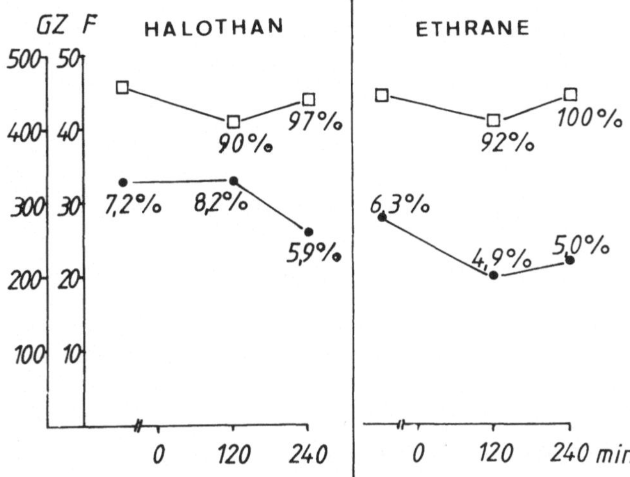

Abb. 3. d2-Test (Aufmerksamkeits-Belastungstest)

Die Ergebnisse dieses Aufmerksamkeits-Belastungstestes lassen erkennen, daß sowohl in der Halothan-gruppe als auch in der Ethrane-Gruppe eine Verminderung der Leistung 2 Stunden nach Narkoseende gegenüber dem präoperativen Ausgangswert aufgetreten ist, daß aber 4 Stunden nach Narkoseende die präoperative Ausgangslage wieder erreicht ist.

Die Fehlerquote in der Halothan-Gruppe hat gegenüber den Ausgangswerten unwesentlich zugenommen, liegt 4 Stunden nach Narkoseende jedoch wieder im präoperativen Ausgangsbereich. In der Ethrane-Gruppe ist insgesamt eine Verminderung der Fehlerhäufigkeit gegenüber den präoperativen Ausgangswerten zu erkennen.

Vergleicht man beide Kollektive hinsichtlich der Ergebnisse des Aufmerksamkeits-Belastungstestes, so sind auch hier keine klinisch relevanten oder statistisch signifikanten Unterschiede zu erkennen.

Abb. 4 zeigt die Mittelwerte der Halothan- bzw. Ethrane-Blutspiegel zu den jeweiligen Meßzeitpunkten in μmol/l, wobei hier wiederum aus Gründen der Übersichtlichkeit die Standardabweichungen ausgelassen wurden. Beim Vergleich beider Eliminationskurven erkennt man, daß diese nahezu identisch verlaufen. Auch die Absolutwerte zu den einzelnen Meßzeitpunkten sind nahezu identisch, ein Aspekt, der zunächst überraschen mag, jedoch durch die differente Referenzgröße μmol/l gegenüber mg/100 ml in anderen Untersuchungen zustande kommt. Auch bei unseren Messungen lagen die Ethrane-Blutspiegelkonzentrationen um 25—50 % über denen der Halothan-Gruppe, wenn in mg/100 ml bezeichnet wurde.

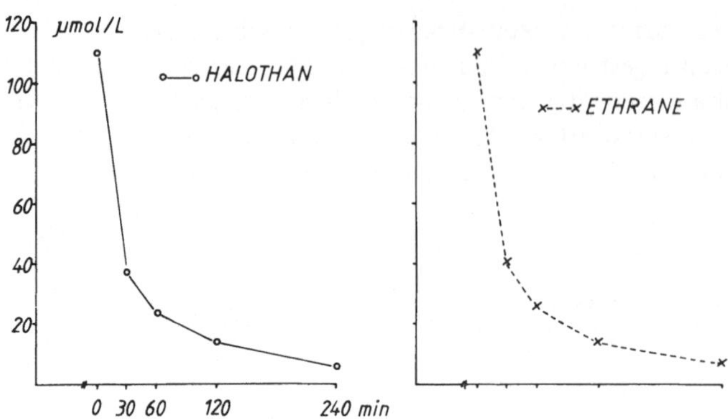

Abb. 4. Konzentration im Vollblut

Diskussion

Die Fragestellung der Untersuchungen läßt sich zusammengefaßt folgendermaßen beantworten:
1. Die beiden Patientenkollektive waren hinsichtlich des Alters, des Körpergewichts, des Narkoserisikos und der Operations- bzw. Narkosedauer vergleichbar.
2. Bei der klinischen Beurteilung des Bewußtseinszustandes fällt auf, daß in der Ethrane-
Gruppe die Zahl der bereits wachen oder annähernd wachen Patienten jeweils deutlich höher
lag als in der Halothan-Gruppe.
3. Die weitgehend objektiven Beurteilungskriterien der Reaktionszeitmessung zeigen jedoch
keinen Unterschied zwischen beiden Kollektiven.
4. Auch die Ergebnisse des Aufmerksamkeits-Belastungstestes ließen keine klinisch relevanten Unterschiede zwischen beiden Gruppen erkennen. Allerdings war in der Halothan-Gruppe zum Zeitpunkt 120 min nach Narkoseende die Leistungsfähigkeit gegenüber dem Ausgangswert leicht vermindert bei leicht erhöhter Fehlerquote. In der Ethrane-Gruppe jedoch
fiel lediglich der leichte Abfall der Leistungsfähigkeit auf, während sich die Fehlerquote gegenüber dem Ausgangswert ebenfalls reduzierte. Das Erreichen der Gesamtzahl von 100%
bereits 4 Stunden nach Narkoseende und insbesondere die Reduktion der Fehlerquote gegenüber den präoperativen Werten ist auch auf einen Lerneffekt zurückzuführen.
5. Das Fehlen meßbarer Unterschiede zwischen beiden Kollektiven sowie hinsichtlich der
Reaktionszeiten als auch der Aufmerksamkeits-Belastungsteste wird im übrigen durch eine
nahezu völlig identische Elimination von Halothan und Ethrane über die Zeit belegt.

Literatur

1. Göthert M (1975) Pharmakologie des Enflurane-Ethrane: Neue Ergebnisse in Forschung und Klinik.
   Symposion am 15. März 1975 in Osnabrück
2. Kessler G, Haferkorn D (1977) Vergleichende Untersuchungen über die postnarkotische Phase nach
   Kurznarkosen mit Halothan und Ethrane. Prakt Anästh 12:269

Komplikationen nach Naloxon

R. Purschke, A. Mangos, I. Dimakos und D. Schemmann

Seit der Einführung von Naloxon sind die Nebenwirkungen der Neuroleptanaesthesie, insbesondere die postoperative Atemdepression beherrschbarer geworden. Folgt man jüngsten Berichten [1, 2, 3], so findet man, daß Naloxon, nach der sogenannten Titrations-Methode gegeben, eine opioidbedingte Atemdepression sicher beseitigen könne, ohne den analgetischen Effekt aufzuheben. Darüber hinaus seien mit dieser Titrationsmethode unerwünschte Nebenwirkungen wie Nausea, hyperkinetisches Syndrom, Herzfrequenzanstiege, Blutdruckanstiege, akute Hyperalgesie, Entziehungssymptome usw. nicht mehr zu beobachten. Es wurde daher empfohlen, nach Kombinationsnarkosen mit Opioiden immer routinemäßig Naloxon zu geben, um eine Atemdepression hintanzuhalten [1, 2].

Anlaß für den folgenden Bericht war die Beobachtung, daß trotz einer vergleichsweise restriktiven Titration von Naloxon doch teilweise schwere Nebenwirkungen auftraten.

Untersuchungsgang

Bei den der Untersuchung zugrunde liegenden Daten wurde Naloxon nicht routinemäßig gegeben, sondern nur nach Bedarf, d.h. nur bei Atemfrequenzen unter 10/Min., unabhängig vom Ausfall der Blutgasanalysen. Die Dosierung erfolgte nach einem Titrationsschema mit Einzeldosen von 0,04 mg bzw. 0,05 mg, die im Bedarfsfall nach 3–4 Min. wiederholt wurden.

In einer zur Hälfte retrospektiven, zur anderen Hälfte prospektiven Analyse wurden die Daten von 943 Patienten ausgewertet, die nach der Narkose Naloxon bekommen haben. Hauptaugenmerk wurde dabei auf das Verhalten des Blutdrucks gelegt, da teilweise kritische Hypertonien unmittelbar nach Gabe von Naloxon aufgetreten waren.

Ergebnisse

In Abb. 1 ist das Blutdruckverhalten des Gesamtkollektives zusammengefaßt. Nach Naloxon findet sich regelmäßig ein Anstieg des Blutdruckes um im Mittel 30 mmHg, nämlich von einem Ausgangswert von 120/70 mmHg auf 150/95 mmHg. Die Herzfrequenz zeigte in diesem Kollektiv keine wesentlichen Änderungen, auf ihre Darstellung wurde daher verzichtet. Im Verlauf der weiteren Beobachtungsperiode bis zu einer Stunde fiel der Blutdruck zwar wieder ab, blieb aber weiterhin deutlich über dem Wert vor der Naloxongabe (Abb. 2). Die Dosierungen von Fentanyl bzw. Naloxon, bezogen auf Körpergewicht und Narkosedauer, zeigten, daß die Fentanylgaben mit durchschnittlich 5 mcg/Kg/h in dem von Tammisto angegebenen unteren Dosierungsbereich liegen [4].

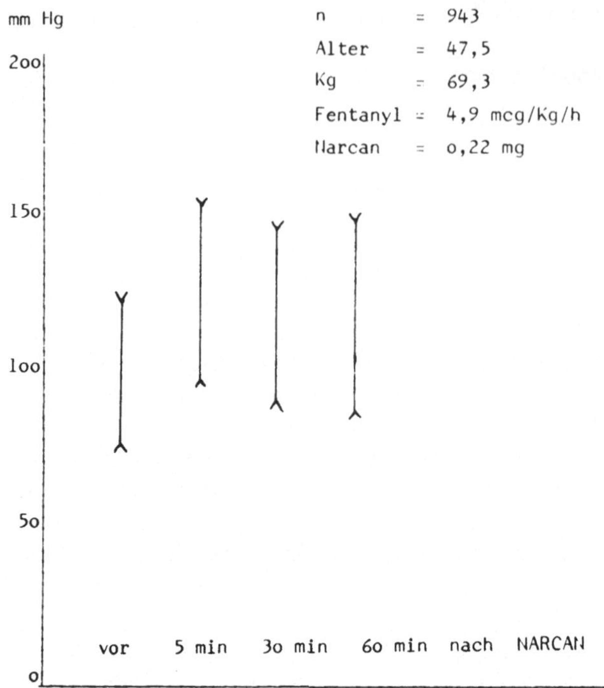

Abb. 1. Durchschnittliches Verhalten des Blutdrucks bei 943 Patienten nach Gabe von Naloxon. Überwachungsperiode 1 Stunde

Stellt man nun gesondert die Patienten zusammen, die präoperativ bereits Blutdruckwerte von systolisch mehr als 150 mmHg aufwiesen, und verfolgt hier das Blutdruckverhalten nach Naloxon, so findet sich auch hier ein Anstieg des Blutdruckes um im Mittel ca. 40 mmHg, ein Änderungswert, der primär nicht besonders auffällig erscheint. Immerhin erreichen aber hier die systolischen Blutdruckwerte Größenordnungen von im Mittel mehr als 200 mmHg, Werte, die man normalerweise nicht mehr tolerieren sollte. Dieses Patientenkollektiv wurde gesondert nach verschiedenen Anaesthesieverfahren analysiert. Es ist festzustellen, daß in allen drei Gruppen praktisch identische Blutdruckreaktionen zu beobachten sind, daß also das Narkoseverfahren selbst die Reaktionsweise nicht beeinflußt (Abb. 3).

Die Schlußfolgerung aus diesem Befund muß daher heißen, daß bei bereits bestehender hypertoner Ausgangslage nach Gabe von Naloxon mit Blutdrucksteigerungen in gefährliche Höhen hinein gerechnet werden muß. Allerdings ist festzustellen, daß unter den insgesamt 79 Patienten, die nach Naloxongaben Blutdrucksteigerungen auf Werte über 200 mmHg systolisch aufwiesen, immerhin 36 vor der Naloxongabe keine hypertone Blutdruckausgangslage hatten. Diese Patientengruppe ist in der Abb. 3 zusammengestellt. Von einem mittleren Ausgangsblutdruck von 130/80 mmHg stieg nach Naloxongabe der Blutdruck auf 210/115 mmHg an und lag auch 60 Min. später immer noch in hohen Bereichen, nämlich annähernd 190/110 mmHg.

Zu dieser Gruppe gehörte auch ein Patient, der ein besonders extremes Verhalten aufwies. Nach Gabe von Naloxon war dieser Patient wach bis mäßig schläfrig, völlig schmerzfrei, und atmete mit einer Frequenz von 10 Atemzügen/Min., bot also ein völlig unauffälliges

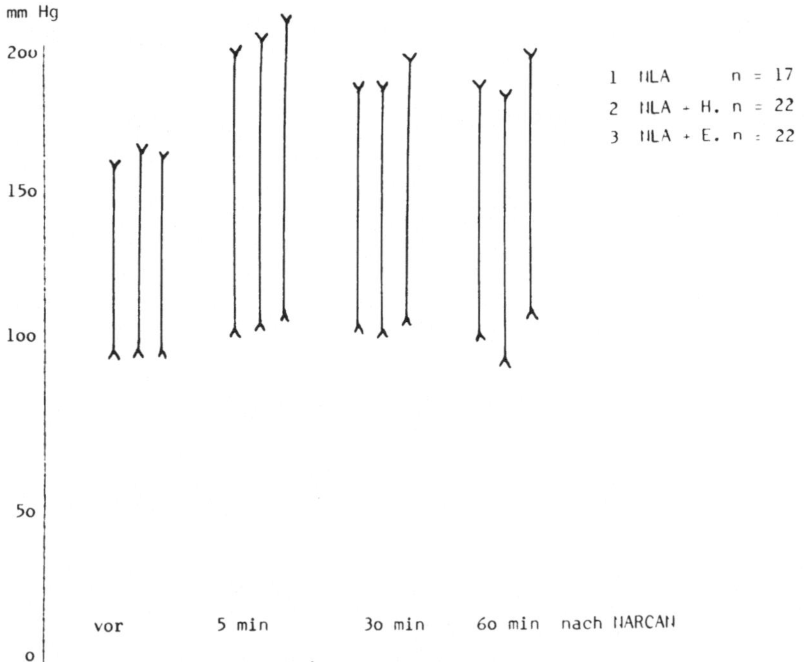

Abb. 2. Durchschnittliches Blutdruckverhalten von Patienten mit Hypertonie nach Naloxongabe. Überwachungsdauer 1 Stunde. Das jeweils 1. Blutdrucksymbol entspricht der Gruppe mit einer reinen Neuroleptanaesthesie, das 2. einer Kombinationsanaesthesie (Neuroleptanaesthesie und Halothan), das 3. einer Kombinationsanaesthesie (Neuroleptanaesthesie und Ethrane)

Bild. Demgegenüber trat unmittelbar nach der Naloxongabe eine Hypertonie auf, die teilweise bis zu 280 mmHg systolisch reichte, ohne daß prä- oder intraoperativ hypertone Blutdruckwerte bestanden hatten.

Faßt man diese Ergebnisse prozentual zusammen, so läßt sich feststellen, daß von 943 Patienten immerhin 79, also 8,3% nach Naloxongabe Blutdrucksteigerungen auf Werte über 200 mmHg, systolisch aufwiesen. Besonders gefährdet sind danach Patienten mit bereits bestehender hypertoner Ausgangslage, denn von den 61 Hypertonikern hatten 43 nach Naloxongabe Blutdruckwerte von mehr als 200 mmHg gezeigt, also mehr als 2/3 des Hypertonikerkollektivs.

Von den 882 Patienten ohne hypertone Ausgangsblutdrucklage zeigten 36 Blutdrucksteigerungen auf über 200 mmHg, das heißt selbst bei „Normal-Patienten" muß in etwa 4% der Fälle mit krisenhaften Blutdrucksteigerungen gerechnet werden, auch wenn man Naloxon vorsichtig titriert und die erwünschte Analgesie postoperativ komplett aufrecht erhält.

Trotz dieser Komplikation halten wir aber Naloxon weiterhin für das praktikabelste Medikament zur Beseitigung einer fentanylbedingten Atemdepression, das gegenwärtig zur Verfügung steht. Der Vorschlag allerdings, Naloxon routinemäßig nach jeder mit Opioiden kombinierten Anaesthesie einzusetzen, ist unseres Erachtens wegen dieser Komplikationsmöglichkeit jedoch nicht gerechtfertigt.

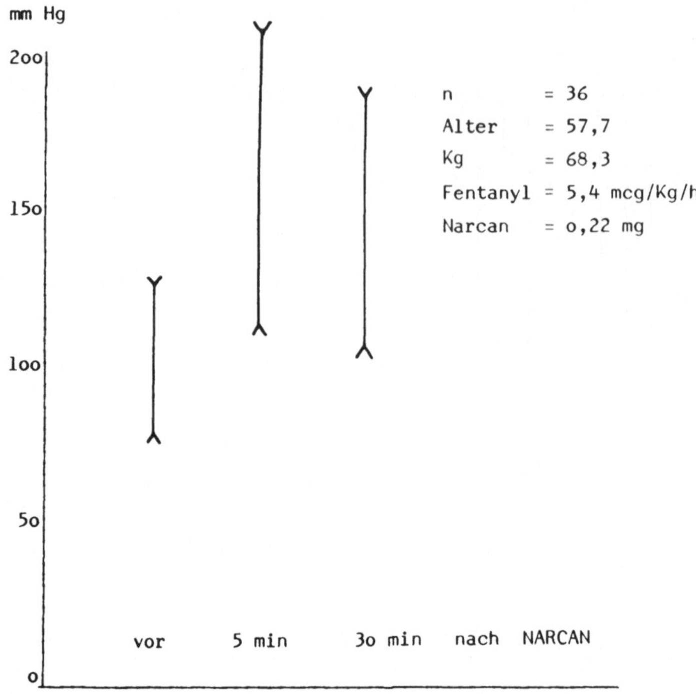

Abb. 3. Durchschnittliches Blutdruckverhalten von 36 Patienten, die nach Naloxongabe eine Hypertonie entwickelten. Überwachungsperiode 30 Min

Darüberhinaus muß betont werden, daß mit Naloxon eine opioid-bedingte Atemdepression nicht immer mit absoluter Sicherheit beseitigt werden kann. Das vielfach empfohlene Schema, nach einer halben Stunde den Patienten mit einer intramuskulären Repetitionsdosis auf die Station zu entlassen, „da jetzt ja nichts mehr passieren könne", halten wir für gefährlich. Wir konnten eine Reihe von Beobachtungen machen, nach denen trotz geringer Fentanylgaben bis zu 6 Stunden nach der Narkose immer wieder Nachinjektionen von Naloxon erforderlich waren, um eine Atemfrequenz von mindestens 8–10 Atemzügen/Min. aufrecht erhalten zu können. Gerade *nach* Naloxon sollte die sorgfältigste Überwachung gewährleistet sein, bis die Atemfrequenz sicher und ohne Naloxon bei mindestens 10 Atemzüge/Min. bleibt.

Literatur

1. Dick W, Milewski P, Knoche E, Traub E (1978) Zur klinischen Anwendung von Naloxon nach Kurznarkosen mit Opiatanalgetika. Anaesthesist 27:272–279
2. Patschke D (1978) Naloxon (Eine klinische Untersuchung zur Frage der Dosierung). Prakt Anästh 13: 81–90
3. Schaer H, Baasch K, Reist F (1978) Die Atemdepression nach Fentanyl und ihre Antagonisierung mit Naloxon. Anaesthesist 27:259–266
4. Tammisto T (1977) Anwendung von Naloxone nach N_2O-O_2-Fentanyl-Kombinationsnarkosen. Anaesth Inform 19:465

The Value and Effects of Neurotropin on the Control of Postoperative Pain

T. Momose

Introduction

Neurotropin is a preparation containing active principles extracted from inflamed skin tissue of rabbits inoculated with vaccinia virus. So far it has been used as an anti-allergy preparation, but in recent years an outstanding sedative and analgesic effect has been observed in animal experiments, and especially a rise in analgesic-threshold and prolonging of the analgesic action when it was used with pentazocine. These actions of Neurotropin are unique in that they are minimal in normal healthy animals but marked in animals in a diseased or stressed state. These effects seen in basic studies are in good agreement with the clinical effects and features of Neurotropin observed so far, in that Neurotropin exerts little effect on healthy subjects but a marked effect on patients, because it restores the extremely excited nerves to normal, thus reversing the disease process.

Table 1. In the study, we observed the effect of Neurotropin on postoperative pain (Table 1). A comparative study was made of the use of Neurotropin and pentazocine combined (N), a physiological saline solution as inactive placebo and pentazocine (S), and of hydroxyzine (now in common use in Japan) and pentazocine (H), respectively, in a double blind situation.

Table 1

Group N	Neurotropin 3 ml + Pentazocine 15 mg
Group S	Saline Solution 3 ml + Pentazocine 15 mg
Group H	Hydroxyzine 100 mg (3 ml) + Pentazocine 15 mg

Methods

The cases were 178 patients complaining of a high degree of pain after laparotomy given under GOF anaesthesia; 143 cases were used in a comparison between N and S, and 36 cases in a comparison between N and H.

The method of administration was limited to a one time dose of the chosen drug when the patient complained of severe pain (Table 2). The degree of pain in patients was measured 30 minutes after administration and every hour thereafter, and the analgesic effect was evaluated according to the "pain score". In the case of insufficient analgesia after the administration of the chosen drug, another analgesic agent was used, but only one hour after initial administration.

Table 2. Criteria used in judging the degree of pain

(3) Severe:	Intolerable pain, administration of analgesics necessary.
(2) Mild:	Patient wants analgesics but can tolerate pain without.
(1) Slight:	Slight pain.
(0) None:	No pain.

Results

Comparison of N and S (Table 3)

Table 3. Comparison of the number of cases with PI of zero

Time	Group	Number of cases PI (0)	Number of cases other than PI (0)	Test
30 min.	Group N	41	41	N.S.
	Group S	35	46	
1 hour	Group N	49	33	$x^2 = 4.4661*$
	Group S	35	46	3.8287
2 hours	Group N	31	51	N.S.
	Group S	28	53	
3 hours	Group N	20	62	N.S.
	Group S	19	62	

* $P < 0.05$

1. Comparison of the degree of pain in the initial stages after administration

Concerning the number of cases whose degree of pain was zero, that is complete analgesia at 1 hour, we found the number in group N was significantly higher than in group S.

2. Comparison of the need for administration of additional analgesic agent (Table 4)

Table 4. Comparison of the need for administration of additional analgesic agent within 24 hours

	Additional administration (−)	Additional administration (+)	Total
Group N	31	51	82
Group S	18	63	81

$x^2 = 4.7062*, 3.9942*$
* $P < 0.05$

The number of cases which did not require any additional analgesic agent within 24 hours of the administration of the subjected drug was higher in group N than in group S and a significant difference ($p < 0.05$) in the duration of analgesic effect was observed. Similarly, the number of cases needing no additional agent within 12 hours of administration of the subjected drug was significantly higher in group N (Table 5).

Table 5. Comparison of the need for administration of additional analgesic agent within 12 hours

	Additional administration (−)	Additional administration (+)	Total
Group N	33	49	82
Group S	18	63	81

$\chi^2 = 6.1559^*, 5.3461^*$
* $P < 0.05$

3. *Comparison of the duration of analgesic effect* (Table 6)

Table 6. Comparison of the duration of analgesic effect and the need for additional administration within 24 hrs

	Duration of analgesic effect mean time (min.)	freedom	F-value	t-value
Group N	736.90	81	1.3908	2.1172*
Group S	557.62	80		

* $P < 0.05$

The interval between the administration of the subjected drug and the initial administration of additional analgesic agents, that is the duration of analgesic effect of the subjected drug, was observed. At the point of 24 hours after administration of the drugs, a significant prolonging of analgesic effect was found statistically in group N, but at the point of 12 hours no such difference between the groups was observed (Table 7).

Table 7. Comparison of the duration of analgesic effect and the need for additional administration within 12 hrs

	Duration of analgesic effect mean time (min.)	freedom	F-value	t-value
Group N	455.67	81	1.3752	1.5360
Group S	397.62	80		

4. *Criteria used in judging the analgesic effects and the evaluation of results* (Table 8)

Table 8. Criteria used in judging the analgesic effects

	Degree of pain at 4th hour	Degree of pain at 5th hour
Excellent	0	0
	0	1
	0	2
Good	1	1
	1	2
Fair	0	3
	1	3
	2	3
None	2	3
	3	

By considering the average duration of action of pentazocine to be 3 hours, the analgesic effect was evaluated based on previously established criteria, after examining the change in the degree of pain after 3 hours.

This was done in the cases which did not require additional analgesic agents after the administration of the subjected drug. The scale of efficacy, that is, "excellent", "good", "fair" and "poor" was determined from the change in the degree of pain, by taking into consideration the degree of pain at the 4th and 5th hours, respectively.

As a result of this evaluation, it was observed (Table 9) that group N was significantly superior to group S in the U test ($p < 0.05$), Mann-Whiteney. Also group N was significantly superior to group S in the χ^2 test ($p < 0.01$) using the following grouping 1) "excellent and good" 2) "poor and none" (Table 10).

Table 9. (1) Evaluation of analgesic effects using criteria

	Total	Excellent	Good	Fair	None	Simple efficacy
Group N	63	18 (28.6)	29 (46.0)	2 (3.2)	14 (22.2)	74.6%
Group S	64	10 (15.6)	23 (35.9)	17 (26.6)	14 (21.9)	51.5%

$Z = 2.1346^*$

$$\text{Simple Efficacy} = \frac{\text{"Excellent" cases} + \text{"Good" cases}}{\text{Total Cases}} \times 100$$

Comparison of N and H

A comparative study of the analgesic effects in N and H groups was made, but no significant difference was observed statistically, although there was a tendency for group N to be superior to group H.

Table 10. (2) Evaluation of analgesic effects using criteria

	Excellent + Good	Fair + None	Total
Group N	47	16	63
Group S	33	31	64
Total	80	47	127

χ^2 = 7.2298**; 6.2752*
* $P < 0.05$
** $P < 0.01$

Side effects (Table 11)

Perspiration, nausea, vomiting, thirst and hypertension were observed but of a transient nature, and in no way severe. These symptoms have previously been considered to be side effects of pentazocine, and there was no significant difference between the two groups concerning these side effects. No effect resulting from the combined use of Neurotropin was observed.

Table 11. Side effects

	Group N (82 cases)	Group S (81 cases)	Total
Perspiration	3	2	5
Nausea	2	0	2
Thirst	0	1	1
Vomiting	0	1	1
Hypertension	0	1	1
Total	5	5	10

Conclusions

After conducting a clinical study of the combined use of Neurotropin and pentazocine (N) and, of a physiological saline solution as inactive placebo and pentazocine (S), and of hydroxyzine and pentazocine (H), respectively, in a double blind situation, the following results were obtained:
1. In group N, the number of cases of "no pain (0)" at one hour after the administration of the subjected drug was higher than in group S. Statistically, there was a significant difference between the groups.
2. Statistically, in group N, the number of cases of "no administration" of additional analgesics was significantly higher than in group S.

3. So far as the duration of the analgesic effects is concerned, a prolongation was observed in group N and a significant difference was observed within 24 hours of administration.
4. Group N was significantly superior in the test based on measuring the degree of pain after 3 hours, in the cases which did not require additional analgesics.
5. No significant side effects were observed.

Verhalten der freien Fettsäuren bei der Primärversorgung von Femurfrakturen durch Marknagelung in der prä-, intra- und postoperativen Phase

H.-J. Hartung, P.M. Osswald, R. Spier und R. Klose

Einleitung

Zahlreiche Studien zeigen, daß bei der Primärbehandlung unfallchirurgischer Patienten der posttraumatischen respiratorischen Insuffizienz besondere Bedeutung zukommt. Die Oberschenkelschaftfraktur stellt dabei das Paradebeispiel einer schweren Allgemeinverletzung dar und kann das Auftreten einer sogenannten Schocklunge durch hohen Blutverlust mit konsekutivem Schock, sekundärer Fetteinschwemmung sowie Aktivierung des Gerinnungssystems fördern. Die Versorgung der Oberschenkelschaftfraktur durch die geschlossene Marknagelung ist daher bei diesen Patienten nicht unwidersprochen geblieben [1, 6, 7]. Die Fetteinschwemmung, insbesondere in die pulmonale Strombahn und damit das Auftreten eines Fettemboliesyndroms als Epiphänomen der Schocklunge, wird als schwer einschätzbares Risiko beim Einschlagen des Marknagels gefürchtet.

Ziel der vorliegenden Untersuchung ist es, den Einfluß der primären Nagelung eines langen Röhrenknochens auf die Konzentration der freien Fettsäuren und den eventuell bestehenden Zusammenhang zwischen der primären Frakturfixation und posttraumatischen Komplikationen im Hinblick auf die posttraumatische respiratorische Insuffizienz aufzuzeigen.

Patienten und Methode

Die Untersuchungen wurden an 18 frisch verunfallten Patienten im Alter von 16 bis 82 Jahren (mittleres Alter 46,4 Jahre) durchgeführt. Keiner der Patienten hatte ein begleitendes Thoraxtrauma.

Folgende Meßwerte wurden ermittelt, bzw. errechnet: Der arterielle Druck wurde mittels eines Stathamdruckwandlers (P23) über die Arteria radialis blutig gemessen, der Mitteldruck wurde elektronisch errechnet. Über die Vena jugularis interna wurde ein Swan Ganz-Katheter (93a – 118 – 7s) in die Pulmonalarterie eingeschwemmt, in adäquate Wedgeposition gebracht und der Druck im Pulmonalkreislauf kontinuierlich gemessen. Aus dem arteriellen Blut des Systemkreislaufs sowie dem gemischt-venösen Blut des Pulmonalkreislaufes wurden folgende Bestimmungen durchgeführt: Blutgasanalysen, Säurebasenhaushalt, freie Fettsäuren, Thrombozyten, Fibrinogen, Quick, PTT und PTZ. Die Entnahme der Blutproben erfolgte 60 Minuten nach Klinikaufnahme (Punkt 1), nach Narkoseeinleitung (Punkt 2), am Ende der erfolgten Nagelung (Punkt 3) 2, 6 und 24 Stunden nach Beendigung der Operation (Punkt 4, 5 und 6).

Die Narkose wurde unter kontrollierter Beatmung in Neuroleptanalgesie durchgeführt.

Ergebnisse

Die Serumkonzentration der freien Fettsäuren (Abb. 1) liegt unmittelbar nach Klinikaufnahme mit 0,76 mval/L im arteriellen Blut und mit 0,80 mval/L im gemischt-venösen Blut im Normbereich. 2 Stunden nach Marknagelung kommt es zu einem leichten Konzentrationsabfall im arteriellen Blut auf 0,54 mval/L und im gemischt-venösen Blut auf 0,44 mval/L. 6 Stunden nach Marknagelung kommt es wiederum zu einem geringfügigen Anstieg, gefolgt von einem mäßigen Abfall der Fettsäurekonzentration arteriell sowie gemischt-venös. Insgesamt liegen die Fettsäuren immer im Normbereich. Die Schwankungen zu den einzelnen Punkten sind statistisch nicht signifikant, ebenso bleibt die arterio-gemischt-venöse Konzentrationsdifferenz praktisch konstant.

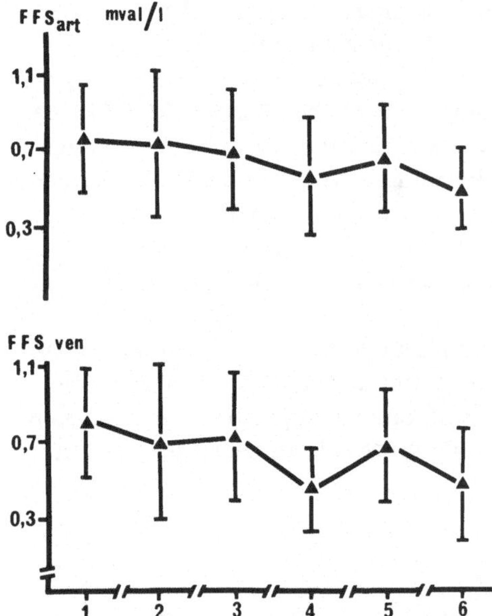

Abb. 1. Konzentrationsverlauf der freien Fettsäuren, arteriell und gemischtvenös

Arterieller Blutdruck und Herzfrequenz (Abb. 2) zeigen über den gesamten Untersuchungszeitraum nur mäßige Schwankungen. So liegen die Mittelwerte der Herzfrequenz immer zwischen 95 und 100 pro Min. Der arterielle systolische Druck zwischen 115 und 135 mmHg.

Der Pulmonalarteriendruck (Abb. 3) zeigt während der gesamten prä-, intra- und postoperativen Periode einen statistisch nicht verifizierbaren Anstieg von 22 mmHg bei Klinikaufnahme bis auf 24 mmHg 24 Stunden postoperativ. Der Pulmonalarterienmitteldruck läßt ein simultanes Verhalten erkennen. Die arterio-venöse Sauerstoffgehaltsdifferenz (Abb. 4) zeigt bei unserem Patientengut vom ersten Meßzeitpunkt nach Klinikaufnahme bis 2 Stunden nach Nagelung einen kontinuierlichen Anstieg auf 3,9 ml O_2/100 ml Blut, fällt dann aber signifikant bereits 6 Stunden nach Nagelung auf 2,9 ml O_2/100 ml Blut ab.

Die Thrombozyten (Abb. 5) vermindern sich über den gemessenen Zeitraum kontinuierlich von 137 000 präoperativ auf 107 000 24 Stunden postoperativ.

Die Mittelwerte des Säurebasenhaushaltes und der Blutgase zeigen keine relevanten Veränderungen.

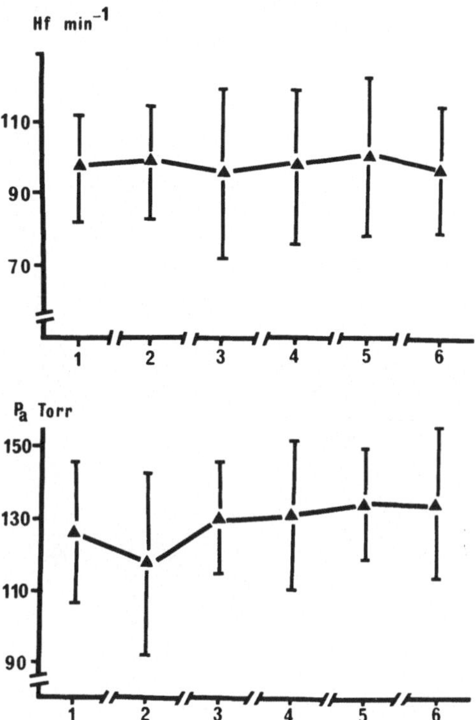

Abb. 2. Arterieller Blutdruck (syst.) und Herzfrequenz während des Untersuchungszeitraumes

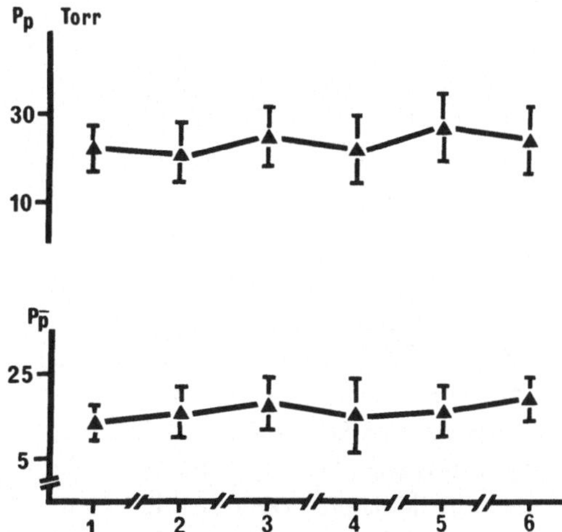

Abb. 3. Pulmonalarteriendruck (syst.) und Mitteldruck

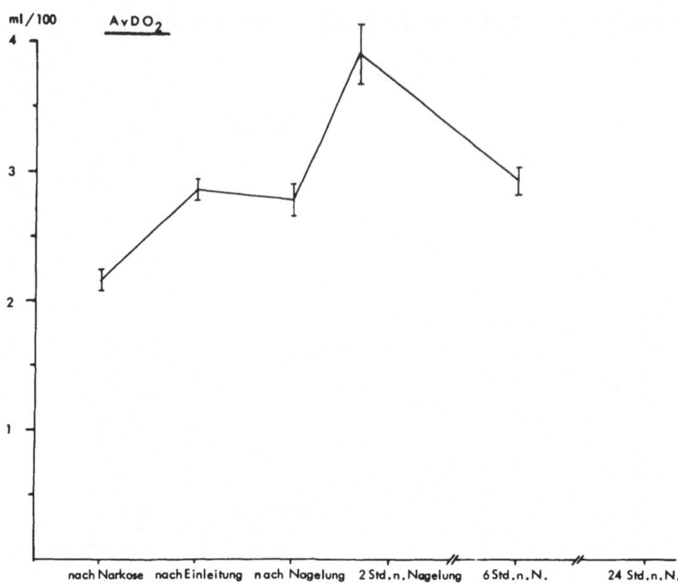

Abb. 4. AVDO$_2$ in ml O$_2$/100 ml Blut

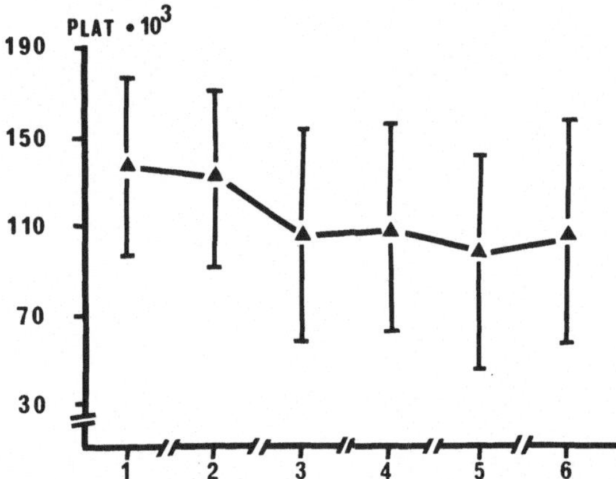

Abb. 5. Verlauf der Thrombozyten prae-, intra- und postoperativ

Diskussion

Der Verlauf der freien Fettsäuren im Serum zeigt, daß die Freisetzung der Fettsäuren durch das Operationsereignis nicht verändert wird. Die im Mittel auftretende Erhöhung der Gesamtkonzentration liegt innerhalb der üblicherweise auftretenden Schwankungen. Hinsichtlich einer möglichen Fettemboliegefährdung bei der geschlossenen Marknagelung einer Oberschenkelfraktur scheint uns dieses Ergebnis besonders bemerkenswert. Die beschriebenen Konzentrationsschwankungen charakterisieren die sympathikotone Situation, in der sich die Patienten perioperativ befinden.

Die beobachtete Konzentrationsdifferenz im arteriellen und gemischt-venösen Blut kann durch eine Filterwirkung der Lungenstrombahn auf Fett erklärt werden [7], wobei die Konzentrationsdifferenz praktisch konstant bleibt.

Das untersuchte Patientenkollektiv zeigte bei den sogenannten einfachen Kreislaufparametern während der gesamten perioperativen Periode eine im Normbereich liegende Hämodynamik. Der gleichzeitig gemessene Pulmonalarterien- und Pulmonalarterienmitteldruck lassen im Gesamtverlauf postoperativ einen leichten Anstieg erkennen. Dies kann als Zunahme des Widerstands der Lungenstrombahn gewertet werden. Die 2 Stunden postoperativ erhöhte arterio-venöse Sauerstoffgehaltsdifferenz weist ebenfalls auf Veränderungen vom Sauerstoffangebot, Sauerstoffextraktionsrate und Sauerstoffverbrauch als wichtigste Parameter des Sauerstofftransportes in der posttraumatischen Phase hin. Als korrelierend zu diesen Befunden könnte der Abfall der Thrombozyten gewertet werden, wird doch der Zusammenhang zwischen Thrombozytenabfall und Veränderungen in der pulmonalen Strombahn auch von anderen Autoren beschrieben [1, 2, 3, 4, 5]. Dieser Zusammenhang ist allerdings inkonstant, respiratorische Konsequenzen können durchaus ausbleiben [2, 4].

Jedoch kommt den Thrombozyten bei der Entwicklung von Komplikationen verunfallter Patienten eine nicht unwesentliche Bedeutung zu. Die kontinuierliche Aktivierung des Gerinnungssystems in der perioperativen Phase kann über eine Verminderung gerinnbarer Substrate und funktionstüchtiger Thrombozyten Anlaß einer Gerinnungsstörung bei Unterschreiten einer kritischen Grenze einer Verbrauchskoagulopathie sein. Zusätzliche Mechanismen, wie metabolische Entgleisung im Sinne einer Acidose, sowie die Freisetzung von Gewebsthrombokinase sind zu berücksichtigen. Außer dem Thrombozytenabfall ließ sich bei unserer Untersuchung für einen Aufbrauch des Hämostasepotentiales kein Anhalt gewinnen.

Postoperativ zeigten 3 Patienten eine beginnende respiratorische Insuffizienz, wobei die differenzierte Betrachtung der erhobenen Laborwerte dieser 3 Patienten eine deutliche Verschlechterung der arteriellen Sauerstoffwerte und der Hämoglobinsauerstoffsättigung erkennen ließen. Bei keinem dieser Patienten war jedoch eine Erhöhung der Konzentrationswerte der freien Fettsäuren im Serum über den gesamten Untersuchungszeitraum meßbar. Werte von 0,81 mval/L wurden zu keinem Zeitpunkt überschritten. Die klinische Symptomatik war nach konsequenter Physiotherapie voll rückbildungsfähig innerhalb von 24 Stunden. Aufgrund der vorliegenden Untersuchungsergebnisse kann gefolgert werden, daß die primäre geschlossene, intramedulläre Frakturfixation ohne Aufbohren bei Oberschenkelschaftfrakturen auf den Konzentrationsverlauf der freien Fettsäuren im Serum keinen Einfluß hat.

Posttraumatische Komplikationen im Sinne einer posttraumatischen respiratorischen Insuffizienz oder Fettembolie als Ausdruck des Epiphänomens einer Schocklunge wird durch die primäre Versorgung kein Vorschub geleistet. Sämtliche gemessenen Parameter zeigen im Hinblick auf das Entstehen einer respiratorischen Insuffizienz bei unserem Patientengut keine prognostische Relevanz.

Zusammenfassung

Bei 18 Patienten mit posttraumatischer Femurfraktur werden in der perioperativen Phase die freien Fettsäuren, Thrombozyten, $AVDO_2$, Pulmonalisdrucke sowie einfache Kreislaufparameter gemessen. Die Serumkonzentrationen der freien Fettsäuren zeigen über den gemessenen Zeitraum keine mit dem Operationsereignis korrelierenden signifikanten Veränderungen. Die Hämodynamik des Systemkreislaufes läßt keine Abweichungen vom Normbereich erkennen. Die postoperativ gemessenen Werte der Pulmonalisdrucke liegen im oberen Normbereich. Die gemessenen Kreislaufgrößen und die laborchemischen Parameter werden unter besonderer Berücksichtigung ihrer prognostischen Relevanz für das Entstehen posttraumatischer respiratorischer Insuffizienz analysiert. Die operative Primärversorgung von Femurfrakturen durch die geschlossene Marknagelung wird diskutiert.

Literatur

1. Bachofen-Porchert M, Bachofen H (1973) Lungenveränderungen nach Trauma und Schock: Das Respiratory Distress Syndrome des Erwachsenen. Schweiz Med Wschr 103:1
2. Baltensweiler J (1977) Fettembolie-Syndrom. Verlag Hans Huber, Bern Stuttgart Wien
3. Bergentz SE, Lewis D, Ljungqvist U (1971) Die Lunge im Schock. Thrombozytenanhäufung nach Trauma und intravasaler Gerinnung. Langenbecks Arch klin Chir 329:658
4. Feldmann F, Kent E, Green WM (1975) The fat embolism syndrome. Diagnostic Radiology, März 1975
5. Kaith RG, Mahoney LJ, Garvey MB (1971) Disseminated intravascular coagulation: An important feature of the fat embolism syndrome. Cand med Ass J 105:74
6. Magerl F, Tscherny H (1966) Zur Diagnose, Therapie und Prophylaxe der Fettembolie. Langenbecks Arch clin Chir 314:292
7. Waldströhm L (1959) Plasma lipid and surgical trauma. Acta chir Scand 238

Panel 5
Anaesthesieletalität

Vorsitz: E. Rügheimer

Einleitung

E. Rügheimer

Bruno Haid äußerte am Ende seiner Antrittsvorlesung anläßlich der Errichtung und Übernahme des Instituts für Anästhesiologie der Universität Innsbruck seinen Zuhörern gegenüber die Hoffnung:

„Das gewählte Thema — Vom „Narkosetod" zur „Wiederbelebung" — sollte nicht die Operationssituation, in die wir alle kommen können, dramatisieren, um etwa gar Angst auszulösen, im Gegenteil: es würde mich freuen, wenn Sie weggingen mit einem Gefühl erhöhter Sicherheit, welches aufgrund der Fortschritte auf allen medizinischen Gebieten und nunmehr auch dank der modernen Anästhesie und Wiederbelebung wirklich gerechtfertigt ist."

Damit wird ohne Überheblichkeit zum Ausdruck gebracht, daß die spektakulären Fortschritte in der operativen Medizin ohne die Weiterentwicklung leistungsfähiger und risikoarmer Anästhesieverfahren undenkbar sind. Eine Narkose ist — wie Opderbecke sagt — heute für den Patienten im Regelfall kein Wagnis mit ungewissem Ausgang mehr, sonderen ein medizinisches Verfahren, dessen Risiko in Abhängigkeit vom Alter und Zustand des Patienten und der Dauer und Ausdehnung des operativen Eingriffs kalkulierbar geworden ist (Opderbecke). Mit dieser Feststellung soll zugleich zum Ausdruck gebracht werden, daß es auch heute kein Anästhesieverfahren gibt, das als gänzlich risikolos bezeichnet werden könnte. Im Gegenteil, statistische Erhebungen zeigen, daß an der heutigen Operationsletalität das angewandte Betäubungsverfahren keineswegs unbeteiligt ist. Gründe für dieses paradoxe Phänomen sind, daß ein Teil des anästhesiologischen Fortschritts durch die fortwährende Ausweitung der Operationsindikation kompensiert wird, und daß andererseits die Perfektionierung moderner Anästhesieverfahren zu einer vermehrten Gefahr technischer Pannen oder menschlicher Fehler führt. Der Anästhesist ist wie kaum ein anderer medizinischer Fachvertreter damit ein Opfer der Perfektion seiner eigenen Methoden geworden. Ein unerwarteter Exitus in tabula wird in der Regel zunächst einmal dem Anästhesisten angelastet. Erst wenn es ihm gelingt glaubhaft zu machen, daß kein Sorgfaltsmangel, kein ärztlicher Kunstfehler vorliegt, ist der medizinische Laie bereit, die Komplikation als schicksalsbedingt oder mit dem operativen Grundleiden im Zusammenhang stehend anzuerkennen. Das ist eine ganz gravierende Tatsache. Schließlich ist die Anästhesie nur in den seltensten Fällen Heilmittel per se, so z.B. beim Status asthmaticus oder Status epilepticus. In den meisten Fällen ist sie eine zwar notwendige, sicher auch segensreiche, aber letztlich doch nur akzessorische Maßnahme, um den eigentlichen Heileingriff, die Operation durchführen zu können. Mit anderen Worten, nur wenn Leib und Leben des Patienten in Gefahr sind und nur ein operativer Eingriff diese Gefahr beseitigen kann, ist auch die mögliche Anästhesiekomplikation zu vertreten. Häufig ist aber die Operation nicht ohne Alternative, sondern ein nicht unerheblicher Anteil steht mit anderen Heilmaßnahmen in Konkurrenz. Damit kommt der Wertung des Anästhesierisikos bei der Abwägung des Gesamtrisikos entscheidende Bedeutung zu.

Meine Damen und Herren, unsere Patienten haben begriffen, daß ihr Gegenüber kein Halbgott ist, sondern ein Mensch, der eine allerdings schwierige und wissensintensive Kunst vertritt und sie haben begriffen, daß ihr Arzt wie jeder andere Mensch in der Perfektion seiner Arbeit einer gewissen Limitierung unterliegt. Die Patienten beginnen deshalb nach Kriterien für seine Zuverlässigkeit zu fragen. Die Zuverlässigkeit eines Arztes hängt ganz entscheidend von der Sorgfalt ab, mit der er sein medizinisches Wissen in Diagnose und Therapie einsetzt. Wenn es uns also gelingt, einen Verhaltenskodex anästhesiologischer Sorgfaltsregeln zu formulieren, der sowohl die ärztlichen Verrichtungen als auch die technisch apparativen und personellen Voraussetzungen umfaßt, müßte es uns auch gelingen, die Brücken des Vertrauens zu unseren Patienten, die allem Anvertrauen vorausgehen, wieder zu festigen.

Lernen ohne zu denken, ist verlorene Mühe, ist eitel. Denken ohne zu lernen, ist gefährlich. Wenn wir diese Spruchweisheit von Konfuzius zur Prämisse für unser heutiges Gespräch über Anästhesieletalität machen, dann kann aus der zumindest primavista Negativdarstellung unseres Fachgebietes durchaus etwas absolut Positives entstehen. Wir müssen nur, wie gesagt, bereit sein, über unsere Fehler nachzudenken und daraus zu lernen. Diese Forderung auszusprechen ist sicherlich leichter, als sie in die Tat umzusetzen. Ich bin mir bewußt, daß die Behandlung dieses äußerst brisanten Themas sehr viel Fingerspitzengefühl verlangt, den Teilnehmern am Panel aber eine emotionslose Betrachtungsweise, Besonnenheit der Argumentation, vor allem aber Offenheit in der Darlegung unserer Fehler abverlangt.

Nun, meine Damen und Herren, Themen und Referenten sind mit größter Sorgfalt ausgewählt. Jeder der Panelisten hat sich über viele Jahre mit der von ihm vorgetragenen Problematik auseinandergesetzt. Jeder urteilt aus einem reichen Erfahrungsschatz. Jeder lebt von seinen glasklaren Formulierungen und ist deshalb als Diskutant geschätzt. Jeder lebt mit jedem in Harmonie, gleichwohl ist keiner bereit, sein Argument bloßer Harmonisierung zu opfern. Wir dürfen deshalb gespannt sein auf die Referate und die anschließende Diskussion.

Statistik der Anästhesieletalität

D. Langrehr

Zur Statistik der Anästhesieletalität will ich versuchen, in der kurzen vorgegebenen Zeit einen Eindruck zu vermitteln über Art, Häufigkeit, Vorhersehbarkeit und Vermeidbarkeit von lebensbedrohlichen und tödlichen Anästhesiekomplikationen. Die zu ziehenden Schlußfolgerungen sollten Anlaß zu Diskussion und weiterer Dokumentation sein.

Komplikationsgruppen (Tabelle 1)

Tabelle 1. Anaesthesie – Komplikationen

$\emptyset$	Zahn, Schleimhaut, Haut, Nerven (thermisch, elektrisch, mechanisch)	
„lebens-bedrohlich"	Tod innerhalb 24 Std. Bezug zur Anaesthesie 1 : 81	Th. Gordh anaesthesie: chir = 6 : 1? neurosurgery 1 : 1? cardiac surg. 0 : 1?
	Kardialer arrest (Asystolie, Flimmern) zirkulatorischer arrest (weak contraction) fulminantes Lungenoedem massives Erbrechen – Aspiration Ventilationsstörung – Hypoxie (IT, Cuff, Dekonn., Nachschub, Leck, Blockade, Broncho-Laryngospasmus, Fremdkörper, Pneu) postoperative pulmo-cardiale Insuffizienz anaphylactoide Reaktion toxische Reaktion, indiv. Überdosierung, Unterdos. → stress (Hyperthermie, andere seltene Zustände) postoperative (Organtoxizität) Insuffizienz (Leber, Niere) (rasch zunehmende Zahl von Stoffen) Fehlinjektion, -infusion Luftembolie, toxische Gase, Explosionen, Katheterembolie	

a) Thermische, elektrische und mechanische Schäden an Zahn, Schleimhaut, Haut und Nerven führen nicht selten zu Dauerschäden, sind jedoch nur in Ausnahmefällen lebensbedrohliche Komplikationen.

b) Jeder Tod innerhalb von 24–48 Stunden nach Anästhesieende sollte besonders eingehend auf einen Zusammenhang mit der Anästhesie untersucht werden, auch wenn während der Anästhesie keine Komplikation aufgetreten war. Die von Th. Gordh gemachte Angabe über das Verhältnis von Anästhesie – zu Chirurgie – bzw. Grundkrankheit-bedingtem Tod 6 : 1 (Neurochirurgie 1 : 1, Cardiochirurgie 10 : 1) soll nach seinen Worten weltweit anerkannt sein, entbehrt nach unserer Meinung aber jeder Grundlage, wenn man hier Todesfälle katalogisiert, die primär keine Anästhesiekomplikation boten. Im eigenen Material ist das Verhältnis dementsprechend 1 : 81.

c) Kardialer Stillstand und zirkulatorischer Stillstand (sogenannte weak contraction) sollten gesondert aufgeführt werden wegen der grundsätzlich differenten Prognose. Hier ist in jedem Falle eine sorgfältige Diskussion einer möglichen primären oder kontributiven Anästhesiebeteiligung nötig. In diesen beiden Gruppen finden sich auch die Problemfälle wie: „Kein anästhesiologischer oder chirurgischer Fehler im Licht der derzeitigen Kenntnisse“, wofür die Hyperthermie vor ihrer Entdeckung ein gutes Beispiel ist. Hier wird aber auch die Behauptung (1970, Special Committee Investigating Death under Anesthesia, New South Wales): „Anästhesiesubstanzen selbst sind nicht tödlich, nur ihr Mißbrauch“ fragwürdig, wenn sowohl ein Katecholaminabkömmling wie Atropin in kleinen Dosen gegen plötzliche schwere Reflexbradycardie in einem Fall von unbehandelter Mitralstenose zu Lungenoedem, Ventrikelfibrillieren und Tod führt. Die ungelöste Frage nach der optimalen Behandlung einer zunächst nicht tödlichen Komplikation ist hier die Grundlage der Schwierigkeit zur Einordnung: Anästhesiefehler oder Risiko unerwartet heftiger adverser Substanzreaktion.

Gerade in Fällen, in denen ein vermuteter, nicht auf Fehlern beruhender Myocardinfarkt oder eine vermutete massive Lungenembolie wegen Sectionsverweigerung der letzten Bestätigung entbehrt, wird die Zuordnung schwierig. Anästhesisten sollten solche Fälle in ihre Statistik gesondert aufnehmen. Beim gleichen Zusammenhang, der durch Section gesichert werden konnte, muß oft zugegeben werden, daß ohne Operation und Anästhesie dieses Ereignis wahrscheinlich zumindest nicht in diesem Augenblick eingetreten wäre, immer vorausgesetzt, es liegt keine anästhesiologische oder chirurgische Komplikation vor.

Dabei wird meist die überhaupt selten diskutierte Tatsache außer Acht gelassen, daß sich z.B. für ca. 200 Millionen Amerikaner bei 16 Millionen Operationen jährlich 32 Millionen Patienten-Gefahrentage ergeben, an denen etwa 350 000 Fälle von „plötzlichem Tod innerhalb einer Stunde aus offenbarer Gesundheit“ geschehen müssen, d.h. an jedem 100. Tag 1 Fall, wenn man 2 vulnerable Tage um die Operation herum annimmt. Keats [4], der diesen Zusammenhang diskutiert, fragt mit Recht: „Sind diese Fälle von Sekunden-Herztod auf dem Tisch wirklich Anästhesietote?“

d) Nachdem in den beiden vorausgehenden Gruppen die besonders problematischen Zusammenhänge angedeutet wurden, bieten die nun folgenden Gruppen keine Schwierigkeiten der Interpretation. Neben dem fulminanten Lungenoedem und dem Erbrechen mit Aspiration ist es vor allem die große Gruppe von Ventilationsstörungen mit Hypoxie, die immer wieder häufige Ursache für fatale Zwischenfälle bei sonst leidlich gesunden Patienten zur elektiven Chirurgie ist, und die Gemüter zu Recht erregt. Hier wie bei der postanästhetischen pulmocardialen Insuffizienz, der mittelschweren und schweren anaphylactoiden Reaktion, der mehr oder weniger substanzspezifischen individuellen toxischen Reaktion im Sinne inzwischen bekannter oder auch noch nicht bekannter Zusammenhänge (z.B. Hyperthermie, Sauerstoff und Bleomycin, individuelle Über- und Unterdosierung), der Fehlinjektion oder Infusion und der postanästhetischen Organtoxizität durch bekannt gewordene, rasch an Zahl zunehmende Substanzen, bedarf es der ganzen Umsicht und erheblicher Kenntnisse erstklassig ausgebildeter Anästhesisten, um die Komplikation rechtzeitig aufzufangen und bleibenden Schaden für den Patienten zu vermeiden.

Aus der kurzen Übersicht geht schon hervor, daß die Feststellungen von Robert MacIntosh [7]: „Jeder Anästhesietod ist vermeidbar, jeder Anästhesietod beruht auf einem Fehler, postmortale Untersuchungen führen nicht zur Klärung von Anästhesietodesfällen und Anästhesisten erzählen über einen Zwischenfall nicht die Wahrheit" zumindest in dieser Form nicht mehr haltbar sind. Auf der anderen Seite muß betont werden, daß eine einheitliche Definition des Anästhesietodes bisher fehlt.

Häufigkeit (Tabelle 2)

Tabelle 2. Anaesthesie-Letalität

---

primär − kontributiv, 1950−1979
USA, Australien, Canada, Dänemark, Deutschland, Frankreich, Südafrika, Schweden, Großbritannien

---

17 Autoren, 5 Mill. Anaesthesien, 2500 † = 0.05%, ~1 : 2000

---

1 : 259 (USA 1961) bis *1 : 9614* (Dänemark 1967)

Demnach ist es auch nicht verwunderlich, daß die Angaben über die Anästhesieletalität aus den Publikationen der letzten 30 Jahre so erstaunliche Unterschiede zwischen 1 : 259 und 1 : 9614 aufweisen. Ist die daraus resultierende Letalität von ca. 1 : 2000 d.h. 0,05% hoch oder niedrig? Der Versuch diese Angaben etwa mit älteren Statistiken, selbst dem Beecher-Todd-Report mit der Frage nach dem Erfolg der modernen Anästhesiologie zu vergleichen, muß scheitern, da es sich hier um in mehrfacher Hinsicht völlig Unvergleichbares handelt.

Im Zusammenhang mit der Frage, ob diese Letalität hoch oder niedrig sei, mögen die Zahlen der Mortalität im Krankenhaus im eigenen Erfahrungsbereich herangezogen werden. Daraus ergibt sich: (Tabelle 3)
1. Die Mortalität chirurgischer Patienten (1,8−5,07 %) differiert nur wenig von der Mortalität aller im Krankenhaus behandelten Patienten (4,65%).
2. Spezielle Risikodisziplinen wie Cardiochirurgie und Neurochirurgie haben demgegenüber keine auffallend hohe Mortalität mehr (2,2−4,6 %), selbst die moderne Intensivtherapie liegt nicht höher (4%). Die Absterberate der Bevölkerung von ca. 1% legt die Vermutung nahe, daß die konzentriert selektierte kranke und moribunde „Krankenhausbevölkerung" insgesamt mit einer Vervierfachung der Mortalität rein rechnerisch nur die „konzentrierte Absterberate" darstellt. So nimmt es nicht wunder, daß die Anästhesieletalität der Bundesrepublik nach Lutz (1975) mit 1 : 4255 oder 0,02%, d.h. 705/anno 250x niedriger liegt.

Während für einzelne Gruppen von Komplikationen (Hyperthermie, anaphylactoide Reaktion, Relaxansabbaustörungen) stark variierende Häufigkeitsangaben gemacht werden, fehlen solche für andere Anästhesiekomplikationen nahezu vollständig. Gestatten Sie mir daher wiederum auf die eigene Erfahrung zurückzugreifen. Die Tabelle 4 zeigt Verteilung und Häufigkeit der verschiedenen Gruppen von lebensbedrohlichen Anästhesiekomplikationen (112 309 Anästhesien aus 16 Jahren). Bei jedem 183. Fall kam es zu einer solchen lebensbe-

Tabelle 3. Krankenhaus − operative − Mortalität

		†	
ZK HB Nord 1964−1977	alle stat. Pat. (155 943)	7257	4,65%
	allg. chir. Pat. (41 067)	2082	5,07%
AZG Groningen 1978/79	chir. Pat. (11 898)	219	1,8%
	Thorax Pat. (1163)	53	4,6%
	Neurochir. Pat. (1960)	42	2,2%
	IC Pat. (1978 = 975)	39	4,0%
Bevölkerung Mortalität	~1,0%/anno; Deutschland − Lutz (1975) ~600 000/anno; 1 : 4255		
Anaesthesie Letalität	~0,01% ~3 Mill. Anaest. = 705/anno		

Tabelle 4. ZK-HB-Nord. AZG-Groningen (1964−1979) 112 309 Anaesthesien

∅	Komplikationsgruppen	nicht anaesth.	primär o. kontributiv anaesth.	† nicht anaesth.	anaesth.
lebens- bedrohlich	Zahn, Schleimhaut, Haut, Nerven		46		
	† innerhalb 24 Std.	81	1	81	1
	kardialer Stillstand	65	13	59	6
	zirkulator. Stillstand	55	57	16	
	Lungenoedem		17		
	Erbrechen-Aspiration		74		
	Ventilation-Hypoxie		83	2	
	postanaesth. pulm. card. Insuff.		75	3	
	anaphylaktoide Reaktion		257	1	2
	toxische Medik. Reaktion Hyperthermie		3		
	postop. Organtoxizität Leber-Niereninsuff.		16	4	
	Fehlinjektion, -infusion Luftembolie		17	1	
	Total		860	176	
	Anaesthesie		659	9	

613 lebensbedr. Anaesth. Kompl.   1 : 183 → 0,55%
9 „Anaesthesie" Tote   1 : 12478 → 0,01%
davon 5mal Embolie-Verdacht → keine Sektion
4 Anaesthesie Tote   1 : 28077

drohlichen Komplikation, d.h. in 0,55% aller Anästhesien. Von 9 Anästhesietodesfällen, d.h.
1 : 12478 = 0.01% konnte 5× der Embolieverdacht nicht endgültig durch Section geklärt
werden. Nur in 4 Fällen (1 : 28077) war der Zusammenhang des Todes mit der Anästhesie
klar. Von 613 lebensbedrohlichen Komplikationen während der Anästhesie verließen 604
Patienten ohne jeden Schaden die Klinik.

Eine seltene Mitteilung über Häufigkeit von Anästhesiekomplikationen findet sich bei
B. Smalhout, er teilt 203 lebensbedrohliche Komplikationen bei 35 171 Anästhesien (1973–
1976) mit, d.h. 1 : 173 oder 0,58%. Eine Vielzahl von Schwierigkeiten, die nicht direkt le-
bensbedrohlich sind, haben wir nicht aufgeführt, bei Smalhout ist die Gesamtzahl 3776, d.h.
1 : 10, wobei die Verteilung in leichte, mäßig schwere und lebensbedrohliche 55 : 40 : 5% ist.

Vorhersehbarkeit (Tabelle 5)

Es hat nicht an Bemühungen gefehlt, das anästhesiologische Risiko im Rahmen der Voruntersuchung des Patienten in Maß und Zahl zu bringen. Dabei hat sich gezeigt, daß sowohl für

Tabelle 5. Präoperative Risiko-Erfassung

ASA Dripps, Eckenhoff 1963	MIC (Multifact. ind. card. risk) Goldman alii 1977		Lungenformel Wassner, Timm 1976
I healthy patient	Age > 60	5	pulm.-card. insuff.- Wahrscheinlichkeit
	Myoc. infarction 6 Mo.	10	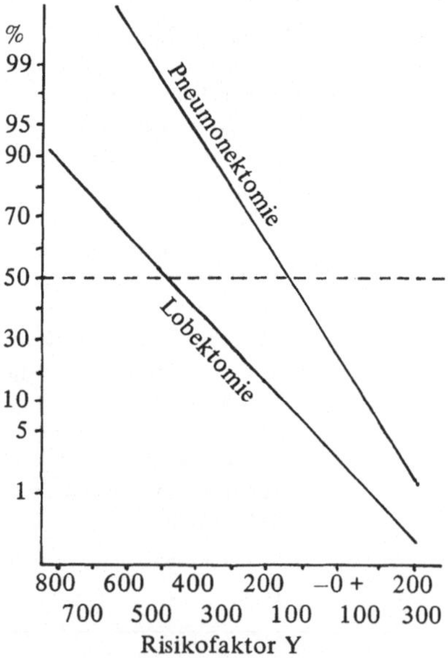
	Gallop. Jug. V. dist.	11	%
	Valv. aort. sten.	3	99
II mild disease	Rhyth other than sinus	7	
	> 5 premat. atr. contr./min.	7	95
	PO_2 < 60 PCO_2 > 50 Torr		90
III severe systemic	K < 3,0 mmol/l		
limited	Rest-N > 50 mg/dl	3	70
activity not	Abnormal SGOT		
incapacitating	Chron. liver dis.		50
	Intraperit. thoracal.	3	
	Aorten – op		30
IV incapacitating syst.	Emergency	4	
			10
const. threat to life	total points	53	5
			1

V moribund pat. not expected to survive	ASA	Points	MGH-class
	I	0–5	I
	II		
	III	6 12	II
	IV	13–25	III
additional E = Emergency	V	> 26	IV

MGH = Mass. Gen. Hosp.
ähnlich wie:
N.Y. Heart Ass. funct. class.

$Y = 2,4$ (VT max) $+ 2,5$ (VT max/sec)
$+ 0,7$ (Vent max) $- 4,3$ (V pulm.min)
$+ 1,7$ (PO_2) $- 5,3$ (PCO_3)
$- 100$ (Herzrisikozahl 1–5)
$- 3,8$ (Alter/Jahre)

die relativ einfache ASA-Klassifikation, deren Bestimmungen Lutz durch einen umfangreichen Wertekatalog sicher bestimmbar und reproduzierbar gemacht hat, wie auch für die speziell auf myocardiale Risikofaktoren abgestellte MIC-Klassifikation (unten in der Mitte der Abbildung 5 sehen Sie die Relation der 53 MIC-Punkte zu ASA- und MGH-Klassifikation) sichere Relationen zur postoperativen Mortalität herzustellen sind. Auch das von Wassner und Timm aus 1000 retrospektiv untersuchten Lungenresektionen gewonnene Wahrscheinlichkeitsnomogramm ermöglicht sehr zuverlässig aus relativ einfachen präoperativen Ventilationswerten, Blutgasen und Herzrisikowerten mit Hilfe einer multivariablen Faktorenanalyse vorauszubestimmen, wie groß die Überlebenschance eines Patienten ist.

Es erhebt sich die Frage, ob die meist von Anästhesisten inaugurierten Risikoklassifikationen neben ihrer zuverlässigen Prognose über das per- und postoperative Mortalitätsrisiko hinaus auch das gefragte Risiko der Anästhesie anzugeben vermögen.

Tabelle 6. Risiko-Verteilung

Patienten	ASA I	II	III	IV	V	Σ let. III, IV, V
11. US Naval Hosp. Study						
Vacanti v. Houten, Letalität (%)	0,08	0,27	1,8	7,8	9,4	5084
68 588 Anaesthesien (%)	74,2	18,4	5,3	1,2	0,9	7,4%
ZK HB Nord (Zahl)	65 373	22 969	2292	3726	1146	7164
95 506 Anaesthesien (%)	68,5	24,0	2,4	3,9	1,2	7,5%
† innerhalb 24 Std. (Zahl)	23	21	36	68	124	
cardialer + zirkul. arrest						
272 Fälle (%)	8,5	7,7	13,2	25,0	45,6	
übrige lebensbedrohliche						
Anaesthesie Komplik. (Zahl)	340	64	57	52	29	
542 Fälle (%)	62,7	11,8	10,5	9,6	5,4	

Die Tabelle 6 gibt in der oberen Zeile die Verteilung von ASA-Gruppen auf 68 388 Anästhesien durch Vacanti und Van Houten wieder, sowie die Zuordnung der entsprechenden Krankenhaus-Gesamtletalität. Die zweite Zeile gibt dieselben ASA-Gruppen Prozente des eigenen Bremer Gesamtmaterials (95 506 Anästhesien) und zeigt eine gute Übereinstimmung der Risikogruppenverteilung mit der 11 US-Naval-Hospital Study. In der dritten Zeile sind in gleicher Weise die 3 Gruppen: Tod innerhalb 24 Stunden, cardialer und zirkulatorischer Arrest aufgeschlüsselt. Hier wird deutlich, daß diese 272 Fälle ganz deutlich ein starkes Überwiegen der ASA Klassen III, IV und V aufweisen.

Demgegenüber entsprechen die übrigen 542 lebensbedrohlichen Anästhesiekomplikationen (unterste Zeile) der Normrisikoverteilung weitgehend, d.h. diese Komplikationen sind zumindest durch die praeoperative Risikoerfassung üblicherweise nicht vorhersehbar.

Darüberhinaus ist nach unserer Meinung, auch aus anderen Erfahrungen, die Feststellung gerechtfertigt, daß die praeoperative Risikoerfassung in der angeführten Art kaum eine schlüssige Relation zu anästhesiologischen Schwierigkeiten, Komplikationen und fatalen Zwischenfällen ergibt, somit also für die Gesamtbetrachtung per- und postoperativer Überlebenschancen wertvoll für die prospektive Erfassung von zu erwartenden Anästhesieschwierigkeiten aber von geringer Bedeutung ist.

Bedenkt man, daß für Risikoeingriffe meist versiertere Anästhesisten mit größerer Sorgfalt arbeiten, so wird unsere Erfahrung mit 2 Kollektiven über 60jähriger gynäkologischer Patienten (637 Fälle, 37,5% ASA III—V) und Eingriffen an den Gallenwegen (227 Fälle, 72% ASA III—V) verständlich, wo bei deutlichen Unterschieden in Komplikations- und Mortalitätsrate (Gyn = 90% ohne Komplikationen, 1,1% Tote; Gallen = 53% ohne Komplikationen, 19% Tote) anästhesiologische Schwierigkeiten oder Komplikationen in keinem Fall beider Kollektive zu registrieren waren.

Vermeidbarkeit

Wenn eine sorgfältige präanästhetische Befunderhebung zwar von unbestreitbarem Wert, aber nicht geeignet ist, die Mehrzahl anästhesiologischer Komplikationen vorauszusagen, müssen sich die Bemühungen um Vermeidung und Beherrschung solcher Komplikationen in erster Linie auf zwei Zusammenhänge konzentrieren.
1. Sorgfältigste Beobachtung des Patienten mit Zuhilfenahme von allen Möglichkeiten eines modernen Monitoring, wobei allerdings die Vielzahl von Monitoren nicht die kontrollierende Aufmerksamkeit des Anästhesisten ersetzen kann, ein Übermaß ihn sogar eher vom direkten Beobachtungskontakt mit dem Patienten ablenkt.

Der noch vielerorts verbalisierten Vorstellung, ein Anästhesist könne ohne Zweifel mit mehreren Hilfskräften an mehreren Tafeln verantwortlich anästhesieren, kann in diesem Zusammenhang gar nicht heftig genug widersprochen werden. Die Notsituation kann nie Regelfall sein. Der Hinweis auf Anästhesien geringer Risikoklassifizierung erweist sich nach den Darlegungen als ebenso unsinnig wie die Vorstellung, daß ein Chirurg mehrere Operationen gleichzeitig durchführt.
2. Da die Mehrzahl der unvorhersehbar auftretenden lebensbedrohlichen Anästhesiekomplikationen erfahrungsgemäß durch Anästhesisten mit hohem Ausbildungsstand und großer Erfahrung ohne bleibenden Schaden für den Patienten beherrscht werden kann, muß alles nur mögliche getan werden, um jeden Patienten in den Genuß eines solchen Anästhesisten zu bringen. Gerade Mitteilungen über ganze Serien auf den ersten Blick vermeidbarer fataler Zwischenfälle auf dem Boden banaler Vorkommnisse, durch welche die Bevölkerung beunruhigt wird und dann entsprechende Briefe an ihre Patienten heftet, zeigen, daß solche Komplikationen bei weitgehend gesunden Patienten unbedingt in Zukunft vermieden werden müssen. Das rupturierte Aortenaneurysma beim polytraumatisierten, moribunden Unfallopfer nachts auf dem Tisch oder wenige Stunden danach zu verlieren, ist nicht Gegenstand der Diskussion. Gerade hier leistet die moderne Anästhesiologie Erstaunliches.

Die gesunde Intervall-Appendizitis jedoch durch massive Aspiration oder unbemerkte Ventilationsdekonnektion verloren zu haben, wiegt schwer.

Zusammenfassung

1. Hohes Lebensalter und schwere Vorschädigung verschiedener Organsysteme bieten für erfahrene Anästhesisten hinsichtlich der Anästhesie per se kein merklich gesteigertes Risiko. Die präoperative Klassifizierung: „hohes Risiko" bezieht sich weit mehr auf Grundkrankheitsverlauf und operative Komplikationen.
2. Hinsichtlich der Häufigkeit lebensbedrohlicher Anästhesiekomplikationen bietet die präoperative Risikoklassifizierung keine verläßliche Voraussage, wenn auch schwerere Herz-

Kreislaufkomplikationen per- und postoperativ ohne Anästhesiefehler deutlich mit der Risikoklasse korreliert sind.

3. Bei bedeutenden methodologischen Fortschritten der Anästhesiologie führen potente Pharmaka, komplizierte, störanfällige Techniken und erhebliche Erweiterung der Indikation zum operativen Eingriff zu einer Rate von lebensbedrohlichen Anästhesiekomplikationen bei jeder 170.–180. Anästhesie. Die Häufigkeit nicht direkt lebensbedrohlicher Komplikationen liegt noch weit höher. Eine umfassende nationale Dokumentation ist dringend nötig.

4. Nur ein hoher Ausbildungsstand langjährig geschulter Anästhesisten gibt die Gewähr für eine nahezu vollständige Bewältigung dieser Schwierigkeiten. Die Allgemein- und Leitungsanästhesie ist, mehr denn je, eine fachärztliche Spezialaufgabe, die den vollen Einsatz eines nicht überbelasteten Anästhesisten verlangt.

5. Während in unserem Patientengut trotz zahlenmäßig bedeutender Schwierigkeiten Dauerschäden im Sinne von Defektheilungen nicht vorkommen, liegt die der Anästhesie zuzuordnende Letalität mit 9 Fällen bei 1 : 12 478 = 0,01%. Die Tatsache, daß davon 5× ein Embolieverdacht ohne Anästhesiekomplikation nicht durch Section erhärtet werden konnte, macht die Notwendigkeit einer klaren Definition: primäre und kontributive Anästhesieletalität deutlich, ständige Komplikationskonferenzen sollten an jeder Abteilung mit interdisziplinärer Besprechung obligat werden.

Nur 4 Fälle boten einen klaren kausalen Zusammenhang mit der Anästhesie (1 : 28 077). Ein Vergleich dieser Ergebnisse mit Frühzeiten der Anästhesie ist kaum möglich.

6. Bedenkt man, daß etwa 60% aller im Krankenhaus stationär behandelter Patienten ein oder mehrmals des Schutzes der Anästhesie gegenüber invasiver Diagnostik und Therapie bedürfen, so wird allein von daher klar, daß die höchsten Anstrengungen des Faches zur Vermeidung von fatalen Komplikationen gerechtfertigt sind.

Ganz ohne Zweifel sichert das bisher Erreichte für den Patienten die beruhigende Gewißheit, daß er sich einer wohlorganisierten und funktionsfähigen Anästhesieabteilung jederzeit ohne Furcht anvertrauen kann.

Literatur

1. Beecher HK, Todd DP (1964) A study of the deaths associated with anesthesia and surgery. Ann Surg 140:2
2. Goldman L, Caldera D, Nussbaum S, et al. (1977) Multifactorial index of cardiac risk in noncardiac surgery. New Engl J Med 297:845
3. Gordh T, Mostert JW (1978) Anesthetic accidents case studies. Intern Anesth Clinics 16, No. 3
4. Keats AS (1979) What do we know about anesthetic mortality? Anesthesiology 50:387
5. Langrehr D, Singbartl G, Arnold R, Neuhaus R, Kluge I (1978) Das Risiko der Allgemeinanästhesie. Prakt Anästh 13:345
6. Lutz H, Klose R (1979) Operationsvorbereitung aus anästhesiologischer Sicht. Med Welt 30:639
7. MacIntosh RR (1948) Deaths under anesthetics. Brit J Anaesth 21:107
8. Smalhout B (1978) Safe anesthesia: some general considerations. Acta anesth belg 29:1
9. Vacanti Ch, van Houten R (1970) A statistical analysis of the relationship of physical status to postoperative mortality in 68 388 cases. Anesth Analg Curr Res 49:564
10. Wassner UJ, Timm J (1976) Zur präoperativen Ermittlung der Wahrscheinlichkeit einer pulmocardialen Insuffizienz nach Lungenresektion. Chirurg 47:602

Systematik und Erfassung der Anästhesieletalität

H.W. Opderbecke

Die Fortschritte der operativen Medizin in den letzten beiden Jahrzehnten, ihre Ausdehnung auf extreme Altersgruppen und Risikopatienten, aber auch die breite Anwendung neuer operativer Methoden, sind eng mit Verbesserungen der Anästhesietechnik verbunden. Man sollte meinen, daß diese Verbesserungen auch zu einem Rückgang der Anästhesieletalität geführt hätten. Das läßt sich jedoch durch die Statistik nicht belegen. Für die vergangenen 20 Jahre kann jedenfalls eine statistisch relevante Reduzierung anästhesiebedingter Todesfälle nicht verzeichnet werden [14].

Diese erstaunliche Tatsache verpflichtet uns zu einer eingehenden, fortlaufenden Fehleranalyse durch Erfassung aller anästhesiologischen Risikofaktoren. Eine solche statistisch einwandfreie Erfassung des Anästhesierisikos setzt zunächst einmal seine Abgrenzung gegenüber dem Operationsrisiko im engeren Sinne voraus, die jedoch auf erhebliche Schwierigkeiten stößt [7].

Beim Studium der Literatur läßt sich erkennen, daß es kaum zwei Autoren gibt, die zu einer solchen Abgrenzung die gleichen Kriterien verwenden. Alleine schon die Frage, welche postoperative Zeitspanne der Erfassung von anästhesiebedingten Komplikationen zugrunde gelegt werden soll, wird nicht einheitlich beantwortet. Die meisten Autoren berücksichtigen nur diejenigen Zwischenfälle, die während der Operation und innerhalb der ersten postoperativen 24 Stunden zum Tode geführt haben. Andere legen bis zu 30 Tage zugrunde.

Tabelle 1. Statistik des Anaesthesierisikos 1954–1974 (modifiziert nach Goldstein and Keats [9])

Autoren	Jahr	Anzahl der Anaesthesien	Todesursache ausschließlich anaesthesiebedingt	zusätzlich anaesthesiebedingt	erfaßter Zeitraum in Tagen
Beecher and Todd [1]	1954	599 584	1 : 2680	1 : 1560	
Dornette and Orth [4]	1956	63 150	1 : 2429	1 : 1344	
Phillips [16]	1960		1 : 7700	1 : 3710	1
Dripps et al. [6]	1961				
Spinal-Anaesth.		18 737	1 : 1560	1 : 780	30 (!)
Allg.-Anaesth.		14 487	1 : 536	1 : 259	
Clifton and Hotten [2]	1963	205 640	1 : 6048	1 : 3955	intraoperativ
Memery	1965	69 291	1 : 3145	1 : 1082	
Harrison [8]	1968	177 928	–	1 : 3007	1
Lutz et al. [10, 11]	1972	30 126	–	1 : 3063	28
Marx et al. [12]	1973	34 145	–	1 : 1265	7
Harrison [8]	1974	141 000	1 : 5550	1 : 4555	1

In Tabelle 1 sind einige wesentliche Arbeiten zum Thema „Anästhesieletalität" aus den Jahren 1954 bis 1974 zusammengestellt. Man erkennt die zahlenmäßige Abhängigkeit von der für die Erfassung zugrunde gelegten postoperativen Zeitspanne. Darüber hinhaus liegt auf der Hand, daß bei der Beurteilung, ob die vorliegende Todesursache „ausschließlich" anästhesiebedingt oder „zusätzlich" anästhesiebedingt gewesen ist, ein weiter, subjektiver Ermessensspielraum besteht.

Mit derartigen pauschalen statistischen Aufschlüsselungen, vor allem wenn sie als retrospektive Studie erfolgt, kann somit u.E. keine verwertbare Risikoanalyse durchgeführt werden. Vielleicht läßt sich dieses Ziel eher erreichen, wenn man eine grundsätzlich andere Systematik anwendet, die Einteilung der anästhesiologischen Risikofaktoren in zwei Gruppen, in

1. biologisch-medizinische Risikofaktoren und
2. methodisch-technische Risikofaktoren.

Biologisch-medizinische Risikofaktoren

Diese hängen vom Alter und Zustand des Patienten im Verhältnis zu Art und Schwere des operativen Eingriffes ab. Mit der ständigen Ausweitung der Operationsindikation auf immer extremere Risikogruppen müßte natürlich — statistisch gesehen — auch die Anästhesieletalität ansteigen. Dieser Anstieg wird jedoch weitgehend durch die Perfektionierung der anästhesiologischen Technik kompensiert. Das heißt, in dem Maße, in dem die modernen Anästhesieverfahren an Sicherheit dazugewinnen, wird die Operationsindikation automatisch ausgeweitet bis zur Grenze einer gerade noch vertretbaren Risikoquote.

Wenn man davon ausgeht, daß die operative Medizin auch in den kommenden Jahrzehnten weiter fortschreiten und stets bestrebt sein wird, bis an die äußersten Grenzen der nach dem jeweiligen Stand der Anästhesiologie möglichen Bedingungen zu stoßen, ist immer mit einer gewissen, anästhesiebedingten, gerade noch als tragbar erscheinende Letalitätsrate zu rechnen, es sei denn, man wollte durch eine Einschränkung der Operationsindikation einen Stillstand der operativen Medizin inkauf nehmen.

Statistische Zahlenangaben über diese durch biologisch-medizinische Risikofaktoren bedingte Anästhesieletalität sagen somit nichts aus über die Letalität bestimmter Anästhesieverfahren, sondern allenfalls über die Letalität bestimmter Patientengruppen in bezug auf das Gesamtrisiko von Operation und zugehörigem Anästhesieverfahren.

Methodisch-technische Risikofaktoren

Ganz andere Voraussetzungen bestehen im Hinblick auf die zweite Kategorie von Risikofaktoren, den methodisch-technischen. Diese sind weitgehend unabhängig vom Zustand des Patienten und der Schwere des operativen Eingriffes. Vielmehr besteht hier ein unmittelbarer Zusammenhang mit der angewandten Verfahrenstechnik. Bei dieser Gruppe geht es somit nicht um die Letalität bestimmter Patientenkollektive, sondern umgekehrt bestimmter Anästhesiemethoden.

Schon eine der ersten großen Statistiken von Beecher und Todd [1] aus dem Jahre 1954, die sich auf ein Gesamtkollektiv von rund 600 000 Fällen aus 10 Hospitälern stützt, ist hierfür ein gutes Beispiel (Tabelle 2). Die Untersuchung kommt nämlich zu dem Ergebnis, daß die Häufigkeit anästhesiebedingter Todesfälle bei Narkosen unter Verwendung von Muskelre-

Tabelle 2. Vergleich der Rate anaesthesiebedingter Todesfälle mit und ohne Verwendung von Muskelrelaxantien (Beecher u. Todd 1954)

Table XIII	Total incidence of "Curare" use and associated Death
Total number anaesthesias	599 500
Number Anaesthesias in which "Curare" used (1 : 14)	44 100
Frequency of death related to Anaesthesia	
Anaesthesias which did not include "Curare" (266)	1 : 2100
Anaesthesias which include "Curare" (118)	1 : 370

laxanzien auf 1 : 370 gegenüber 1 : 2100 bei Anästhesien ohne Verwendung von Muskelrelaxanzien ansteigt. Ein wesentlicher Grund für dieses frappierende, zur damaligen Zeit aufsehenerregende Zahlenverhältnis dürfte darin zu suchen sein, daß man vor mehr als 20 Jahren die mit der Anwendung von Muskelrelaxanzien verbundenen Probleme der Intubation und Beatmung noch nicht mit der heutigen technischen Perfektion beherrscht hat.

Das bedeutet aber nicht, daß methodisch-technische Risikofaktoren heute keine Rolle mehr spielen, im Gegenteil! Gerade die Intubationsnarkose bietet zwar gegenüber älteren, überholten Verfahren dem Patienten — vor allem dem durch biologisch-medizinische Risikofaktoren gefährdeten Patienten — ein hohes Maß an Sicherheit, beinhaltet aber zugleich die vermehrte Möglichkeit technischer Fehler und Gefahren. Angefangen von der ortsgebundenen zentralen Narkosegasversorgung bis hin zum Trachealtubus ist eine Fülle von technischen Mängeln oder Pannen infolge Verkettung unglücklicher Umstände, mangelhafter Aufmerksamkeit bei der Überwachung oder sogar ausgesprochener Sorgfaltsmängel denkbar, die den Patienten, und zwar auch den organgesunden Patienten, von einer Minute auf die andere in unmittelbare Lebensgefahr bringen können [3]. Einen solchen technisch bedingten Zwischenfall kann man somit geradezu als „Anästhesieunfall" bezeichnen.

Die Bedeutung solcher Anästhesieunfälle läßt sich am Beispiel einer britischen Zusammenstellung von 204 intraoperativen Herzstillständen ablesen (Tabelle 3). Von diesen überlebte nur 1 Patient den Zwischenfall ohne jede Folgen. 22% überlebten ihn länger als eine Woche mit mehr oder weniger schweren neurologischen Ausfallerscheinungen. Ein großer Teil dieser Zwischenfälle ereignete sich bei Patienten in gutem Allgemeinzustand, aus Anlaß

Tabelle 3. Analyse von 204 intraoperativen Herzstillständen 1964 bis 1973 in Großbritannien (Lancet 1975; Wylie, 1975)

Analyse von 204 intraoperativen Herzstillständen 1964–1973, davon 29 durch technische Mängel bedingt	
Ursachen:	
Sauerstoffmangel aus verschiedener Ursache	17
Diskonnektion von Patient und Gerät	5
Unsachgerechte Gerätebedienung	3
Kohlensäureüberschuß	2
Lachgasüberschuß	2

einer wenig eingreifenden Operation und unter der Verantwortung eines gut ausgebildeten Anästhesisten. In der Hälfte der Fälle hätte der Herzstillstand verhindert werden können; in 12 Fällen konnte Fahrlässigkeit nachgewiesen werden [20].

Dies weist auf eine weitere Schwierigkeit einer zuverlässigen Erfassung anästhesiebedingter, tödlicher Zwischenfälle hin; sie steht eng mit der Frage strafrechtlicher Konsequenzen in Zusammenhang.

Es besteht kein Zweifel, daß der Anästhesist, dem ein Fehler unterlaufen ist, alleine schon deswegen verpflichtet ist, alles zur Aufdeckung des Sachverhaltes beizutragen, um berechtigten zivilrechtlichen Ansprüchen des Patienten oder seiner Angehörigen entgegenzukommen. Ob diese Verpflichtung allerdings so weit zu gehen hat, durch den Antrag auf eine gerichtliche Sektion ein strafrechtliches Ermittlungsverfahren gegen sich in Gang zu setzen, möchte ich hier offen lassen. Kein Staatsbürger ist zu einer Selbstanzeige verpflichtet; dieser Grundsatz müßte auch für den Arzt gelten [15].

Die Gefahr strafrechtlicher Sanktionen verhindert sicher auch in vielen Fällen die offene Publikation von Anästhesietodesfällen und die freimütige Erörterung ihrer Ursachen. Auch die Realisierung eines an sich begrüßenswerten Vorschlages von Lutz [9] dürfte nicht zuletzt aufgrund dieser Schwierigkeiten auf Hindernisse stoßen: Die Schaffung eines zentralen Registers für tödliche Anästhesiezwischenfälle zum Zwecke einer systematischen Fehleranalyse. Dieses könnte nicht außerhalb des geltenden Rechtes eingerichtet werden und wäre somit im Zuge eines strafrechtlichen Ermittlungsverfahrens dem Zugriff der Staatsanwaltschaft ebenfalls nicht entzogen [19].

Wir Anästhesisten haben die wissenschaftliche Pflicht, uns um die Erfassung von Risikofaktoren zu bemühen, Fehler und Gefahren zu analysieren und daraus die notwendigen Konsequenzen für unser Fachgebiet zu ziehen. Aus den gemachten Ausführungen geht hervor, daß eine solche Erfassung aus den verschiedenen Gründen bisher unvollständig und unsystematisch und damit unbefriedigend erfolgt ist. Wir sollten uns daher bemühen, diese für uns elementare Aufgabenstellung einer Lösung zuzuführen. Hierzu möchten wir abschließend zwei Vorschläge machen:

1. In Anlehnung an einen Vorschlag des Rechtsmediziners Pribilla [17, 18] sollte die Deutsche Gesellschaft für Anästhesiologie und Intensivmedizin für den Bereich der Bundesrepublik Deutschland eine Kommission von Juristen, Rechtsmedizinern und Anästhesisten mit der Aufgabe ins Leben rufen, sämtliche tödlichen Anästhesiezwischenfälle zu erfassen und sie im Einvernehmen mit der zuständigen Staatsanwaltschaft und ohne Verletzung rechtlicher Vorschriften durch außergerichtliche Sektion und Begutachtung abzuklären. — Dabei könnten vielleicht die in Österreich gemachten Erfahrungen mit der gesetzlich vorgeschriebenen Obduktion operativer Todesfälle Berücksichtigung finden. Die Kommission hätte die Verpflichtung zur regelmäßigen Publikation der Ergebnisse ihrer Arbeit.

2. Eine gemeinsame Arbeitsgruppe der drei deutschsprachigen Anästhesiegesellschaften sollte die Aufgabe erhalten, für den deutschen Sprachraum einheitliche Kriterien zur Erfassung der Anästhesieletalität zu erarbeiten. Hierzu gehört eine Definition der Begriffe „Anästhesierisiko" bzw. „Anästhesiekomplikation" und ihre Abgrenzung gegenüber operativen Risiken und Komplikationen, ferner Grundsätze für ihre statistische Auswertung. — Vielleicht wäre es eine verdienstvolle Aufgabe der neugegründeten „Europäischen Akademie für Anästhesiologie", die gleiche Aufgabe für den europäischen Raum zu übernehmen.

Literatur

1. Beecher HK, Todd DP (1954) A study of deaths associated with anesthesia and surgery. Ann Surg 140:2–34
2. Clifton BS, Hotten WIT (1963) Deaths associated with anaesthesia. Brit J Anaesth 35:250–259
3. Cooper JB, Newbower RS, Long ChD, McPeek B (1978) Preventable anesthesia mishaps: as study of human factors. Anesthesiology 49:399–406
4. Dornette WHL, Orth OS (1956) Death in the operating room. Anesth Analg Curr Res 35:545–569
5. Dotzauer G (1978) Mors in tabula. Prakt Anästh 13:345–351
6. Dripps RD, Lamont A, Eckenhoff JE (1961) The role of anaesthesia in surgical mortality. J Amer med Ass 178:261–266
7. Goldstein A, Keats AS (1970) The risk of anesthesia. Anesthesiology 33:130–143
8. Harrison GG (1974) Anaesthetic associated mortality. S Afr Med J, S 550–554
9. Lutz H (1970) Sorgfalt bei der Voruntersuchung und Vorbehandlung. Anästh Intensivmed 20:31–35
10. Lutz H, Klose R, Peter K (1972) Untersuchungen zum Risiko der Allgemeinanästhesie unter operativen Bedingungen. Dtsch med Wschr 97:1816–1820
11. Lutz H, Peter K (1973) Das Risiko der Anaesthesie unter operativen Bedingungen. Langenbecks Arch Chir 334:672–679
12. Marx GF, Mateo CV, Orkin LR (1973) Computer analysis of postanesthetic deaths. Anesthesiology 39:54–58
13. Memery HN (1965) Anesthesia mortality in private practise: a ten-year-study. J Amer med Ass 194:1185
14. Opderbecke HW (1977) Risikofaktoren der Anästhesie. Anästh Inform 18:561–567
15. Opderbecke HW (1978) Anästhesie und ärztliche Sorgfaltspflicht. Anaesthesiologie und Wiederbelebung, Bd. 100; Springer, Berlin Heidelberg New York
16. Philips OC, Frazier TM, Graff TD, de Kornfeld TJ (1960) The Baltimore Anesthesia Study Committee: Review of 1024 postanesthetic deaths. J Amer med Ass 174:2015–2019
17. Pribilla O (1964) Der Tod in Narkose. Anaesthesist 13:340–345
18. Pribilla O (1979) Natürlicher und nicht natürlicher Tod in der Anästhesie. Anästh Intensivmed 20, im Druck
19. Wagner H-J (1979) Sorgfaltspflicht aus rechtsmedizinischer Sicht. Anästh Intensivmed 20:85–88
20. Wylie WD (1975) There but for the grace of God. Ann Roy Coll Surg Engl 56:171–180

Rechtsmedizinische Aspekte des tödlichen Anaesthesiezwischenfalls

W. Schwerd

Meine kurzen Gedanken zu diesem Thema betreffen zwei Aspekte.
1. Wann hat sich der Rechtsmediziner mit tödlichen Anaesthesiezwischenfällen zu befassen?
2. Welche Feststellungsmöglichkeiten hat er?

Zu Punkt 1

Aufgabe des *Rechtsmediziners* ist es, *bei nicht-geklärten und nicht-natürlichen Todesfällen* Untersuchungen zur Feststellung der Todesursache vorzunehmen. Die Bearbeitung der *Todesfälle aus natürlicher Ursache* ist *Sache des Pathologen.* Diese Abgrenzung wird jedenfalls dort zu finden sein, wo vernünftige Pathologen und Rechtsmediziner nebeneinander arbeiten.

Damit ergibt sich aber zunächst auch die Frage nach der *Definition des natürlichen bzw. nicht-natürlichen Todes,* eine Definition, die merkwürdigerweise immer wieder Schwierigkeiten zu bereiten scheint. Interessant ist vielleicht schon die Tatsache, daß man in den meisten Lehrbüchern meines Fachgebiets vergeblich nach einer einfachen Definition des natürlichen Todes sucht. Anscheinend wird dieser Begriff als so klar angesehen, daß er einer weiteren Definition nicht bedarf.

Allerdings hat die Begriffsbestimmung auch ihre Tücken: Strenggenommen wäre ein *natürlicher Tod* nur ein Tod an reiner *Altersschwäche.* Wir wissen heute, daß gerade dieser Tod nur extrem selten vorkommt, denn auch der alte Mensch stirbt meist nicht an reiner Altersschwäche. Deshalb könnte man den *natürlichen Tod* als den *Tod eines Menschen* definieren, *der von äußeren Faktoren unabhängig* also *allein aus innerer (krankhafter) Ursache eingetreten* ist. Diese einfache Definition wird aber nicht allen Gegebenheiten der Praxis gerecht; denn bei der Bewertung der „äußeren Faktoren" gibt es nicht immer eine scharfe Grenze zwischen natürlichem und nicht-natürlichem Tod. Wenn man eine bakterielle Infektion als äußere Ursache ansieht, dann ist der Tod infolge einer Infektionskrankheit ex definitione *kein* natürlicher Tod.

Andererseits gilt ein Tod durch „Zivilisationsschäden", z.B. ein Koronartod bei Nikotinabusus als natürlicher Tod, obwohl er diese Qualifikation sicher nicht verdient. Das gleiche gilt auch für einen Tod an den Folgen einer Lebercirrhose bei chronischem Alkoholismus. Ein Tod an Pneumonie darf *nicht* als natürlicher Tod gelten, wenn die Pneumonie beispielsweise während eines aufgezwungenen — unfallbedingten — Krankenlagers aufgetreten ist.

Daraus ergibt sich als Fazit: Der Begriff „natürlicher Tod" ist ein aufgrund praktischer, d.h. vor allem rechtlicher Bedürfnisse zusammengedrechseltes Kunstprodukt. Somit unsere Definition: *„Natürlicher Tod" ist ein Tod aus krankhafter Ursache, der völlig unabhängig von rechtlich bedeutsamen äußeren Faktoren eingetreten ist.*

Ein „Exitus in tabula" *kann* ein natürlicher Tod sein, in vielen Fällen ist aber die Narkose ein ausschlaggebender Faktor für den Todeseintritt. Dies bedeutet noch lange nicht, daß dem Anaesthesisten ein Vorwurf zu machen ist. Eine Klärung kann nur durch eine Obduktion erfolgen und es dürfte wohl aus ärztlich-ethischer Sicht kein Zweifel daran bestehen, daß eine solche Klärung in jedem Falle erfolgen muß, das gebietet schon die Wahrheitspflicht des Arztes. Die weitere Frage ist dann: Gerichtliche oder nicht-gerichtliche Obduktion?

Die gerichtliche Obduktion hat eine Verständigung des Staatsanwalts zur Voraussetzung und — für den Fall des Nachweises einer Verletzung der Sorgfaltspflicht — die Einleitung eines Strafverfahrens zur Folge.

Als Rechtsmediziner stehe ich wahrscheinlich im Verdacht, es für selbstverständlich zu halten, daß es in jedem Falle einer Fehlleistung zu einem Strafverfahren kommen muß. Diese Meinung ist sicher falsch: Wir Rechtsmediziner sind keine Büttel des Staatsanwalts, im Gegenteil, wir empfinden es als echtes Erfolgserlebnis, wenn wir dem Staatsanwalt sagen können, daß der Verdacht einer Fehlleistung nicht berechtigt ist.

Selbstverständlich gehört es zu unseren besonderen Berufspflichten, daß wir unparteiisch urteilen. Gestatten Sie mir deshalb die Bemerkung, daß wir diese Unparteilichkeit in klinischen Stellungnahmen oftmals vermissen. Sollte es nicht ein selbstverständlicher Bestandteil ärztlicher Ethik sein, daß der Satz „salus aegroti suprema lex" auch dann noch gilt, oder für den Fall seines Todes noch nachwirkt, wenn etwas schiefgegangen ist. Man braucht sich nur in die Situation des Opfers bzw. seiner Angehörigen hineinzudenken, um zu wissen, was gemeint ist. Diese werden kaum Rachegefühle haben und deshalb nach dem Staatsanwalt schreien, aber sie werden wohl immer ein berechtigtes Interesse an einer sachlichen Aufklärung des Zwischenfalls als entscheidende Voraussetzung für einen etwaigen „Schadensersatz" haben.

Ich bin von jeher der Meinung, daß es in unserem Recht höchst unglücklich ist, daß dem Arzt bei der Bekanntgabe einer möglichen Fehlleistung die Gefahr eines Strafverfahrens droht. Mancher ärztliche Kunstfehler wird deshalb vertuscht und dem Opfer bzw. seinen Angehörigen damit keine Entschädigung zuteil.

Ein Ausweg aus der bisherigen Situation wäre vielleicht dadurch möglich, daß der Gesetzgeber beim ärztlichen Kunstfehler eine strafrechtliche Verfolgung nur auf Antrag (Strafantragserfordernis) zuläßt.

Ich hielte jedenfalls jede Lösung für besser, die eine Sicherstellung etwaiger zivilrechtlicher Ansprüche gewährleistet, ohne daß in jedem Fall ein strafrechtliches Ermittlungsverfahren anläuft. Dies ist aber nur eine Vorbemerkung zu meiner grundsätzlichen Einstellung zu diesem Problem. Jedenfalls halte ich den Hinweis von Herrn Opderbecke, daß der Arzt wie jeder andere Bürger nicht zur Selbstanzeige verpflichtet ist, für keine gute Lösung des Problems. Aus ärztlich-ethischen Gründen ist das deshalb bedenklich, weil es eben gerade in eindeutigen Fällen von Fehlleistungen Anwendung finden dürfte und hierbei die Gefahr besonders groß ist, daß Opfer und Angehörige benachteiligt werden oder, wie man es auch ganz grob und unjuristisch ausdrücken könnte, daß Opfer und Angehörige doppelt bestraft werden:
a) durch die Schädigung und
b) durch die ausbleibende Entschädigung.

Im übrigen sollte man bei der Prüfung der Frage, der auch sonst fehlenden staatsbürgerlichen Pflicht zur Selbstanzeige daran denken, daß es davon eine wichtige Ausnahme gibt, nämlich die Unfallflucht (§ 142 StGB). Es besteht kein Zweifel daran, daß ein wesentlicher Gesichtspunkt für den § 142 die Sicherung zivilrechtlicher Ansprüche des Geschädigten ist und ich meine, daß Parallelen zum ärztlichen Kunstfehler insoweit unübersehbar sind.

Aber zurück zur Frage der gerichtlichen Obduktion: Ich gehe davon aus, daß es zu den selbstverständlichen Pflichten des Arztes gehört, bei der Narkose ein Höchstmaß an Sorgfalt anzuwenden, weil ihm der Mitmensch so vollkommen ausgeliefert ist. Wenn es trotzdem zu einem Zwischenfall kommt, dann kann der Arzt, der seine Sorgfaltspflicht beachtet hat, der Aufklärung der Todesursache gelassen entgegen sehen. Geschieht sie im Rahmen einer gerichtlichen Obduktion, so wird der so häufig von Laien erhobene Vorwurf der Unparteilichkeit im Keime erstickt. Im übrigen sehe ich derzeit keine rechtlich vertretbare Möglichkeit *im Falle einer klaren Fehlleistung ein staatsanwaltschaftliches Ermittlungsverfahren* — sprich: gerichtliche Obduktionen und weitere Untersuchungen — zu umgehen, ohne gleichzeitig die zivilrechtlichen Ansprüche der Angehörigen in Frage zu stellen. Nach nichtgerichtlichen Obduktionen wird oft der Verdacht geäußert, daß aus „kollegialen" Gründen eine zuverlässige Protokollierung der Befunde unterblieben ist.

Sollten wir uns aber insoweit einig sein, daß die Vertuschung einer Fehlleistung weder zu billigen noch zu unterstützen ist, so bleiben in keinem Falle Vorbehalte gegen eine gerichtliche Obduktion. Wenn der Arzt sich nicht selbst anzeigt, so mag man ihm dies zubilligen. An seine Stelle tritt dann der Leichenschauer oder gegebenenfalls der Pathologe oder Rechtsmediziner. Diese Personen sind — wie wir an anderer Stelle ausgeführt haben — nicht durch die ärztliche Schweigepflicht gedeckt; denn die Schweigepflicht besteht zum Schutz des Patienten und nicht zum Schutz des behandelnden Arztes (Schwerd u. Strubel).

Zu Punkt 2

Welche Feststellungsmöglichkeiten hat der Rechtsmediziner beim tödlichen Anaesthesiezwischenfall?

Diese Frage im Rahmen eines Kurzreferates zu behandeln, ist fast unmöglich. Ich kann nur stichwortartig einige Punkte herausgreifen.

Ohne Kenntnis der Vorgeschichte ist es sicher nicht in jedem Falle möglich, die Feststellung eines Todes während oder im direkten Zusammenhang mit einer Narkose zu treffen. Ich kann aber wohl davon absehen, hierzu detaillierte Ausführungen zu machen, weil diese Fragestellung in der Praxis nicht zu erwarten ist oder anders ausgedrückt: man wird wohl kaum dem Pathologen oder Rechtsmediziner eine Leiche auf den Sektionstisch legen und ihn darüber im unklaren lassen, daß es sich um einen Exitus in tabula handelt.

Die nicht ganz seltenen Todesfälle durch nichtasphyktischen Sauerstoffmangel sind mit den derzeitigen Methoden nicht zu erkennen. Asphyktische Formen von Sauerstoffmangel, also echte Erstickungen nach dem bisherigen Sprachgebrauch, kommen kaum in Betracht. Bei ihnen wären die üblichen Erstickungszeichen (Cyanose, petechiale Blutaustritte, flüssiges Leichenblut) zu erwarten.

Die toxikologische Untersuchung zum Nachweis des Narkosemittels kommt dann in Betracht, wenn Überdosierungen in Frage stehen. Sie bietet im Prinzip keine Schwierigkeit, wenngleich sie technisch sehr aufwendig sein kann. Die Auswertung der Befunde ist aber u.U. problematisch, weil z.B. flüchtige Narkosemittel bei Reanimationsmaßnahmen abgeatmet worden sein können. Bei nichtflüchtigen Mitteln ist zu bedenken, daß eindeutige Beziehungen zwischen der Konzentration im Blut und dem Wirkungsgrad nicht immer gegeben sind.

Trotzdem sollte eine solche Untersuchung bei unklaren Zwischenfällen aus 2 Gründen erfolgen:
1.) Weil der Verdacht einer Fehldosierung gegebenenfalls entkräftet werden kann und

2.) weil sie die Möglichkeit bietet, eine bei Narkosebeginn bestehende, dem Anaesthesisten jedoch verschwiegene Prämedikation, evtl. auch das Vorhandensein von Suchtmitteln und dadurch bedingte fatale Potenzierungen der Narkosemittel aufzudecken, oder andere Nebenwirkungen zu erklären. Auch Blutalkoholbestimmung kann ein überraschendes Ergebnis haben. Zum Schluß möchte ich noch anhand einer Beobachtung aus meinem Institut die Wichtigkeit der Obduktion beim Exitus in tabula unterstreichen.

Bei einer 50jährigen Frau kam es in der Narkose, die wegen eines kleinen gynäkologischen Eingriffs vorgenommen wurde, beim Lagewechsel der Patientin zum plötzlichen Herzstillstand. Das zunächst völlig unerklärliche Herzversagen war — wie sich bei der Obduktion herausgestellt hat — offensichtlich bedingt durch einen hühnereigroßen Tumor (histologisch ein Myxom) im linken Vorhof (Abb. 1), der anscheinend teils mechanisch, teils dynamisch (verminderte Druckverhältnisse im Herzen) ventilartig den Durchgang zwischen Kammer und Vorhof verlegt hat. Ein solcher Zwischenfall ist nicht vorhersehbar.

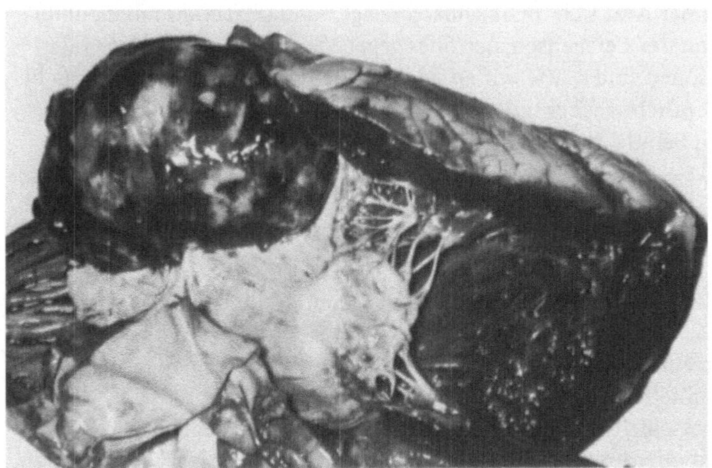

Abb. 1. Tumor im linken Vorhof (Myxom) bei einer 50jährigen Patientin (Obd.: Prof. Schulz, Institut für Rechtsmedizin der Univ. Würzburg)

Rechtliche Wertung des tödlichen Anästhesiezwischenfalls

W. Weissauer

Schließen wir uns der von Opderbecke vorgeschlagenen Systematik an, unterscheiden wir also zwischen biologischen und methodisch-technischen Ursachen des tödlichen Anästhesiezwischenfalls, so gewinnen wir damit auch einen guten Ausgangspunkt für die rechtliche Wertung. Allein wegen des Mißlingens einer Leistung, das zu Schäden an Leib oder Leben führt, hat der Arzt weder strafrechtliche, noch zivilrechtliche Sanktionen auf sich zu nehmen. Forensische Konsequenzen ergeben sich nach einem tödlichen Anästhesiezwischenfall erst dann, wenn der für das Betäubungsverfahren verantwortliche Arzt den Tod des Patienten durch einen schuldhaften Behandlungsfehler verursacht hat.

Ist der ärztliche Eingriff aus der Sicht ex ante lege artis indiziert und wurde er — mit Einwilligung des Patienten — lege artis ausgeführt, so trifft den Arzt kein Verschulden, wenn es aus nicht vorherberechenbaren und nicht beherrschbaren, also schicksalhaften biologischen Abläufen zu einem tödlichen Zwischenfall kommt. Sinn der Eingriffsaufklärung ist es, den Patienten zu informieren, daß es solche schicksalhafte Risiken gibt, und seine Entscheidung herbeizuführen, ob er sie bei Abwägung der für und gegen den Eingriff sprechenden Faktoren in Kauf nimmt.

Die Abgrenzung zwischen schicksalshaft und schuldhaft sollte, so meinen wir, zugleich das entscheidende Kriterium für die Zuordnung zum Begriff des natürlichen und des nicht natürlichen Todes sein. Die durch die ärztliche Kunst nicht beherrschbaren Risiken indizierter ärztlicher Behandlung sind Teil des biologischen Krankheitsrisikos. Dies wird deutlich gerade bei Eingriffen mit hohem Mortalitätsrisiko, wie etwa der Osteosynthese bei einem hochbetagten Patienten mit Schenkelhalsbruch. Ist die Überlebenschance ohne den Eingriff deutlich geringer, so darf, ja muß der Arzt dem Patienten den Eingriff trotz seiner hohen Risiken vorschlagen. Das unvermeidbare Behandlungsrisiko liegt hier in der Natur der Verletzung und in den vorgegebenen biologischen Fakten, also dem hohen Lebensalter und in Begleitkrankheiten.

Aus dem vorgegebenen biologischen Risiko wird ein methodisch-technisches, wenn es darum geht, den spezifischen Erfordernissen des konkreten Falles bei der Prüfung der Anästhesiefähigkeit, bei der Vorbehandlung, bei der Wahl der Anästhesiemethode und der Anästhetika, bei der Überwachung der Vitalfunktionen und bei der Fülle aller anderen Vorsichtsmaßnahmen Rechnung zu tragen, die das Bild der modernen Anästhesie prägen. Offenbar ist es oft gerade die Summierung kleiner und kleinster Fehler und Mängel, beginnend bei der Anamnese und bei der Auswertung der Untersuchungsbefunde, die zu den schweren Anästhesiezwischenfällen führt.

Der Vorwurf eines Verschuldens darf freilich nicht schon dann erhoben werden, wenn sich das methodisch-technische Vorgehen des für die Anästhesie verantwortlichen Arztes nach der Beurteilung des Sachverständigen im Zeitpunkt der Erstattung des Gutachtens, also

aufgrund der Erkenntnisse ex post, als falsch erweist. Der Richter und der Sachverständige
müssen sich vielmehr in die Situation ex ante versetzen. Beurteilungsmaßstab ist das Verhalten eines gewissenhaften Arztes bzw. Facharztes in gleicher Situation. An den Anästhesisten
sind bei Verrichtungen im Rahmen seines Faches höhere Anforderungen zu stellen als an
einen Operateur, der das Betäubungsverfahren selbst durchführt; für den Operateur kann sich
aber der Vorwurf des Übernahmeverschuldens ergeben, wenn er einen Anästhesisten hätte
zuziehen können.

Auch von Anästhesieabteilung zu Anästhesieabteilung sind die personellen und apparativen Voraussetzungen verschieden. Selbst in gut besetzten Abteilungen ist es jedoch heute
und in absehbarer Zeit völlig ausgeschlossen, auf den Einsatz der in fachlicher Weiterbildung
stehenden Ärzte für die Durchführung von Allgemeinanästhesien zu verzichten. Je weiter entfernt der ärztliche Mitarbeiter von der Facharztreife ist, desto mehr muß freilich der leitende
Arzt durch Anleitung und Überwachung dafür sorgen, daß Leistungsdefizite ausgeglichen
werden.

Für den Kenner der Materie gleicht diese Aufgabe leider allzu oft der Quadratur des
Kreises. Die Planstellen für Ärzte sind aufgrund überalterter Anhaltszahlen für die Besetzung von Anästhesieabteilungen meist streng limitiert. Andererseits soll der Operationsbe-
trieb aufrechterhalten werden. Kommt es zu einem schweren Zwischenfall, so prüfen die Gerichte, wenn sie sich überzeugt haben, daß die personelle Situation eine andere Besetzung des
Operationstisches nicht zuließ, ob nicht die eine oder die andere Operation auf eine spätere
Tageszeit oder auf den nächsten Tag hätte verschoben werden können. Da nicht alle Eingriffe dringlich sind, kann diese Frage mit schöner Regelmäßigkeit bejaht werden.

Ex post sind wir uns einig, daß es bei diesem einen von hunderten Fällen, bei dem es zu
schweren Komplikationen kam, besser gewesen wäre, das Operationsprogramm im Interesse
einer optimalen Besetzung des Tisches zu kürzen. Ex ante läßt sich dies nicht vorhersehen
und auch nicht so verfahren, weil es damit zu schwersten Behinderungen und Reduzierungen
des Operationsbetriebes im eigenen Haus, aber auch in allen anderen Häusern käme, die vor
gleichen oder ähnlichen Problemen stehen. Man darf zu Lasten des Anästhesisten keine Forderungen ex post für den konkreten Fall an die Organisation des Anästhesiebetriebes stellen,
die aus personellen und finanziellen Gründen generell nicht erfüllbar sind.

Ob der leitende Anästhesist seinen Organisations-, Leitungs- und Überwachungspflichten
genügt hat, kann der Richter nicht ohne Hilfe der medizinischen Sachverständigen beurteilen. Der Sachverständige hat sein Gutachten objektiv zu erstatten. Sie kennen die Kritik am
sogenannten Krähenkomment, der in der Öffentlichkeit lautstark erhoben wird, aber auch
die dezenteren, jedoch unüberhörbaren Hinweise der Rechtsprechung.

Was die Öffentlichkeit und ebenso die Gerichte wegen fehlender medizinischer Sachkun-
de nicht registrieren, ist eine diametral entgegengesetzte Erfahrung, die man gerade auch bei
der Durchsicht anästhesiologischer Gutachten gewinnt: Die Sachverständigen neigen sehr oft
dazu, der Beurteilung von Zwischenfällen die Sicht ex post und ihre eigenen günstigeren Ar-
beitsvoraussetzungen zugrunde zu legen; vor allem aber erliegen manche Sachverständige der
Gefahr, ihre eigene Auffassung über das zweckmäßige Verfahren zum Dogma zu erheben,
statt deutlich zu machen, daß andere die gegenteilige Auffassung vertreten, von einer allgemeinen Meinung und einer Kunstregel also nicht die Rede sein kann. Was solche apodiktische
Aussagen für den betroffenen Kollegen gerade im Strafverfahren bedeuten können, brauche
ich nicht näher zu erläutern. Nicht der Krähenkomment kommt hier zum Zuge, sondern offenbar ist gelegentlich im gerichtlichen Verfahren „der Kollege des Kollegen größter Feind",
obwohl er dies keineswegs beabsichtigt.

Ein Gutachten, das eindeutig ein menschliches Versagen als Ursache eines tödlichen Anästhesiezwischenfalles feststellt, entspricht naturgemäß weit mehr der Erwartungshaltung der Öffentlichkeit, als die ebenso objektive wie ernüchternde Erklärung des Sachverständigen, daß er sich im Hinblick auf die unübersehbare Vielfalt der biologischen Komponenten in seinen Aussagen über die Kausalzusammenhänge oft mit größeren oder geringeren Graden an Wahrscheinlichkeit begnügen müsse.

Ziehen wir noch einmal die systematische Unterscheidung zwischen den biologischen und den methodisch-technisch bedingten Zwischenfällen zu Rate, so wird die Zuordnung zu dieser letzteren Gruppe — jedenfalls in den Augen der Öffentlichkeit — freilich um so wahrscheinlicher, je geringer die biologische Vorbelastung des Patienten und je weniger eingreifend die Operation ist. Bei einem jungen, organgesunden Menschen, der bei einem Eingriff ohne einen erkennbaren operativen Zwischenfall stirbt, muß der Anästhesist heute die Einleitung eines strafrechtlichen Ermittlungsverfahrens und Schadensersatzansprüche der Angehörigen in Rechnung stellen.

Die Angabe „natürlicher Tod" auf dem Leichenschauschein könnte unter diesen Prämissen noch die Annahme verstärken, daß bei dem Zwischenfall menschliches Versagen im Spiele steht. Das richtige Verfahren erscheint auch mir in der Benachrichtigung der Polizei oder der Staatsanwaltschaft zu bestehen und in dem Vermerk „Todesursache ungeklärt". Nach meiner Auslegung fällt — wie bereits ausgeführt — unter den Begriff des „natürlichen Todes" auch der exitus in tabula, der auf den eingriffsimmanenten, durch ärztliche Sorgfalt nicht beherrschbaren Risiken beruht. Bis zur Feststellung, ob menschliches Versagen vorliegt, bleibt danach die Todesursache ungeklärt. Auch mit dieser Eintragung setzt der Anästhesist ein Verfahren zur Ermittlung der Todesursache in Gang.

Ordnen die Gerichte oder die Strafverfolgungsbehörden die Sektion nicht an, so sollte m.E. der Anästhesist, der den Verdacht kunstfehlerhaften Verhaltens und die Gefahr zivilrechtlicher Schadensersatzansprüche abwenden will, von sich aus die Angehörigen des Patienten um die Einwilligung in die Obduktion bitten.

In Österreich wird die Obduktion ohne Rücksicht auf etwaige Verdachtsmomente vorgenommen, die für einen ärztlichen Kunstfehler sprechen können; auch aus meiner Sicht spricht viel für eine solche Lösung. Sie ermöglicht die Klärung der Todesursache, ohne daß der Arzt sich durch seine eigene Mitteilung dem Verdacht eines Kunstfehlers auszusetzen braucht.

Um auch die unterschiedliche prozessuale Situation kurz zu skizzieren: Im Strafverfahren trägt der Arzt keine Beweislast. Kann ihm ein schuldhafter Behandlungsfehler und dessen Ursächlichkeit für den Tod des Patienten nicht mit an Sicherheit grenzender Wahrscheinlichkeit nachgewiesen werden, so muß er nach dem strafprozessualen Grundsatz „in dubio pro reo" freigesprochen werden.

Im Zivilprozeß ist die Ausgangssituation im Prinzip ähnlich. Der Kläger, hier also die Angehörigen des Patienten, muß dem Arzt den schuldhaften Behandlungsfehler und den Ursachenzusammenhang mit dem tödlichen Anästhesiezwischenfall beweisen. Zu seinen Gunsten gibt es jedoch eine Reihe von Beweiserleichterungen, vom prima facie Beweis bis hin zur Beweislastumkehr.

Beim prima facie Beweis kann von einem Behandlungsmißerfolg auf Grund allgemeiner Erfahrungssätze auf die Ursachen dieses Mißerfolgs und auch auf das Verschulden des Arztes geschlossen werden (und umgekehrt). Es ist dann Sache des Arztes, besondere Umstände darzutun, die im konkreten Fall gegen diese Schlußfolgerung sprechen.

Allein die Tatsache, daß es bei einem organgesunden jungen Menschen und einem relativ harmlosen Eingriff zu einem tödlichen Zwischenfall gekommen ist, rechtfertigt aber noch nicht die Schlußfolgerung auf einen schuldhaften Anästhesiefehler. Die medizinische Erfahrung, auf die hier abzustellen ist, weist vielmehr darauf hin, daß eine schicksalhafte Verkettung unglücklicher Umstände auch ohne menschliches Versagen zu schweren Anästhesiezwischenfällen führen kann. Die Vorstellung, daß es möglich sein müßte, durch eine alle denkbaren Risikofaktoren erfassende Voruntersuchung und Vorbehandlung die Gefahr solcher Verkettungen auszuschließen, scheitert an den Realitäten. Wer die Wahrung jeder erdenklichen Sorgfalt fordern wollte, würde den Stillstand der operativen Medizin provozieren und eine Gesamtbelastung des Patienten durch eine Vielzahl von Voruntersuchungen in Kauf nehmen, die letztlich deren Erkenntniswert für die Risikominderung überstiege.

Die Tendenz, die Beweissituation des Patienten oder seiner Angehörigen unter dem Schlagwort der „Waffengleichheit" zu verbessern, ist freilich beim Bundesgerichtshof, unserer höchsten Instanz in Zivilsachen, unverkennbar. Nach den grundlegenden Aussagen des „Dammschnitturteils" hat der Arzt dem Gericht den ordnungsgemäßen Behandlungsverlauf darzulegen und ihn, soweit dies anhand einer ordnungsgemäß geführten Dokumentation möglich ist, auch zu beweisen. Dieser Beweis hat sich darauf zu erstrecken, daß die Dokumentation nicht nachträglich angefertigt oder verfälscht worden ist.

Von vielleicht noch größerer Tragweite ist für die anästhesiologische Versorgung der Patienten eine weitere grundlegende Aussage in diesem Urteil. Der Bundesgerichtshof bestätigt zunächst, daß von einem Behandlungsmißerfolg — im konkreten Fall war es die Verletzung des Schließmuskels — noch nicht auf einen schuldhaften Behandlungsfehler geschlossen werden könne. Er meint dann aber, an die Feststellung, daß ein Arzt als Verrichtungsgehilfe des Krankenhausträgers einem Patienten pflichtwidrig Schaden zugefügt habe, dürften keine allzu strengen Anforderungen gestellt werden, „denn auch Zwischenfälle und Mißerfolge, die im Einzelfall nicht mit voller Sicherheit zu vermeiden sind, unterlaufen einem erfahrenen und fähigen Arzt in zahlreichen Gebieten um ein Vielfaches seltener als einem weniger geübten und geschickten". Der Bundesgerichtshof schließt daran die Folgerung, der Krankenhausträger habe nachzuweisen, daß der in gynäkologischer Weiterbildung stehende Arzt nach verläßlichen Kontrollen im Bereich der Geburtshilfe, insbesondere in Bezug auf den Dammschnitt und dabei zu gewärtigende Komplikationen, über das erforderliche Maß an Wissen und Erfahrung verfügte.

Diese Aspekte lassen sich nahezu nahtlos auf die Anästhesie übertragen. Für den in Weiterbildung stehenden Mitarbeiter kann dies zu einer nahezu vollständigen Umkehr der Beweislast führen, soweit er selbst auf Schadensersatz in Anspruch genommen wird.

Zu einer partiellen Verschiebung der Beweislast speziell für den Bereich der Anästhesie kam der Bundesgerichtshof bei der Entscheidung über einen auf einem Gerätefehler beruhenden Zwischenfall. Danach muß der Anästhesist beweisen, daß die Anästhesiegeräte ordnungsgemäß gepflegt und gewartet waren sowie vor ihrem Einsatz auf ihre Funktionsfähigkeit geprüft wurden.

Abgesehen von diesen speziellen Bereichen, die ich hier nur in einem engen Ausschnitt ansprechen kann, wird es zur Umkehrung der Beweislast im Zivilprozeß stets dann kommen, wenn der Arzt dem Patienten die Beweisführung schuldhaft erschwert, etwa indem er Gegenstände in Kenntnis ihres Beweiswertes vernichtet, oder wenn er keine Behandlungsaufzeichnungen dort führt, wo dies bei einer ordnungsgemäßen Dokumentation zu erwarten wäre.

Deshalb auch heute wieder mein dringender Rat: Führen Sie ein ordnungsgemäßes Anästhesieprotokoll. Fehlen Eintragungen dort, wo sie an sich zu erwarten wären, vor allem aber bei der Kontrolle der Vitalfunktionen, so weckt dies doch immer auch den Zweifel, ob die fehlenden Werte überhaupt erhoben wurden und ob es nicht daran lag, daß eine sich abzeichnende tödliche Komplikation zu spät erkannt wurde. Bleiben bei der Ermittlung der Ursache eines exitus in tabula Zweifel, so gehen sie im Zivilprozeß zu Lasten dessen, der die Darlegungs- und Beweislast trägt. Dies wird, so fürchte ich, in zunehmendem Maße der Anästhesist sein.

Sorgen Sie nach einem schweren Zwischenfall für die optimale Therapie und insbesondere auch hier für eine sorgfältige Dokumentation. Es mag oft zweifelhaft sein, ob selbst die optimale Nachbehandlung den Tod des Patienten nach einem Zwischenfall abgewendet hätte. Können aber grobe Mängel bei der Zwischenfallstherapie und der unmittelbar anschließenden Nachbehandlung nachgewiesen werden, so liegt die Umkehr der Beweislast zum Nachteil des Anästhesisten nahe, wenn es um die Frage der Ursächlichkeit dieser Mängel für die Schäden an Leib oder Leben geht.

Sehen Sie mir bitte nach, daß ich im wesentlichen auf die Beurteilung nach deutschem Recht abgestellt habe. Die Erfahrung lehrt, daß die Rechtsprechung im Bereich der Arzthaftung trotz bedeutsamer Unterschiede in den Rechtsgrundlagen und in den dogmatischen Ansätzen doch zu ähnlichen Ergebnissen tendiert. Schon der Vergleich der veröffentlichten Entscheidungen zeigt, daß das hohe forensische Risiko des Anästhesisten heute offenbar selbst das der operativen Fächer übersteigt. Andererseits müssen wir einräumen, daß die Anästhesie als selbständige medizinische Disziplin geschaffen wurde, um die Sicherheit im Operationssaal zu erhöhen. Die Sicherung einer hohen Qualität der anästhesiologischen Leistung gerade unter den Aspekten der Risikominderung ist deshalb die vornehmste Aufgabe des Fachgebietes. Nur auf diesem Wege kann letztlich auch das forensische Risiko des Anästhesisten auf ein tragbares Maß reduziert werden. Dazu muß aber auch die Gesellschaft ihren Beitrag leisten. Es geht nicht an, daß der Anästhesist forensisch büßen dafür muß, daß er ein Übermaß an Arbeit mit einer unterbesetzten Abteilung zu leisten hat.

Technische und organisatorische Sicherheitsmaßnahmen zur Prophylaxe von Anaesthesie-Zwischenfällen

V. Feurstein

Wenn über Sicherheit gesprochen werden soll, muß von zwei allgemein unumstößlichen Tatsachen ausgegangen werden, einmal, daß der Mensch an sich nicht fehlerfrei handeln kann, und zum zweiten, daß auch die ausgereifte Technologie niemals vollkommene Sicherheit bietet. In der anaesthesiologischen Praxis sind Mensch und Maschine eng miteinander verwoben. Fehlleistungen beider erhöhen nicht nur, sie potenzieren das Risiko für den Patienten. Hinzu kommt, daß letzterer unter Umständen schon sich sich aus aufgrund seiner Erkrankung besondere Probleme bietet. So steht der Anaesthesiologie im Hinblick auf die Prophylaxe von Anaesthesie-Zwischenfällen vor drei klar definierten Aufgaben:
1. Ihm obliegt die ständige Kontrolle der Sicherheit seines Gerätes und der Sicherheitsvorkehrungen seines Arbeitsplatzes,
2. er hat die Eigenkontrolle seiner fachlichen Leistungsfähigkeit vorzunehmen, d.h. Selbstkritik zu üben,
3. er hat die klinische Kontrolle des ihm anvertrauten Patienten, insbesondere vor Durchführung einer Anaesthesie wahrzunehmen.

Wenn in diesem Kreise die Sicherheitsfragen von Gerät und Arbeitsplatz an erster Stelle gereiht wurden, dann deshalb, weil der Kliniker — fast müßte man sagen in naiver Bescheidenheit — dazu neigt, der modernen Technologie ein allzugroßes Maß an Vertrauen zu schenken, oder die Gewährleistung sicherer technischer Funktionen lieber jenen anderen zu überlassen, die es meistens nicht gibt. Welcher Routine-Anaesthesist hat sich schon intensiv mit den physikalischen Grundlagen der Brand- und Explosionsgefahr jener Gase und Dämpfe befaßt, mit denen er täglich arbeitet, wer kennt schon genauer die Erweiterung der Zündgrenzen durch ein Lachgas-Sauerstoffgemisch, das unter bestimmten Umständen auch sogenannte nicht brennbare Inhalationsanaesthetika explodieren läßt. Wer weiß, daß schon beim Platzen eines 3-Volt-Endoskopielämpchens die Mindestzündenergie dazu frei wird?

Seitdem Äther und einige hochexplosible Gase nicht mehr en vogue sind, glaubt man die Brandgefahr gebannt zu haben, in Wirklichkeit aber besteht sie nach wie vor. Zündfähige Flüssigkeiten und Dämpfe, z.B. ein 4% Halothan-Luftgemisch, Methoxyfluran, komprimierte Gase, endogene physiologische Gase, wie Methan oder Wasserstoff, Reinigungs-, Entfettungs- und Desinfektionsmittel, schränken auch heute noch die Feuersicherheit erheblich ein. Daß hierbei Funkenbildungen jeglicher Art, vor allem durch ungeschützte bzw. schadhafte elektrische Apparaturen, ebenso aber auch durch statische Elektrizität eine Katastrophe auslösen können, liegt nahe. 50% der registrierten Schadensereignisse haben ihre Ursache in nicht operationssicheren beweglichen medizinischen Geräten, 25% werden der Entladung statischer Elektrizität zugeschrieben. Dazu sollte man auch wissen, daß sich das Zündrisiko über den Operationssaal hinaus erstreckt, denn Narkosegase bleiben in der Lunge bis 30 Minuten, im Magen sogar bis 60 Minuten zündfähig.

Der Umgang mit reinem Sauerstoff erfordert besondere Vorsicht, da an sich harmlose Oxydationsvorgänge unter bestimmten Bedingungen zur Explosion ausarten können. Als Grundregel gilt:

Langsames Aufdrehen der Ventile, kein Fett, kein Schmutz, kein Staub, in sauerstoffreicher Atmosphäre keine elektrischen Anlagen.

Das Narkosegerät selbst, aber auch seine Zusatzapparaturen wie Respiratoren, Verdampfer, Meßgeräte bedürfen der täglichen Kontrolle ihrer Betriebssicherheit bzw. ihrer einwandfreien Funktion. Bei modernen Geräten ist die berüchtigte Möglichkeit der Verwechslung von Gasen auf Grund der DIN-Normen bzw. des Pin-Index-Systems praktisch ausgeschlossen. Ältere Geräte, mit aufschiebbaren Schlauchverbindungen zwischen Reduzierventil und Rotameter bieten noch immer diese Gefahr. In keinem Fall ausgeschlossen ist die Unterbrechung der Sauerstoffzufuhr durch unbemerkt leer gewordene Sauerstoff-Flaschen. Hiergegen schützen relativ preiswerte, einfach montierbare Alarmanlagen, die auch den anaesthesierten Anaesthesisten akustisch in die Wirklichkeit zurückrufen sollen. Jeder im Operations- und Intensivbereich Erfahrene kennt den gelegentlich geradezu kriminellen Spieltrieb einzelner Dummköpfe, die es nicht lassen können, an Schrauben und Hebeln aus Neugierde zu hantieren. Gegen dieserart verstellte Regulationen, fehlende Schlauchverbindungen, oder offene Ventile nicht benutzter Gasanschlüsse (z.B. Kohlendioxyd) durch die, dem Venturi-Prinzip gleich, Raumluft angesaugt und die Sauerstoffkonzentration entsprechend verringert wird, gibt es nur eine Sicherheitsmaßnahme: Die sture Kontrolle des Gerätes vor jeder Narkose! Dazu gehört selbstverständlich auch das Laryngoskop, sowie der intratracheale Tubus, in dessen Lichtung sich schon mancher Fremdkörper verborgen hat.

Wenn es dennoch — aus welchem Grunde immer — Funktionsstörungen gibt, die nicht mit einem Blick, mit einem Griff, in einer Sekunde behoben werden können, dann muß als Notmaßnahme die gesamte Apparatur entfernt werden. Die Weiterführung der Narkose kann provisorisch mit einfachen Mitteln, gegebenenfalls unter Ambu-Beatmung, vorgenommen werden, bis die technische Störung behoben ist.

Ein Wort zu elektrischen Unglücksfällen, die nicht nur das Personal, sondern ebenso den Patienten betreffen können. Auch wenn der Anaesthesist außer gelegentlichem Monitoring mit elektromedizinischen Geräten nicht unmittelbar befaßt ist, spielt für ihn die elektrische Sicherheit im Operationssaal eine große Rolle, da der plötzliche „unerklärbare" Todesfall — worin immer er seine Ursache haben mag, — zunächst der Narkoseführung angelastet wird. Weit mehr als die Hälfte elektrischer Unfälle sind auf Unwissenheit, der Rest auf Schlamperei zurückzuführen. Der Anaesthesist sollte daher:
● Die Grundbegriffe der Elektrizitätslehre kennen,
● Besondere Aufmerksamkeit den Sicherheitsvorschriften schenken (keine Doppelstecker, keine Verlängerungskabel, keine VDE-ungeschützten Geräte),
● Unabdingbaren Wert auf einwandfreie Schutzleiter, besser noch Schutzleitungssysteme legen,
● Die richtige Anlage der inaktiven Elektrode bei HF-Chirurgiegeräten überprüfen, damit nicht durch Nebenschlüsse Verbrennungen, unter Umständen sogar Explosionen innerhalb der Atemschläuche herbeigeführt werden. Die Notwendigkeit, ein HF-Gerät zur Verstärkung der Stromdichte hochregeln zu müssen, ist bereits ein Alarmzeichen und bedeutet Gefahr.
● Schließlich sollte der Anaesthesist eng mit dem sicherheitstechnischen Personal zusammenarbeiten.

Die österreichischen gesetzlichen Vorschriften sehen die Bestellung von Sicherheits-Ingenieuren und des weiteren Sicherheits-Beauftragten im Krankenhaus vor, die nicht nur die tägliche aktuelle Überwachung zur Aufgabe haben, sondern auch alle medizinisch-technischen

Geräte in bestimmten Zeitabständen überprüfen müssen, wenn für sie kein Wartungsvertrag abgeschlossen ist. Wir haben in unserem Bereich neben einer umfassenden Prüfungs-Kartei das „Pickerlsystem" eingeführt, d.h. jedes überprüfte Gerät bekommt eine Marke, die auf den nächst fälligen Prüftermin hinweist (Abb. 1). Soviel zur Technologie.

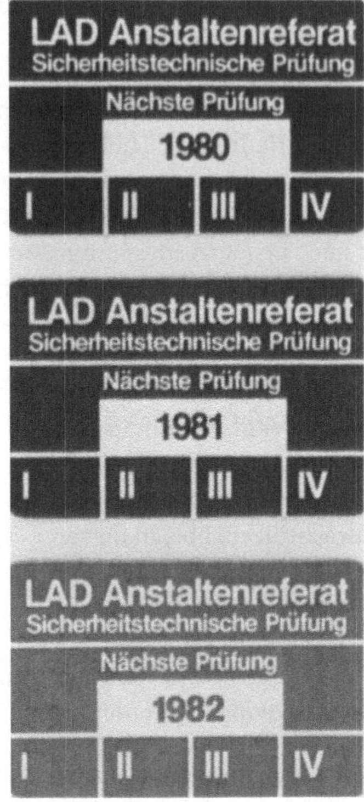

Abb. 1

  Welche Bedeutung hat nun die Persönlichkeit des Anaesthesisten im Hinblick auf die Vorbeugung von Zwischenfällen? Es hieße Eulen nach Athen zu tragen, hier neuerlich die Feststellung zu machen, daß eine fundierte Ausbildung der beste Schutz gegen Fehlleistungen darstellt. Dennoch, gerade die moderne Anaesthesie ist ein Fachgebiet mit großen Entwicklungstendenzen, die zweifellos gutes, aber ebenso auch wieder verwerfbares hervorbringen. So beschränke sich auch der erfahrene Facharzt vor allem auf bewährtes, insbesondere aber auf jene Methoden, die sich in seiner Hand als verläßlich und sicher erwiesen haben. Die Versuchung ist groß, im Neuesten auch gleich das Beste sehen zu wollen, besonders dann, wenn eine erfolgsträchtige Literatur die dringend nötige Selbstkritik vermissen läßt. Das heißt nun nicht, daß man sich dem Reiz des vermeintlichen Fortschritts entziehen soll, sondern daß man Vor- und Nachteile kritisch abwägt, daß man sozusagen auch den Fortschritt lernt. Der Weise hat längst erkannt, daß man auf dieser Welt nichts geschenkt bekommt und daß man in der Regel den neuen Bonus auch mit einem neuen Malus bezahlen muß.

  Neben der eigentlichen Ausbildung spielt auch die physische und psychische Verfassung des Narkosearztes eine entscheidende Rolle. Dies sei eine sehr bewußt gemachte Feststellung, denn nicht selten verlangt man von ihm in einer von Gasen und Dämpfen verseuchten Atmosphäre ein stundenlanges Arbeiten, während sich die Operationsmannschaften abwechseln können. Die Übermüdung durch Dauerleistung einerseits und Intoxikation andererseits, stellt eine nicht zu unterschätzende Gefahr dar. Auch das Narkoseteam muß daher die Möglichkeit der Ablösung haben, besonderer Wert ist aber auf die Einrichtung von Gasabsauganlagen für alle an einem operativen Eingriff beteiligten zu legen.

Nicht zuletzt ist die Profilierung des Anaesthesiologen gegenüber anderen Fachbereichen für die Sicherheit des Kranken von Bedeutung. Auf der Kapitänsmentalität des Operateurs und der Bootsmannmeuterei des Narkotiseurs läßt sich keine erfolgreiche Chirurgie aufbauen. Der Operationssaal ist kein Schiff, der Patient kein Passagier, weder Chirurgie noch Anaesthesiologie an sich tun not. Beide haben sich heute zu respektieren, beider Erfahrungen sind abzuwägen, beide tragen eine Verantwortung, die zu eng verwoben ist, um sie unverletzt trennen zu können.

Wenn hier vor allem auf Bildung und Ausbildung des Fachmannes eingegangen wurde, dann muß es sich erübrigen, auf weitere Zwischenfallsmöglichkeiten einzugehen, die durch offensichtliche Unkenntnis bedingt sind, wie Überdosierungen, massive Bolus-Injektionen, oder fälschliche Anwendung von Medikamenten.

Ein besonderes Kapitel aber stellen allergische Reaktionen dar, die von der eher harmlosen Urticaria bis zum anaphylaktischen, lebensbedrohenden Schock bei Anwendung von Plasma-Expandern auftreten können. Wenn auch an der Vorbeugung solcher Zwischenfälle, im besonderen auf dem Sektor der Dextrane, intensiv gearbeitet wird, so muß man doch festhalten, daß Sicherheit nicht nur ein Problem der Prophylaxe, sondern in gleichem Maße eine Frage der Beherrschung des möglichen und eben nicht auszuschließenden Zwischenfalls ist. Problematisch hierbei bleibt allerdings vorerst die meist unvorhersehbare Komplikation der „Malignen Hyperthermie", die trotz aller bekannter therapeutischer Bemühungen häufig nicht in den Griff zu bekommen ist. Vielleicht eröffnet die neuerdings vorgeschlagene Behandlung der malignen Hyperthermie mit Dantrolene erfolgversprechendere Wege.

Die dritte Sicherheitsaufgabe des Anaesthesisten betrifft schließlich den Patienten selbst. Sie ist dessen klinische Voruntersuchung, die sogenannte präoperative Visite und gegebenenfalls eine entsprechende Vorbehandlung. Ein eigenes Panel dieses Kongresses hat sich mit diesen Fragen im Rahmen der „präoperativen Anaesthesie-Ambulanz" beschäftigt. Wie immer man diese Kontrolle des Kranken durchführen will, fest steht, daß auf sie keinesfalls verzichtet werden kann. Wir haben im vergangenen Jahr anläßlich eines einschlägigen Rundtischgespräches der Salzburger Ärztegesellschaft über „Die Vorbereitung des Patienten zur Operation in Klinik und Praxis", die notwendige präoperative Untersuchung entsprechend dem Allgemeinzustand des Kranken und der zu erwartenden Größe der Operation in vier Punkte gegliedert:
1. Die Anamnese des Patienten
2. Die physikalische Basis-Untersuchung mit Harnbefund
3. Die erweiterte klinische Untersuchung bei größeren Eingriffen (Röntgen, EKG, Jonogramm etc.)
4. Die klinische Spezialuntersuchung, wenn erhobene Befunde oder besondere Hinweise weitere Abklärung erfordern.

Die beiden ersten Punkte müssen jedoch als klinische Grundlage jeder Narkoseanwendung angesehen werden.

Beachtet der verantwortungsbewußte Anaesthesist die ihm gestellten Sicherheitsaufgaben sowohl im technischen, als auch im menschlichen Bereich, dann dient er, je nachdem, ob er nun Humanist oder ein Anhänger der Anglistik ist, dem „nil nocere" oder dem „safety first".

Anaesthesiologie und Intensivmedizin

Anaesthesiology and Intensive Care Medicine

Herausgeber: H. Bergmann (Schriftleiter),
J.B. Brückner, R. Frey, M. Gemperle,
W.F. Henschel, O. Mayrhofer, K. Peter

Band 120
E.G. Star

Äthylenoxid-Sterilisation

1979. 2 Abbildungen, 4 Tabellen. VIII, 43 Seiten
DM 26,-
ISBN 3-540-09294-3

Band 121
H.P. Siepmann

Zur Herzwirkung von Inhalationsanaesthetica

Der isolierte Katzenpapillarmuskel als Myokard-Modell
1979. 14 Abbildungen, 5 Tabellen,. VIII, 63 Seiten
DM 39,50
ISBN 3-540-09230-7

Band 122

Coronare Herzkrankheit

Physiologische, kardiologische und anaesthesiologische Aspekte. Weiterbildungskurs für Anaesthesieärzte am 10. Juni 1978 in Wuppertal
Herausgeber: J. Schara
1979. 61 Abbildungen, 15 Tabellen. IX, 97 Seiten
DM 48,-
ISBN 3-540-09416-4

Band 123
H. Kämmerer, K. Standfuss, E. Klaschik

Pathologische pulmonale Kurzschlußperfusion

Theoretische, klinische und tierexperimentelle Untersuchungen zur Variabilität
1979. 23 Abbildungen, 8 Tabellen. VIII, 71 Seiten
DM 37,-
ISBN 3-540-09498-9

Band 124

Neue Aspekte in der Regionalanaesthesie 1

Wirkung auf Herz, Kreislauf und Endokrinum
Postoperative Periduralanalgesie
Herausgeber: H.J. Wüst, M. Zindler
1980. 97 Abbildungen, 37 Tabellen.
XIV, 196 Seiten
DM 68,-
ISBN 3-540-09500-4

Band 125

Kreislaufschock

Herausgeber: J.B. Brückner
1980. 407 Abbildungen, 96 Tabellen.
XXIV, 646 Seiten
DM 168,-
ISBN 3-540-09660-4

Band 127

Mehrfachverletzungen

Herausgeber: H.-J. Streicher, J. Rolle
1980. 97 Abbildungen. XI, 217 Seiten
DM 79,-
ISBN 3-540-09658-2

Band 128
P. Lemburg

Künstliche Beatmung beim Neugeborenen und Kleinkind

Theorie und Praxis der Anwendung von Respiratoren beim Kind
1980. 85 Abbildungen. X, 146 Seiten
DM 63,-
ISBN 3-540-09659-0

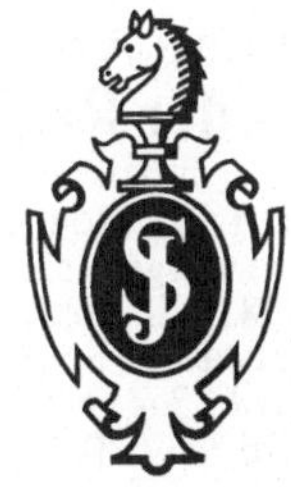

Springer-Verlag
Berlin
Heidelberg
New York

Band 129

25 Jahre Anaesthesiologie und Intensivtherapie in Österreich

Herausgeber: K. Steinbereithner, H. Bergmann
1979. 54 Abbildungen, 40 Tabellen. X, 149 Seiten
DM 69,-
ISBN 3-540-09777-5

Anaesthesiologie und Intensivmedizin

Anaesthesiology and Intensive Care Medicine

Herausgeber: H. Bergmann (Schriftleiter),
J. B. Brückner, R. Frey, M. Gemperle,
W. F. Henschel, O. Mayrhofer, K. Peter

Band 130
25 Jahre DGAI
Jahrestagung in Würzburg, 12.–14. Oktober 1978
Herausgeber: K. H. Weis, G. Cunitz
1980. 689 Abbildungen, zahlreiche Tabellen.
XXXVIII, 1012 Seiten
DM 158,–
ISBN 3-540-10140-3

Band 131
Akute respiratorische Insuffizienz
Herausgeber: K. Peter
1980. 83 Abbildungen, 12 Tabellen.
IX, 131 Seiten (18 Seiten in Englisch)
DM 58,–
ISBN 3-540-10185-3

Band 132
Endocrinology in Anaesthesia and Surgery
Editors: H. Stoeckel, T. Oyama
With the Co-operation of G. Hack
1980. 101 figures, 45 tables. XI, 203 pages
DM 94,–
ISBN 3-540-10211-6

Springer-Verlag
Berlin
Heidelberg
New York

Band 133
Lormetazepam
Experimentelle und klinische Erfahrungen mit
einem neuen Benzodiazepin zur oralen und intra-
venösen Anwendung
Herausgeber: A. Doenicke, H. Ott
1980. 98 Abbildungen, 14 Tabellen.
XXI, 133 Seiten
DM 59,–
ISBN 3-540-10387-2

Band 134
Thrombose und Embolie
Herausgeber: H. Vinazzer
Mit Beiträgen zahlreicher Fachwissenschaftler
1981. 124 Abbildungen, 48 Tabellen.
XII, 345 Seiten
DM 118,–
ISBN 3-540-10393-7

Band 135
P. Sefrin
Polytrauma und Stoffwechsel
1981. 28 Abbildungen, VIII, 90 Seiten
DM 49,–
ISBN 3-540-10525-5

Band 136
W. Seyboldt-Epting
Kardioplegie
Myokardschutz während extrakorporaler
Zirkulation
1981. 36 Abbildungen. IX, 74 Seiten
DM 78,–
ISBN 3-540-10621-9

Band 137
G. Goeckenjan
Kontinuierliche Messung des arteriellen Sauerstoffpartialdrucks
1981. 49 Abbildungen, 11 Tabellen.
IX, 110 Seiten
DM 78,–
ISBN 3-540-10730-4

Band 138
Neue Aspekte in der Regionalanaesthesie 2
Pharmakokinetik, Interaktionen, Thromboembo-
lierisiko, New Trends
Herausgeber: H. J. Wüst, M. Zindler
1981. 70 Abbildungen. Etwa 200 Seiten
(etwa 120 Seiten in Englisch)
DM 78,–
ISBN 3-540-10893-9

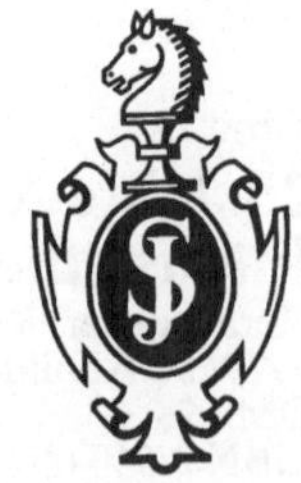